VETERINARY BACTERIOLOGY

a division of
NIPA GENX ELECTRONIC RESOURCES & SOLUTIONS P. LTD.
New Delhi-110 034

Abouth the Author

Dr Indranil Samanta obtained his graduation (BVSc and AH) from West Bengal University of Animal and Fishery Sciences, Kolkata. He post graduated from Indian Veterinary Research Institute (IVRI), Izatanagar, Bareilly, UP in Veterinary Bacteriology. He qualified ICAR-NET twice and CSIR-NET. He joined as Assistant Professor-cum-Junior Scientist at Division of Veterinary Microbiology, S.K. University of Agricultural Sciences and Technology of Kashmir (SKUAST-K), Srinagar, Jammu and Kashmir. After years of service he joined the post of Veterinary Officer, Animal Resource Development Department, Government of West Bengal. He is presently working as Assistant Professor at Department of Veterinary Microbiology, West Bengal University of Animal and Fishery Sciences, Kolkata and he has completed PhD in Veterinary Microbiology. Dr. Samanta has more than 10 years of teaching experience. He has authored four books entitled 'Veterinary Bacteriology' (First edition, NIPA), 'Veterinary Mycology' (Springer), 'Pet bird diseases and care' (Springer-Nature), 'Antimicrobial Resistance in Agriculture' (Academic Press, Elsevier) and 150 research articles in peer reviewed journals with medium to high impact factor associated with prevalence of zoonotic bacteria, antimicrobial resistance in livestock and their transmission dynamics. He is the recipient of National Academy of Agricultural Sciences (NAAS) Associate, American Society of Microbiology travel grant, Indian National Science Academy-Summer Research Fellowship, Best Teacher Award (twice) at faculty and University level of WBUAFS, Elsevier certificate for outstanding contribution in reviewing, P. Madhusudan Gold Medal and several best presentation awards in national or international conferences. He received grants for conducting research from Indian Council of Agricultural Research (ICAR), Medical Research Council (UK), Department of Biotechnology (Government of India) and Department of Science & Technology and Biotechnology (Government of West Bengal). Dr. Samanta acts as Associate Editor and Senior Editorial Board member and reviewer of several international and national journals such as Frontiers in Veterinary Science, BMC Veterinary Research etc. He has delivered numerous talks in television, radio and in different training programmes for the farmers regarding animal and poultry health related issues.

VETERINARY BACTERIOLOGY
2nd Fully Revised Edition

Indranil Samanta
Assistant Professor
Department of Veterinary Microbiology
West Bengal University of Animal & Fishery Sciences
37, K.B. Sarani, Kolkata- 700037
West Bengal, India

a division of
NIPA GENX ELECTRONIC RESOURCES & SOLUTIONS P. LTD.
New Delhi-110 034

a division of
NIPA GENX ELECTRONIC RESOURCES & SOLUTIONS P. LTD.
101,103, Vikas Surya Plaza, CU Block
L.S.C.Market, Pitam Pura, New Delhi-110 034
Ph : +91 11 27341616, 27341717, 27341718
E-mail:newindiapublishingagency@gmail.com
www: www.nipabooks.com

For customer assistance, please contact
Phone: + 91-11-27 34 17 17 Fax: + 91-11- 27 34 16 16
E-Mail: feedbacks@nipabooks.com

ISBN: 978-93-90591-32-9

Composed and Designed by NIPA.

Dedicated to

My Beloved Family

Preface to the Second Edition

Bacteria, the tiny creature inhabiting the earth long before than us, generated oxygen molecule first in the atmosphere by photosynthesis. The oxygen made an environment conducive for the creation of life. The bacteria responsible for inception of our life later became life-threatening and took the leading role in economic losses associated with morbidity and mortality of livestock, poultry and fishes. Antibiotics, the weapon to combat the pathogenic bacteria are also produced by group of beneficial bacteria. Inappropriate use of the weapon is making it blunt although. Throughout my career circling around the pathogenic and beneficial bacterial groups, I felt the importance of these microscopic creatures in our life and society. I wished to disseminate the feelings through the first edition of the book 'Veterinary Bacteriology'.

The second revised edition consists of the general and systematic Veterinary Bacteriology. The book is intended to help undergraduate and post-graduate scholars of Veterinary Microbiology as well as the aspirants of different competitive examinations. The revised edition will also support the person engaged as Government Veterinarian, independent animal health practitioner, or associated with the laboratory for the diagnosis of animal diseases. The book comprises the diagnostic techniques for each bacterial genus ranging from staining parameters to molecular tools with useful photographs. I also tried to keep the language simple as much as possible like the previous edition.

I obtained sufficient 'time', the most valuable requirement to write a text book for which I am grateful to my family. I am also thankful to all the senior and junior colleagues throughout the country who provided me their best photographs of the microbes.

Any suggestion to improve the value of this book will be appreciatively received and will be incorporated in subsequent editions.

Kolkata
2020

Indranil Samanta

Preface to the First Edition

"Never Underestimate the power of bacteria"- J.W. Foster

Veterinary Bacteriology, a branch of Veterinary Microbiology has major importance in diagnosis and treatment of animal diseases. It also provides the basic knowledge for biotechnology related work. During my initial attachment with this subject as a post graduate student and later as a teacher, I felt the necessity of a comprehensive book with update which motivates me to write the present manuscript.

The book is written following the syllabus framed by Veterinary Council of India (VCI). It comprises historical introduction, morphology, classification, resistance, natural habitat, genome, isolation and colony characteristics, biochemical and antigenic properties, pathogenesis, disease produced and diagnosis of each bacterial genus associated with animal and human health. The book is intended to help BVSc and Post Graduate students of Veterinary Microbiology as well as the aspirants of ICAR-JRF, ICAR-NET/ARS examinations. Further it will also help the person engaged as Veterinarian or in the laboratory for the diagnosis of animal diseases. As the book comprises the diagnostic technique for each bacterial genus ranging from staining parameters to molecular tools.

I sincerely thanks to Dr Tapan Kumar Dutta, Associate Professor, Department of Veterinary Microbiology, CAU, Aizawl and Dr Samiran Bandyopadhyay, Scientist, Eastern Regional Station, Indian Veterinary Research Institute, Kolkata for contribution of chapters in this book. I am also grateful to my Departmental colleagues Dr S. N. Joardar, Dr D. P. Isore and my friends Dr G. P. Mandal, Sr. Lecturer, Department of Animal Nutrition, WBUAFS, Kolkata, and Dr T. K. Sar, Sr. Lecturer, Department of Veterinary Pharmacology, WBUAFS, Kolkata for their help. My other friends may forgive me for this insufficient space to recall their immense help.

Moreover, I am highly obliged to my family members for tolerating me and providing me the 'time', the most valuable requirement to write a text book. Specially the mental and technical support by sketching all the illustrations of this book provided by my wife is highly appreciated without which I may not complete this task.

Any suggestion to improve the value of this book will be gratefully received and will be incorporated in subsequent editions.

Kolkata **Indranil Samanta**
2012

Contents

1

Introduction and History of Microbiology

Microbiology is the branch of science which deals with the diverse minute forms of life such as bacteria, archaea, viruses, fungi, prions, protozoa and algae. The study includes structure, classification, growth and nutrition, natural habitat, genome, antigenic characteristics, virulence determinants, types of toxins produced, pathogenesis, diagnosis and ways to combat the infection caused by the microbes.

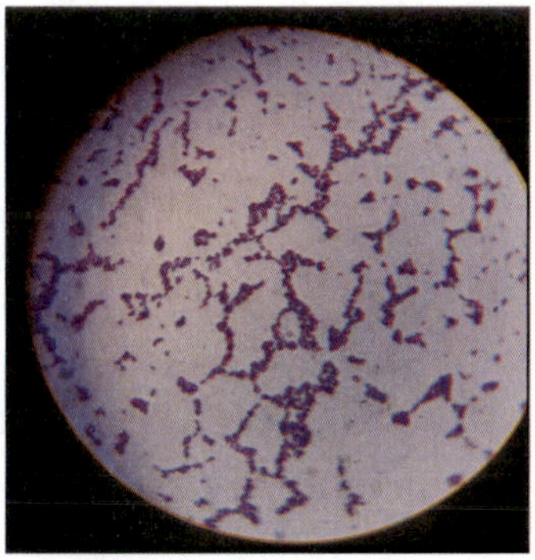

Fig. 1: World of bacteria, *Staphyloccus* spp., Gram stained, 100X

Other than infection oriented study the subject also considers food production, food processing, manufacture of life-saving drugs and biofuels, environmental pollution, climate change, biodegradation etc. under different sub-branches. Microbiological research not only caters the basic needs of human life i.e. safe food and drinking water but also searches few basic human queries such as diversity of life in the earth, presence of extra-terrestrial life in the universe etc. Louis Pasteur (1822-95, France) first coined the term 'microbiology' and for his enormous scientific contribution he is popularly known as 'father of microbiology'.

Veterinary microbiology is associated with the microbes (bacteria, archaea, virus, fungi, prions) having importance in health of livestock, poultry, companion animals, fur bearing animals, and game birds. The curative veterinary medicine cannot offer the precise treatment other than trial and error protocol until the microbial etiology is confirmed. It is the treatment of 'symptoms' not the 'cause' in absence of microbial diagnosis. The knowledge of veterinary microbiology also helps in selection of precise drug for treatment through antibiotic sensitivity assay, development of diagnostics and new vaccines to prevent the infection. According to the study of microbial type veterinary microbiology can be sub-divided into veterinary bacteriology, veterinary mycology and veterinary virology. Veterinary immunology is another branch which concerns with the study of animal or bird immune system, how it works, role of vaccines in prevention of diseases and causes of vaccine failure.

History of Microbiology

The history of microbiology is the story of knowledge about the causes of diseases discovered with the advancement of time.

a) Theurgical theory: The life of early times before scientific advancement throughout the world was governed by superstitions. The disease followed by death occurs due to curse of divine spirit as a punishment of individual sin.

b) Miasmatic (miasma) theory: Hippocrates (460-370 B.C.), the Greek physician and often referred as 'father of medicine' proposed the miasmatic theory of diseases in his book 'On airs, waters and places'. The elements (fire, air, water, earth) and qualities (heat, cold, moisture, dryness) of the world are related to different human body fluids such as blood, phlegm, yellow bile and black bile. Changes of the elements or qualities such as change in temperature, moisture, quality of air ('miasma' or 'bad air') can cause the disease epidemic. Hippocrates although first established the association of natural factors with the causation of disease he did not consider the transferable agents as etiology. Galen (129-210 A.D.), another Greek physician and philosopher supported the miasmatic theory. Galen further classified human temperament on the basis of imbalance in different body fluids such as sanguine (blood), melancholic (black bile), choleric (yellow bile), and phlegmatic (phlegm). The people with 'sanguine' temperaments are extrovert and social, 'choleric' people have energy and passion, 'melancholics' are creative and kind, and 'phlegmatic' people are dependable.

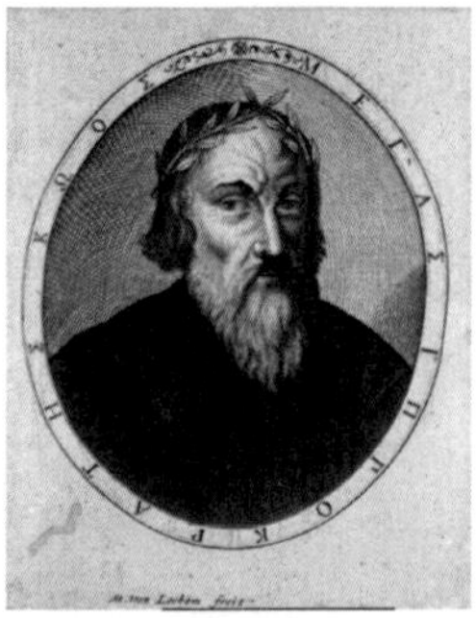

Fig. 2: Hippocrates (Courtesy of the National Library of Medicine)

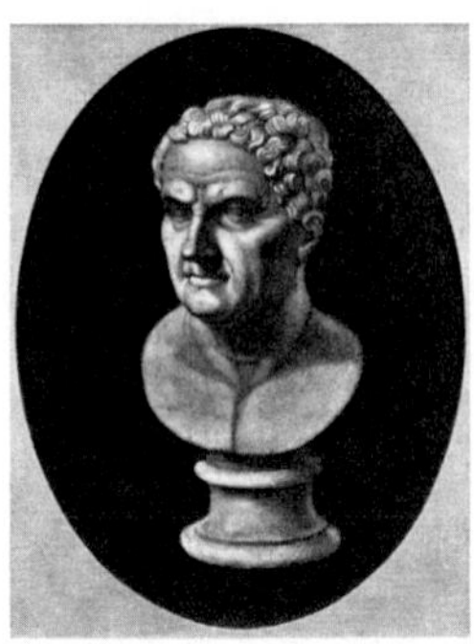

Fig. 3: Galen (Courtesy of the National Library of Medicine)

c) Pore theory: The theory states that the dissymmetry of the pores present in body causes the disease. Asclepiades (124-40 B.C.), a Greek physician and philosopher believed that obstruction of pores with excess corpuscles (atom) causes acute diseases and relaxation of pores due to deficiency of corpuscles produces chronic diseases. Themison of Laodicea (143-23 B.C.), the student of Asclepiades established methodic school of medicine in ancient Greece and Rome based on this theory. Thessalus (A.D. 60) on the other hand proposed that modification of pores present in distressed body parts can cure the disease.

d) Paracelsus hypothesis: During 16th century Philippus Aureolus Theophrastus Bombastus von Hohenheim (1493-1541, Switzerland), an outspoken physician, alchemist with iconoclast nature (a person who works against the beliefs), declared himself superior than Celsus ('Paracelsus'), the renowned Roman physician. Paracelsus had faith on influence of natural factors in disease etiology following Hippocrates.

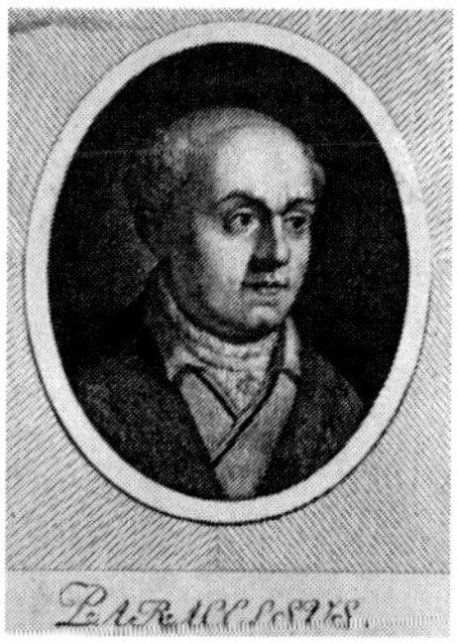

Fig. 4: Paracelsus (Courtesy of the National Library of Medicine)

At the same time he believed in supernatural forces such as influence of planets and stars on different organs and causation of diseases. He first identified the role of minerals and chemicals in treatment of diseases, first identified zinc and its functions, first treated syphilis with mercury and coined the aphorism, 'the dose makes the poison'.

e) Spontaneous generation theory: Aristotle (384-322 B.C., Greece) the great philosopher of ancient Greece proposed the 'spontaneous generation theory'. The theory stated that the animals are originated from soils, plants or other 'unlike' animals if 'pneuma' or 'vital heat' is present. Exposure of meat to the air and heat gives the birth of maggots. It was well accepted in the scientific world till 17th century.

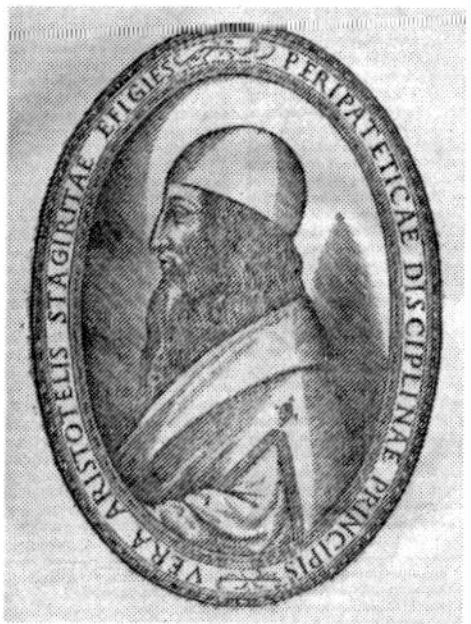

Fig. 5: Aristotle (Courtesy of the National Library of Medicine)

Francisco Redi (1626-97, Italy), a biologist and poet, first observed that maggots are not produced in the meat if covered with a gauze (cloth made of silk or cotton). The maggots and insects were present in the meat kept in an open container. Louis Joblot (1647-1723, France), a naturalist, also showed that heated meat infusions are free of any living creatures. John Needham (1713-81, United Kingdom), a biologist although supported spontaneous generation theory during his experiment with chicken broth. Needham boiled the broth in test tubes with herbs and sealed them but observed the turbidity of broth due to microbial growth after few days. He claimed that the microbes were originated spontaneously from the broth although it actually occurred due to improper boiling of the broth to kill the existing microbes. Lazzaro Spallanzani

(1729-99, Italy), a biologist and physiologist did not agree with Needham and showed that after extensive heating of the broth up to boiling point and sealing the same prevented the turbidity (microbial growth) even after several days. Needham again argued that excess heating destroyed 'life force' present in air required for spontaneous generation of the microbes. Franz Schulze (1815-73) and Theodor Schwann (1810–1882) supported Spallanzani's work by introducing air into the boiled broth after passing through the strong acid solutions. No microbial turbidity was observed even after introduction of air. During 1850, H. Schröder and T. von Dusch (1824-90, Germany) performed the experiment in a sophisticated way. They plugged the test tubes containing heated broth with cotton and allowed the air to pass through the cotton plugs. No microbial growth appeared and thus plugging the culture tubes with cotton was initiated in the microbiology laboratories. The cotton plugs are still used in the laboratories.

The debate continued till 19th century and Paris academy of science declared an award to be given to the scientist who can provide a conclusion. Louis Pasteur (1822-95, France), a chemist and biologist accepted the challenge and started the famous 'swan neck/goose neck flask' experiment. In his experiment Pasteur took broth in a flask having a tortuous neck (Figure 6) and heated thoroughly. He cooled the broth and kept the flask with unplugged neck. No microbial turbidity was observed even after several days. He explained the result that during heating the microbes present in the broth died and although the air entered from outside all the germs present in the air were settled into the swan neck. The air itself has no 'life force' which can help to generate microbes in the heated broth. Thus the spontaneous generation theory was finally disproved.

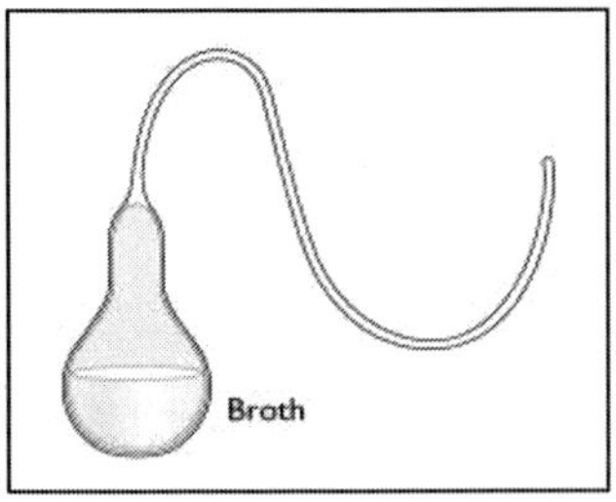

Fig. 6: 'Swan neck/goose neck' flask of Louis Pasteur

f) Germ theory of infectious diseases: Athanasius Kircher (1602-80, Germany) first used a low power microscope to observe 'worms' present in the blood smear of plague patients. During 1590-1610, first compound microscope was developed in Holland (The Netherlands) by Cornelius Drebbel, Hans and Zaccharius Janssen. Galileo (1609) tried to improve the magnification of microscope. Antony Van Leeuwenhoek (1632-1723, The Netherlands) developed a series of microscopes with higher magnification and observed bacteria of different shape and sizes present in pond water. He referred the bacteria as 'animalcule' in his articles submitted to Royal Society of London. In 1720, Benjamin Marten, a London based physician and popular medical author published a book entitled 'a new theory of consumptions: more especially of a phthisis or consumption of the lungs' in which he first wrote about 'inexplicable contagious cause' of tuberculosis.

In 1835, Agostino Bassi (1773-1856, Italy), an entomologist first observed a direct correlation between a fungus (*Botrytis bassiana*) and production of diseases in silkworm. He suggested few hygienic measures and phenolic compounds to prevent the infection in silkworm. In 1839, Johann Lukas Schönlein (1793-1864, Germany) first detected the dermatophyte (*Trichophyton schoenleinii*) as an etiology of tinea favosa, a cutaneous mycosis in human. In 1840, Friedrich Gustav Jacob Henle (1809-85, Germany, in literature known as Jacob Henle), an anatomist and pathologist published a book entitled 'On miasmata and contagia' (*Von den Miasman und Kontagien*) in which he speculated the role of microscopic organisms (*contagia animata*) in production of epidemic diseases. The speculation was based on the works of Agostino Bassi, Schwann and Schleiden's discovery that every living organism has a cellular structure etc. Jacob Henle is credited as 'founder of germ theory'. Reverend Miles J. Berkeley (1846) also detected fungal etiology of 'potato blight' (infection of potato tubers and leaves) in Ireland. In 1847, Ignaz Semmelweis (1818-65, Italy), a physician observed the transmission of childbed fever by the contaminated hands of medical students performing the autopsies.

In 1853, two diseases called 'pebrine' and 'flacherie' ('morts-flats', 'gattine') spread among silkworm nurseries in France and other European countries and produced major economic losses. Jean-Baptiste Dumas (1800-84, France), a chemist requested Louis Pasteur to work on it to save the silkworm industry. During 1865-70, Pasteur worked at Ales, a small French town with silkworm nurseries. He observed that the two diseases were associated with a protozoa ('pebrine') and nutritional deficiency with bacterial superinfection ('flacherie'), respectively. Based on these findings and earlier works of several researchers Pasteur proposed the 'germ theory of the disease' as 'all the contagious and infectious diseases are caused by live organisms (germs)'.

Joseph Lister (1827-1912, Scotland), a physician supported the germ theory with his work on use of antiseptics (phenol) to treat the wounds in 1867.

In 1863-68, Casimir Davaine (1812-1882, France), a physician observed the contagious nature of the germs and coined the term 'bacteria'.

The germ theory was finally established with the classical works of Robert Koch (1843-1910, Germany), a physician, microbiologist and student of Jacob Henle, the founder of the theory. Koch observed that blood from anthrax infected sheep can kill the experimental mice when inoculated. He detected rod shaped bacteria in blood, spleen and lymph nodes of the mice. When he further inoculated the blood of the infected mice into other mice it produced the same results. Thus it was concluded that anthrax is caused by transmission of specific bacteria (germs). Koch presented his findings to Ferdinand Cohn, the renowned botanist of Germany and published the article during 1876.

Individual scientific contributions

Edward Jenner (1749-1823, United Kingdom)

Since the ancient times it was known that survivors of smallpox are resistant to re-infection. A technique known as 'inoculation' (in Latin means 'to graft') or 'variolation' ('variola' means smallpox) was practiced in India, China and Africa to prevent the smallpox. The 'inoculator' used a lancet (surgical knife) to introduce fresh extract of ripe pustule (smallpox lesion) subcutaneously into the arms and legs of the non-immune persons. The technique came to Europe during 18th century with the travellers from Turkey. In 1718, Lady Mary Wortley Montague, the wife of British ambassador in Turkey ordered the embassy surgeon to 'inoculate' her five years old son to protect him from smallpox. After their return to England in 1721 the variolation became popular in the royal family.

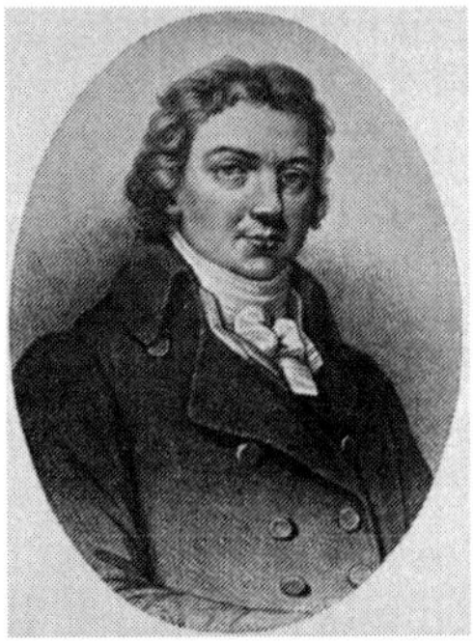

Fig. 7: Edward Jenner (Courtesy of the National Library of Medicine)

Edward Jenner, a country surgeon in Bristol (UK) observed that dairymaid suffered with cowpox never get infected with smallpox. In May 14, 1796 Jenner collected the fresh cowpox lesion extract from a dairymaid (Sarah Nelms) and inoculated into an eight year old boy James Phipps.

In July 1796, Jenner inoculated fresh smallpox lesion extract to the boy and observed that the boy remained healthy. He published the hypothesis that cowpox infection can give protection against smallpox in the form of a booklet. Jenner built a single room hut in the garden of his house (Berkeley, UK) known as 'temple of vaccinia' where he vaccinated the poor free of cost. Gradually vaccination became popular and variolation became prohibited in England in 1840.

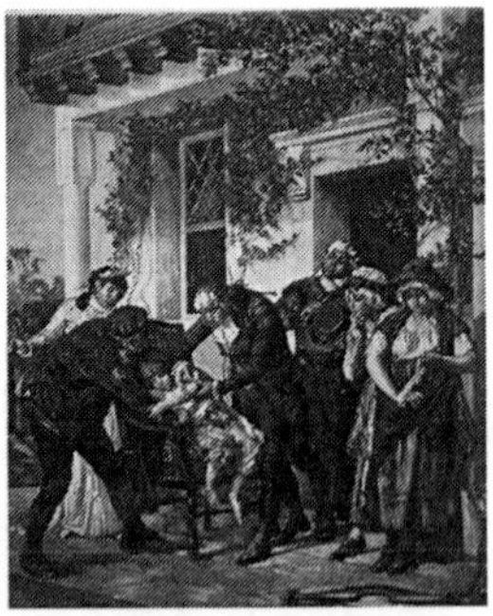

Fig. 8: First vaccination by Edward Jenner (Courtesy of the National Library of Medicine)

Louis Pasteur (1822-95, France)

Pasteur is popularly known as 'Father of microbiology' due to following inventions.

a) Pasteur established that the living organisms (bacteria / yeast) are responsible for process of fermentation ('germ theory of fermentation', 1857-73)

b) He standardized the heating (time and temperature) process of fermentable liquid (beer, wine etc.) to prevent the spoilage. Later the method became popular in milk industry as 'pasteurization'.

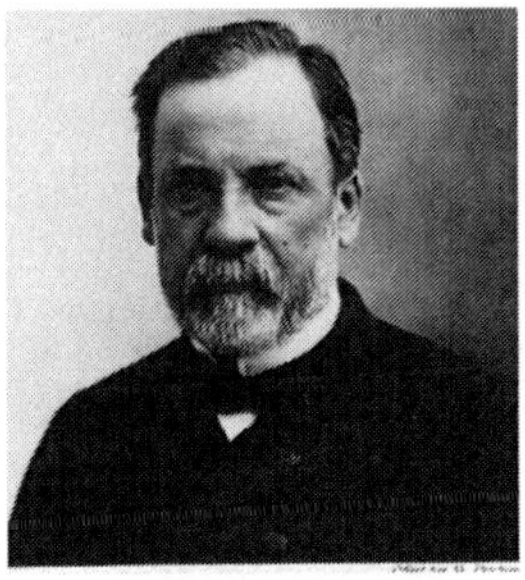

Fig. 9: Louis Pasteur (Courtesy of the National Library of Medicine)

c) He proposed 'germ theory of disease' on the basis of his works on protozoan disease of silkworms (1865-70) and earlier speculations of Jacob Henle

d) In 1879, Pasteur observed that aged cultures of *Pasteurella multocida* lost virulence and inoculation of old cultures into chicken can protect them against fowl cholera, the bacterial infection of chicken caused by *P. multocida*. The phenomenon can be considered as beginning of immunology and Pasteur coined the term 'vaccination' ('vacca' in Latin means cow) in honour of Edward Jenner who first used cowpox virus to prevent smallpox (1796).

e) In 1881, Pasteur tried to reduce the virulence ('attenuation') of *Bacillus anthracis*, the causative organism of anthrax in animals and human. He initially exposed the cultures to oxygen as the method of attenuation. In presence of oxygen, formation of bacterial spores is inhibited and the cultures become non-pathogenic. Pasteur also observed that vaccination with non-pathogenic cultures became more fruitful when a less-attenuated culture was inoculated 12 days after primary inoculation (concept of 'booster'). Finally he attenuated *B. anthracis* cultures with potassium bichhromate and made three passages in mice. On 5th May, 1881 Pasteur inoculated the attenuated culture into 24 sheep, one goat and six cows at Pouilly-le-Fort, a village near Paris. On 17th May he further inoculated the animals a less attenuated culture (booster). On 31st May, all the vaccinated animals and a control group were challenged with a highly virulent bacterial culture. During 2-3 June all the animals of control group died but the vaccinated animals survived. Thus the vaccination against anthrax reduced the livestock mortality to 0.3% in France during the period.

f) In 1883, Pasteur prepared a vaccine against *Erysipelothrix rhusiopathiae* by serial passage of culture into rabbits to protect the pigs from swine erysipelas in Vaucluse, France.

g) Pasteur became interested in rabies with the work of Pierre Galtier (1879), a French veterinarian who first showed that rabies virus can be transmitted into the rabbits through dog saliva. Pasteur successfully transmitted the virus into the rabbits by intracerebral inoculation of infected brain extract. In 1884, he attenuated the virus by passage into unnatural host (dog to monkey). Later in 1885, Pasteur with the help of Emile Roux developed a new technique for rabies virus attenuation. He took the rabies virus infected rabbit spinal cord and dried in air (desiccation). The virus lost its virulence in 15 days. Pasteur prepared emulsions of the rabbit spinal cord and injected daily to the experimental dogs and protected the dogs from the challenge with virulent rabies virus. On 6th July, 1885, a nine year old boy (Joseph Miester) from Alsace (France) met Pasteur for the treatment of dog bite at the hands, legs and hips. The boy was referred by the physician Joseph Grancher. Pasteur was although reluctant but started his treatment on 7th July. The boy received 12 consecutive injections of desiccated rabbit spinal cord and he survived! On the memory of this major scientific triumph against the deadly disease the 6th July is celebrated as 'world zoonosis day'.

Robert Koch (1843-1910, Germany)

Koch is popularly known as 'Father of bacteriology' due to following inventions. Koch was awarded with Nobel Prize in 1905 due to discovery of the causative agent of tuberculosis.

a) Koch first detected that bacteria can propagate by elongation and binary fission

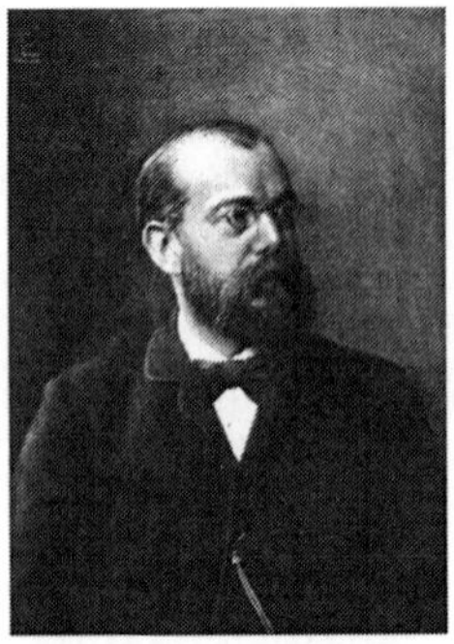

Fig. 10: Robert Koch (Courtesy of the National Library of Medicine)

b) He developed artificial culture technique for isolation of bacteria and observed that aqueous humor can act as effective bacterial culture medium. In 1881 he developed solid plate technique for isolation of bacterial 'pure' culture. Koch tried to produce solid culture media with gelatin. Walter Hesse, the post-doctoral fellow of Koch with the help of his wife Fannie Hesse (Fanny Angelina Eilshemius) detected that agar (a carbohydrate from seaweed) can be used successfully to solidify the culture media. Julius Petri, another student of Koch designed a shallow covered dish where the media can be poured for solidification. It is still used in bacteriology laboratory and is known as 'petri dish'.

c) Koch first detected that the bacteria remain viable in unfavourable condition by producing spores

d) Koch first developed the technique for fixation of bacterial smear in glass slides by air drying

e) Use of light microscopy became a routine practice in bacteriology laboratory after Koch's introduction of oil immersion lens and condenser. Koch was the first scientist in the world who published photographs of bacteria in 1877.

f) Koch discovered the causative bacteria of anthrax (*Bacillus anthracis*, 1876), suppuration (*Staphylococcus*, 1878), tuberculosis (*Mycobacterium tuberculosis*, 1882) and cholera (*Vibrio cholerae*, 1883)

g) On the basis of works done by Jacob Henle (teacher of Koch in Medical school), Loeffler and Klebs, Koch derived a set of 'postulates' for establishing the causation of bacterial diseases (1882). It became famous in medical history as 'Koch's postulates'. The postulates state that:

   i. The specific organism can always be found in association with a given disease

   ii. The organism can be isolated and grown in pure culture in the laboratory

   iii. The organism will produce similar disease when inoculated into an experimental animal

   iv. It is possible to recover the organism in pure culture from experimentally infected animals

h) Koch first observed the importance of water purification in prevention of cholera

i) In 1890, in search of the treatment for tuberculosis, Koch prepared a glycerine extract of *Mycobacterium tuberculosis* which he called 'tuberculin'. The subcutaneous inoculation of tuberculin into guineapigs with tuberculosis produced allergic reaction (Koch phenomenon). Koch failed to show therapeutic potential of tuberculin but it is still in use in a modified form for diagnosis of tuberculosis.

Individual contributions of other scientists associated with microbiology are described in Table 1. The major bacterial diseases, etiology/causative organism and discovery are enumerated in Table 2.

Table 1: Individual contributions of scientists related to microbiology

Year/ Era	Scientist	Contribution
384-322 B.C.	Aristotle	Proposed spontaneous generation theory
1602-80	Athanasius Kircher	First used a low power microscope to observe 'worms' in blood smear of plague patients
1590-1610	Cornelius Drebbel, Hans and Zaccharius Janssen	First use of compound microscope
1632-1723	Antony Van Leeuwenhoek	Developed microscopes with higher magnification and observed bacteria ('animalcule')
1626-97	Francisco Redi	First disapproved spontaneous generation theory
1647-1723	Louis Joblot	Disapproved spontaneous generation theory
1713-81	John Needham	Supported spontaneous generation theory
1720	Benjamin Marten	First gave an idea about contagious germs
1729-99	Lazzaro Spallanzani	Disapproved spontaneous generation theory
1796	Edward Jenner	First vaccination against smallpox
1824-90	H. Schröder and T. von Dusch	First used cotton plugs to cover the test tubes
1822-95	Louis Pasteur	Finally disapproved spontaneous generation theory
1820-1910	Florence Nightingale	Organization of hospitals to reduce cross-infection
1835	Agostino Bassi	First detected that disease in silk worm can be caused by fungus- an infectious agent (germ)
1839	Johann Lukas Schönlein	Tinea favosa in human caused by dermatophyte
1840	Friedrich Gustav Jacob Henle (in literature known as Jacob Henle)	Proposed germ theory of disease
1846	Reverend Miles J. Berkeley	Fungal etiology of 'potato blight'
1847	Ignaz Semmelweis	First advised that hand washing can stop the Spread of infection
1857-73	Louis Pasteur	Germ theory of fermentation
1865-70	Louis Pasteur	Germ theory of disease

Contd.

Year/ Era	Scientist	Contribution
1867	Joseph Lister	antiseptic
1863-68	Casimir Davaine	Coined the term 'bacterium'
1843-1910	Robert Koch	Established 'germ theory of disease' with his Classical works on anthrax
1870	Ernst Abbe	Developed condenser and oil objective of microscope
1876	John Tyndall	Fractional sterilization (tyndallization)
1877	Robert Koch	First photograph of bacteria
1879	Louis Pasteur	Concept of attenuation and coined term 'vaccination'
1881	Louis Pasteur	Concept of 'booster' dose in vaccination
1881	Robert Koch	Solid plate technique for bacterial 'pure culture'
1881	Walter Hesse and Fannie Hesse (Fanny Angelina Eilshemius)	Use of 'agar' for solidification of bacteriological media
1882	Robert Koch	Koch postulate
1882	Paul Ehrlich	Acid fast staining, chemotherapy, development of salvarsan (organo-arsenic compound) against syphilis
1883 (Nobel-1908)	Elie Metchinikoff	Phagocytosis
1884	Hans Christian Gram	Gram's staining technique
1885	Louis Pasteur	First vaccination against rabies
1887	Julius Petri	Invented petri dish for bacterial cultivation
1887	Sergei Nikolaievich Winogradsky	Developed the concept of lithotrophy Based on his works on hydrogen sulphide oxidation
1890 (Nobel-1905)	Robert Koch	Cellular immunity ('Koch phenomenon')
1850-1934	William Henry Welch	Invented Clostridium as etiology of gas gangrene
1859-1934	Theobald Smith	Transmission of Texas fever by cattle tick
1892	Dmitri Iosifovich Ivanovsky (Russia)	First idea of virus (Tobacco Mosaic Virus of Plants)
1894	Simon Flexner	Hypersensitivity
1896	Durham and Grubber	Concept of 'agglutination'
1896	D.E. Salmon	First killed vaccine against Salmonella
1897	Kraus	Concept of 'precipitation'

Contd.

Year/ Era	Scientist	Contribution
1898/99	Martinus W. Beijerinck	Fluid nature of virus ('Contagium vivum fluidum')
1898	F. Loeffler and P. Frosch	Described first animal virus (FMD)
1898 (Von Behring Nobel-1901, first Nobel awardee in Physiology/ Medicine)	Emil Von Behring and Shibasaburo Kitasato	Antitoxin against diptheria; first concept of humoral immunity
1900 (Nobel of Bordet-1919)	Jules Bordet and Octave Gengou	Complement
1900 (Nobel-1930)	Karl Landsteiner	Human blood groups
1902 (Nobel-1913)	Charles Richet	Anaphylaxis
1903	Wright and Douglas	Concept of 'opsonin'
1906	August von Wassermann	Introduction of complement fixation test for syphilis
1915, 1917	F.W. Twort (1915) and F. d'Herelle (1917)	Discovered bacteriophage separately. F. d'Herelle coined the term 'bacteriophage'
1923	Edwards	Developed goat tissue vaccine against rinderpest in India
1928	Alexander Fleming	Discovered first antibiotic-penicillin
1931	Goodpasture	First used embryonated hen egg for virus cultivation
1931	Ruska and Knoll	Electron microscope
1935	Stanley	Purified Tobacco mosaic virus
1935	Gerhard Domagk	Antibacterial activity of Prontosil (sulfanilamide)
1937 (Nobel- 1957)	Daniel Bovet	Antihistamines
1939	René Dubos	Discovered tyrothricin and gramicidin from Bacillus brevis
1949	J.F. Enders, T.H. Weller, P.C. Robbins	Human cell culture for poliovirus
1951	Esther Lederberg	Lambda phage
1957-80	Maurice Ralph Hilleman	Developed vaccines against measles, mumps, chickenpox, meningitis, pneumonia, hepatitis A and B, Haemophilus influenzae, studied antigenic shift/drift in influenza virus, discovered SV40 virus

Contd.

Year/ Era	Scientist	Contribution
1960 (Nobel)	F. Macfarlane Burnet and Peter Medawar	Immunological tolerance
1968	Allan M. Campbell	Insertion of foreign DNA into chromosome (episome)
1972 (Nobel)	Rodney R. Porter and Gerald M. Edelman	Chemical structure of antibody
1976 (Tonegawa Nobel-1987)	Hozumi and Tonegawa	Somatic rearrangement of immunoglobulin genes
1977	W. Gilbert and F. Sanger	Nucleotide sequencing
1970-80	Stanley Falkow	Molecular pathogenesis of bacteria, developed concept of 'molecular Koch's postulates'
1980 (Nobel)	George Snell, Jean Dausset, Baruj Benacerraf	Major histocompatibility complex (MHC)
1984 (Nobel)	Georges F. Köhler and Cesar Milstein	Monoclonal antibody
1985 (Nobel-1993)	Karry Mullis	Polymerase chain reaction (PCR)
1990 (Nobel)	E. Donnall Thomas and Joseph Murray	Organ transplantation
1996 (Nobel)	Peter C. Doherty and Rolf Martin Zinkernagel	Recognition of virus infected cells by immune system (T-cells)
1990-2000	Didier Raoult	Discovered several new bacteria such as *Raoultella planticola* and *Rickettsia raoultii* and large sized 'giant viruses'
1995-2000	Malik Peiris	Diagnosis and prevention strategy of Severe Acute Respiratory Syndrome (SARS) And Middle Eastern Respiratory Syndrome (MERS)
2008 (Nobel)	Luc Montaignier	Human immunodeficiency virus
2014	Kim Lewis	Discovery of teixobactin (new antibiotic in recent times)

Table 2: Major bacterial diseases, etiology/causative organism and discovery

Disease	Organism	Discoverer	Year
Anthrax	*Bacillus anthracis*	Robert Koch	1876
Suppuration	*Staphylococcus*	Robert Koch	1878
Gonorrhoea	*Neisseria gonorrhoeae*	A.L.S. Neisser	1879
Typhiod	Salmonella Typhi	C. J. Eberth	1880
Wound infection	*Staphylococcus aureus*	A. Ogston	1881
Tuberculosis	*Mycobacterium tuberculosis*	Robert Koch	1882
Glanders	*Bacillus mallei (Burkholderia mallei)*	Loeffler and Schütz	1882
Cholera	*Vibrio cholerae*	Robert Koch	1883
Diptheria	*Corynebacterium diptheriae*	Klebs and Loeffler	1883
Swine erysipelas	*Erysipelothrix rhusiopathiae*	Loeffler	1885
Tetanus	*Clostridium tetani*	Nicolaier	1885
Diarrhoea	*Escherichia coli*	T. Escherich	1885
Pneumonia	*Streptococcus pneumoniae*	A. Fraenkel	1886
Meningitis	*Neisseria meningitidis*	A. Weichselbaum	1887
Malta fever	*Brucella melitensis*	Bruce	1888
Strangles	*Strerptococcus equi*	Schütz	1888
Gas gangrene	*Clostridium perfringens*	Welch and Nuttall	1892
Plague	*Yersinia pestis*	S. Kitasato and A.J.E. Yersin (independently)	1894
Fowl typhoid	Salmonella Gallinarum	Moore	1895
Botulism	*Clostridium botulinum*	E.M.P. Van Ermengem	1896
Bang's disease	*Brucella abortus*	Bang	1897
Dysentery	*Shigella dysenteriae*	K. Shiga	1898
Contagious bovine pleuropneumonia	*Mycoplasma mycoides ssp. mycoides SC type*	Nocard and Roux	1898
paratyphoid	Salmonella Paratyphi	H. Schottmuller	1900
Syphilis	*Treponema pallidum*	F.R. Schaudin and E. Hoffmann	1905
Whooping cough	*Bordetella pertussis*	J. Bordet and O. Gengou	1906
Rocky mountain Spotted fever	*Rickettsia rickettsii*	Ricketts	1909
Tularemia	*Francisella tularensis*	McCoy and Chapin	1912

2

Classification and Nomenclature of Bacteria

Taxonomy (biological systematics) is the branch of science which deals with classification of units or individuals on the basis of similarities and differences. The classification, nomenclature, and identification are three interrelated components of bacterial taxonomy (Cowan, 1965).

Classification: Classification is the arrangement of bacteria into groups (taxa) based on the similarities of certain characteristics. Presently 11,000 bacterial species is classified. At the current rate of 600 bacterial species / year it is estimated to take 1000 years to classify all the bacteria!

Nomenclature: It is the assignment of specific names to the taxonomic groups following the regulations mentioned in 'International Code of Nomenclature of Bacteria' (Euzéby, 1997). International committee on systematic bacteriology (International committee on systematics of prokaryotes, ICSP) standardizes the code. The committee is helped by a number of taxonomic subcommittees on different groups of bacteria. The *Code* can be amended by the Judicial Commission. The *Code* contains general considerations, principles, rules and recommendations on the naming of prokaryotes (bacteria) up to the rank of 'Class'.

Identification: It is the practical use of a classification scheme to differentiate certain bacteria from others and to assign them an established taxon or previously unidentified taxon.

Historical perspective of bacterial taxonomy is described in Table 1.

Characteristics of pure culture bacteria

These are the parameters on which classification of bacteria are done. It is not possible to study the characteristics of a single bacterium due to small size. So the characteristics of 'bacterial culture' are considered. The 'culture' can be defined as population of bacteria. The culture composed of single kind of bacterial species is known as 'pure culture'.

The following characteristics of pure culture are considered for bacterial classification.

a) Morphology: Bacterial cellular shape, size, arrangement, staining properties, motility, position of flagella, sporulation can be used

b) Chemical composition: Certain specific group of chemicals is detected in a specific group of microorganisms. Such as teichoic acid and lipopolysaccharide are present in gram-positive and gram-negative group of bacteria, respectively. The viral nucleic acid is composed of either deoxyribose nucleic acid (DNA) or ribonucleic acid (RNA)

c) Cultural characteristics: Nutritional requirements for growth (autotroph/heterotroph), physical conditions (temperature, oxygen) and types of growth on artificial media (smooth/rough colonies, eugonic/dysgonic growth, pellicle/deposit formation in broth, specific colour/smell of bacterial colonies etc.) vary between different groups of microbes. Certain bacterial species requires specific supplements for growth (hoof powder for *Dichelobacter nodosus*) whereas others can grow in a general medium. *Rickettsia* and *Chlamydia* require live cells to propagate. Requirement of temperature also varies between mesophile, thermophile and psychrophile group of bacteria. Most of the bacteria prefer to grow in presence of oxygen (aerobic) whereas oxygen is toxic to others (anaerobic).

d) Metabolic characteristics: The bacteria may differ in source of energy and pathway of synthesis for different cellular constituents

e) Antigenic characteristics: Certain chemical substances (peptidoglycan, lipopolysaccharide, teichoic acid, outer membrane proteins) present in bacterial surface are considered as 'microbial antigen' or 'pathogen associated molecular pattern'. The host body after invasion with the bacteria responses with the production of 'antibody', specific to antigens. The pattern recognition receptors (Toll like receptor, Rig-1, NOD etc.) present in the host body recognize the antigens/patterns and produce the immune response through a complex pathway. As the antibodies are specific to different kinds of microbial antigens, it can be used for classification / identification of bacteria. *Enterobacteriaceae* can be classified into different serogroups based on 'O' / 'H' / 'K' antigens.

f) Genetic characteristics: The deoxyribose nucleic acid (DNA) of each bacterial group has special characteristics specific for the group. Total nucleotide present in DNA is expressed as mol% (G+C). The mol% (G+C) varies between different bacterial species and it can be used for bacterial classification. The sequence of nucleotide present in bacterial DNA is specific for each bacterial strain. Ribosomes are functionally constant ubiquitous molecules. Ribosomal RNAs (5S, 16S, 23S in prokaryotes) are functional unit of ribosome associated with protein synthesis. 16S rRNA is considered as taxonomic marker for classification of bacteria and archaea due to conserved secondary structure. Next generation sequencing (NGS) or Sanger's sequencing of 16S rRNA gene (PCR amplified small subunit) creates thousands of sequences annually. The sequence homology is searched into different algorithms such as basic local alignment search tool (BLAST; https://blast.ncbi.nlm.nih.gov/) and a dendogram is constructed on the basis of similarities with other sequences. The unknown sequences do not match with any of the known sequences in alignment search tool. The new 'species' (or any other taxa) is assigned following a combination of tests such as DNA-DNA hybridization (threshold value 70%), average sequence identities of shared genes (threshold value of 94-96%) etc. In heterologous DNA hybridization, denatured strands of DNA from two different bacterial groups can produce heteroduplexes if they are related (presence of complementary bases). Degree of divergence is calculated by amount of unpaired bases present in two bacterial groups. '*Tm*'-value of heteroduplexes indicates the temperature at which 50% of strand separation occurs. The D*Tm* value of heteroduplex is 0-20°C. The 0°C indicates 'perfect pairing' and each degree of instability indicates about 1% divergence.

g) Pathogenicity: Pathogenic potentiality of the bacteria can be used in classification. Few bacteria are capable to produce diseases in human, animals and plants but others cannot cause any such diseases.

h) Ecological characteristics: Bacterial properties vary with their habitat. Marine bacteria residing in deep sea can tolerate high water pressure whereas the fresh water bacteria living near the surface cannot tolerate such kind of pressure.

'Taxa' (Rank) in bacterial classification

'**Strain**': Basic unit of bacterial taxonomy is a 'strain'. The bacterial strain is a collection of cultures derived from a primary colony. Each strain has a different history and designation (a number). The same bacterial species isolated from different clinical samples will be considered as different strains. The strains are preserved in culture banks with a specific number.

All the microbial culture banks are registered with 'world data center for microorganisms (WDCM, http://www.wdcm.org/)'. It is the official data center of 'world federation for culture collections (WFCC)'. WDCM consists of several databases such as culture collections information worldwide (CCINFO), STRAIN, global catalogue of microorganisms (GCM), reference strain catalogue, GCM type strain genome database etc. The CCINFO/STRAIN is the catalogue of all registered microorganisms which currently consists of 3,150,966 microbes, 789 culture collection centers from 77 countries including India (27 culture collections consists of 1, 52,849 cultures). The global catalogue of microorganisms is the interface where scientists/ academicians and industry people can access the microbial strain information or the cultures. The GCM consists of 4, 47, 781 strains from 48 countries including India.

National collection of type culture (NCTC, UK) is the oldest culture bank (established in 1920) which currently consists of 5100 type and reference bacterial strains available for academic or industrial research. American type culture collection (ATCC, Rockville, Maryland, USA) is another old (established in 1925) culture collection consists of 18,000 bacterial strains, more than 3000 human and animal viruses, and 7600 fungi and yeast.

Major Indian culture collections are enlisted in Table 2.

Table 1: Historical perspectives of bacterial taxonomy

Year	Scientist	Contribution
1735	Carolus Linnaeus	Divided all living organisms into two kingdom such as animals and plants
1786	Otto Friedrich Müller (Denmark)	Classification of minute aquatic creatures such as unicellular algae, protozoa, ciliates, euglenoids etc. ('Infusoria'/ 'Protista')
1838	Christian Gottfried Ehrenberg (Germany)	Introduction of 'bacteria' as a new genus
1866	Haeckel	Classified all unicellular organisms under Kingdom 'Protista' and bacteria under phylum 'Monera'
1872-75	Cohn	Introduced class Schizophyta incorporating bacteria with blue-green algae
1894	Migula	Classified bacteria into Coccaceae, Bacillaceae, and Spirillaceae based on morphology
1913	Vuillemin	Classified bacteria into several new genera such as *Klebsiella, Streptococcus, Neisseria, Clostridium, Bacillus, Spirillum*
1957	Sneath	Numerical classification of bacteria

Table 2: Major Indian microbial culture collections

Culture collections	Coverage / Services	Contact
Microbial Type Culture Collection and Gene Bank (MTCC), Institute of Microbial Technology (IMTECH), Chandigarh (registered with WDCM)	1.Supply of cultures for scientific/industrial research 2. Phenotypical characterization, phylogeny, 16SrRNA analysis, MALDI-TOF analysis, Vitek analysis of cultures	https://mtccindia.res.in/
Division of Standardization, Indian Veterinary Research Institute , Izatanagar, Bareilly (registered with WDCM)	Maintenance and supply of livestock associated bacteria, fungi, yeast, protozoa for scientific/industrial research	http://ivri.nic.in/
National Center for Veterinary Type Cultures, ICAR-National Research Center on Equines, Hisar, Haryana	Maintenance and supply of bacteria, virus, bacteriophage, phage library, recombinant clones, genomic DNA, rumen archeae, fungi, yeast for scientific/industrial research	http://ncvtc.org.in/
National Collection for Dairy Cultures, National Dairy Research Institute, Karnal (registered with WDCM)	Maintenance and supply of bacteria, fungi, yeast, dairy starter cultures for scientific/industrial research	http://www.ndri.res.in/
Culture collection, Microbiology and Cell Biology Laboratory, Indian Institute of Science, Bengaluru (registered with WDCM)	Maintenance and supply of bacteria, virus, fungi, yeast, cell lines scientific/industrial research	http://www.wfcc.info/ccinfo/index.php/search/basic/
National Fungal Culture Collection of India, Maharashtra Association for the Cultivation of Science Agharkar Research Institute, Pune (registered with WDCM)	Maintenance and supply of fungi (3050 strains) for scientific/industrial research	http://aripune.org/
Indian Type Culture Collections, Division of Plant Pathology, Indian Agricultural Research Institute, New Delhi (registered with WDCM)	Maintenance and supply of bacteria and fungi for scientific/industrial research	http://www.iari.res.in/
Microbial Culture Collection (MCC), National center for cell science, Pune (registered with WDCM)	Maintenance and supply of bacteria and fungi for scientific/industrial research	http://gcm.wfcc.info/cc/mcc
National Agriculturally Important Microbial Culture Collection (NAIMCC), ICAR-National Bureau of Agriculturally Important Microorganisms, Mau Nath Bhanjan, U.P. (registered with WDCM)	Maintenance and supply of bacteria, actinomycetes, cyanobacteria and fungi for scientific/industrial research	http://nbaim.org.in/default.aspx
National Collection of Industrial Microorganisms (NCIM), CSIR-National Chemical Laboratory, Pune (registered with WDCM)	Maintenance of non-pathogenic, industry associated bacteria, fungi, actinomycetes, yeast and algae (oldest culture collection in India, established in 1951)	http://www.ncl-india.org/files/NCIM/

'Species': The species is the collection of 'type strain' and other strains having sufficiently similar characteristics to the type strain. 'Type strain' is the permanent reference specimen for the species maintained in different culture collections. The word 'type' does not mean it is typical. For new species the first strain isolated is usually designated as 'type strain'. If the 'type strain' is lost from the culture collection, new strains ('neotype') are prepared following the protocols mentioned in *Code*. On the basis of DNA similarity the members of a bacterial species (genomospecies) should have approximately 70% or greater DNA-DNA relatedness and 5°C or less D*Tm*.

The 'species' can be further sub-divided into 'subspecies' based on phenotypical characteristics and genetic similarities (DNA relatedness and D*Tm*). There is no official guideline to establish the 'subspecies'. Based on morphology, antigenic characteristics etc. few taxa (rank) below the subspecies ('infrasubspecific ranks') are unofficially established (Table 3).

Table 3: Infrasubspecific ranks

Rank	Characteristics
Biovar / Biotype	Bacterial strains having similar biochemical / physiological properties
Morphovar / Morphotype	Bacterial strains having similar morphology
Pathovar / Pathotype	Bacterial strains having similar pathogenicity in a common host
Serovar / Serotype	Bacterial strains having similar antigenic properties
Phagovar / Phage type	Bacterial strains lysed by same phage

'Genus': The 'genus' is the collection of 'type species' and other species having sufficiently similar characteristics to the type species. New genus is established on the basis of 16S rRNA analysis. The 'genus' and 'species' can be written as 'binomen' (binominal name). The genus name is written first with italics and an initial capital letter. It is followed by a species name in italics with all small letters. E.g. *Mycobacterium* (genus) *tuberculosis* (species).

Other taxa / ranks are described similarly in Table 4.

Table 4: Taxa/ ranks in bacterial classification (above genus)

Taxa / Rank	Definition
Family	Collection of genera (plural of genus)
Order	Collection of families
Class	Collection of orders
Division	Collection of classes
Domain	Collection of divisions (Bacteria and Archaea)

Methods of Classifications

a) *Natural classification*: Carolus Linnaeus first developed natural classification system during 18th century. The 'phenetic system' is the best natural classification system of bacteria. It is based on mutual similarities of phenotypic characteristics. It is not dependent on phylogentic analysis. Edward (1962) and Ewing (1986) developed the phenotypic principles for characterization, classification and identification of bacteria. They used a numbers of biochemical tests for characterization of the 'test' organism and expressed the results as percentage. 'Bergey's manual of systematic bacteriology' is the largest resource of bacterial genera and it follows phenetic system of classification. It was first developed by David Hendricks Bergey (USA) in 1923. Currently the book consists of five volumes covering all the classes of bacteria such as Archaea (volume 1), Proteobacteria (volume 2), Firmicutes (volume 3), Spirochaetes and others (volume 4) and Actinobacteria (volume 5).

b) *Numerical taxonomy*: It is the process of grouping of microbes based on similarities of characteristics (morphological / biochemical / physiological) expressed in numerical unit. The 'similarities' between two bacterial strains is expressed as an association co-efficient ('simple matching co-efficient' or 'Jaccard co-efficient'). The coefficients are calculated by checker boards as shown below. Sneath (1957) introduced the numerical techniques for classification of bacteria with Jaccard coefficient (originally developed by Jaccard in 1901). Later simple matching coefficient was developed.

Jaccard co-efficient (S_J): It is a measure of similarity for the two bacterial strains. The similarity is expressed as 0% to 100%. The higher the percentage, the strains are more similar. It does not include the characters absent in both the strains.

$$S_J = \frac{a}{a + b + c}$$

	1	0
1	a	b
0	c	d

a = numbers of characters present in both the bacterial strains (1)

b, c = numbers of characters which differs between two bacterial strains (1,0 or 0,1)

Simple matching co-efficient (S_{SM})

$$\frac{a + d}{a + b + c + d}$$

	1	0
1	a	b
0	c	d

a = numbers of characters present in both the bacterial strains (1)

b, c = numbers of characters which differs between two bacterial strains (1,0 or 0,1)

d = Numbers of characters absent in both the strains (0)

These co-efficient (S_J / S_{SM}) values are placed into a table to calculate 'similarity index'. Each row or column of the table represents one strain. The strains with near value of coefficients are grouped together. Such group is called 'phenon' / 'phenom'. For example, 80 'phenon' is equivalent to bacterial species. It indicates 80% similarities between the bacterial strains compared. The data of numerical taxonomy analysis are summarized in a tree like diagram ('dendogram') similar to genetic analysis.

c) *Genetic relatedness*: The system is based on similarities between the basic hereditary material i.e. deoxyribose nucleic acid (DNA) of organisms. Initially the DNA relatedness between two strains is measured with GC mol% although it is not an exact technique. Two different DNA sequences can be made with same proportion of GC / AT pair. The DNA-DNA hybridization or DNA-RNA hybridization technique can be used to measure genetic relatedness between two strains. The DNA-DNA hybridization study is done in closely related organisms, as no stable hybrid is generated with the sequences having huge dissimilarity. Distantly related organisms are compared with DNA-RNA hybridization study. In DNA-RNA hybridization study, rRNA / tRNA are selected due to their phylogenetically conserved nature. The genome can be directly compared by sequencing of 16S rRNA / 5S rRNA. The sequences are aligned and 'association coefficient (S_{ab})' is calculated. Higher the 'S_{ab}' value the organisms are more closely related.

List of Prokaryotic names with standing in nomenclature (LPSN, http://www.bacterio.net**)**

It is the most authentic source of bacterial nomenclature updated in a regular interval. LPSN was founded by Jean Euze´by, Ecole Nationale Ve´ te´rinaire de Toulouse, Toulouse, (France) in 1997. The LPSN is updated with each issue of International Journal of Systematic and Bacteriology (IJSB), currently known as International Journal of Systematic and Evolutionary Microbiology. It is the official journal of International Committee on Systematic Bacteriology.

'The All-Species Living Tree' Project

It is the collection of 16S rRNA sequences of all validly published species of *Bacteria* and *Archaea*. Currently there are more than 10,950 species. It is created with the collaboration of LPSN, ARB ("arbor"=tree), and SILVA rRNA database project (Microbial Genomics and Bioinformatics Research Group in Bremen, Germany).

3

Microscopy and Micrometry Bacterial Stains and Techniques

Microscope is the primary instrument of a microbiology laboratory and it produces enlarged images of small objects which are invisible by naked eye. With a microscope the operator can get a close view of minute structures which helps in examination and analysis. Examination of minute objects with a microscope is called 'microscopy'. In microbiology, measurement of the microbial dimension observed under microscope is known as 'micrometry'.

Types of microscopes

There are two types of microscopes i.e. light / optical and electron microscope depending on the sources of energy to create the image. The optical microscopes use the lenses and light (artificial or sunlight) to make an image. Following types of optical microscopes are available.

a) Bright field microscope

b) Dark field microscope

c) Phase contrast microscope

d) Interference microscope

e) Ultra-violet microscope

f) Fluorescence microscope

g) Inverted microscope

h) Stereoscopic microscope

i) Polarizing microscope

j) Reflecting microscope

k) Confocal microscope

a) Bright field microscope: The microscopic field is brightly illuminated with artificial light or sunlight and the bacteria appear darker due to absorbance of light. Staining of bacteria increases their light absorbing capacity and it creates a good contrast. Bright field microscope can be classified into simple microscope (single lens) and compound microscope (multiple lenses). A simple microscope can produce 300 × magnification whereas in a compound microscope the magnification varies between 1000× - 2000× (1000-2000 times image magnification). The '×' is algebraic symbol which denotes 'times'. The magnification of microscope is calculated by (Tube length/focal length) × magnification of ocular lens. The tube length is generally adjusted to 160 mm. The focal length is 16 mm (low power objective), 4 mm (high power objective) and 2 mm (oil immersion).

The higher magnification of an optical microscope is not useful until it has a good resolving power. The resolving power of a microscope is its capacity to differentiate two nearby points as distinct and separate. It is the function of numerical aperture of the optical lens and wavelength of the light used for microscopy. The numerical aperture is calculated with the multiplication of refractive index (of the medium between the lens and glass slide) and sine value of half aperture value. The numerical aperture of low, high and oil immersion objectives are 0.25, 0.85 and 1.3, respectively.

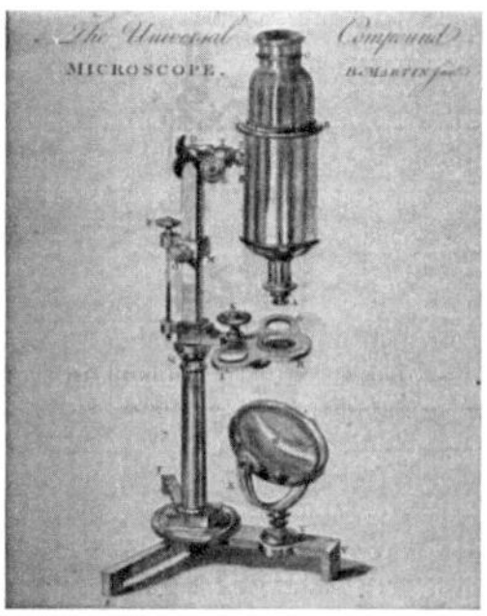

Fig. 1: Universal compound microscope (Courtesy of the National Library of Medicine)

$$d = \frac{\text{wave length of light}}{2 \text{ X numerical aperture}}$$

The 'd' value should be small for better resolution. The resolution can be improved either by using light of shorter wavelength or increasing the numerical aperture. The oil immersion lens has higher refractive index (1.2-1.4) and subsequently higher numerical aperture than dry objective (< 1). So it produces less 'd' value and better resolution than dry objective lens. The resolution is expressed in linear units (preferably 'µm'). The highest resolution of a simple microscope is 1 µm and a compound microscope is 0.2 µm (200 nanometer).

'Photomicrography' is the technique of capturing photograph of the object observed under microscope. Digital trinocular microscope shows the image directly on the computer screen.

Bright field microscope is useful to observe morphology of bacteria, yeasts, moulds, algae and protozoa in both stained and unstained samples.

b) **Dark field microscope:** The objects (bacterial cells) are illuminated against a dark background to create a contrast. The dark background is made with a special condenser which transmits the light in such a way that most of it cannot enter the objective. Only the part of the light which meets the object / bacterial cells on the slide can enter the eye. It is used for observation of unstained bacteria in hanging drop/wet mount preparation.

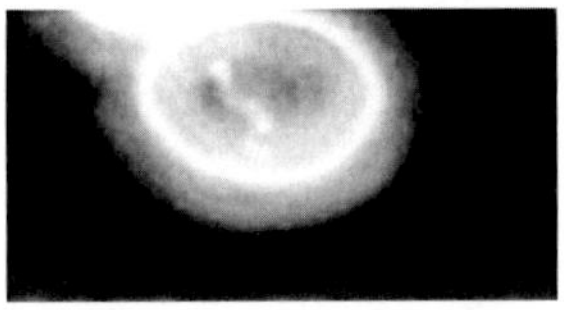

Fig. 2: Dark –field microscopy

c) **Phase contrast microscope:** The biological specimen such as cell nucleus is transparent in comparison to surrounding mounting fluid. It is difficult to observe under normal bright field microscopy due to lack of contrast. Other cell structures vary in refractive index form the surrounding medium. The phase shift can be created with the propagation of light through an object which can make a change in the optical route across the object. This phase shift is converted into variations in intensity to produce an image. This kind of microscope is useful for studying cellular details of larger microbes such as yeasts, algae, protozoa and few bacteria.

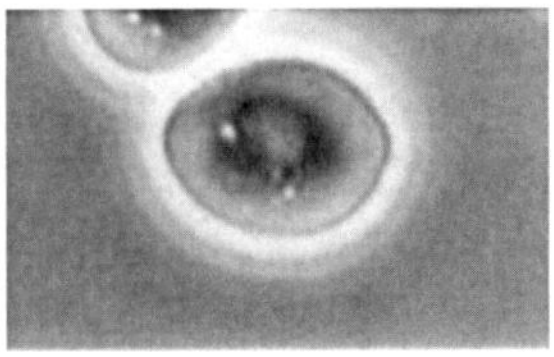

Fig. 3: Phase contrast microscopy

d) **Interference microscope:** It makes the image using the difference between an interfering beam passing through the specimen and an otherwise identical beam that illuminates it. The beams are separated by a beam splitter (Wollaston prism). This microscopy can measure the differences in density within the cells but the resolution is poor.

e) **Ultra-violet (UV) microscope:** It produces higher resolution than other microscopes due to shorter wave length of ultra-violet light. This kind of microscope needs specially made quartz lenses. The lamps in the range from deep blue to near UV are used. The images are made visible by recording on a photographic plate.

f) **Fluorescence microscope:** The chemical substances ('fluorescent') absorb high-energy ultra violet rays and emit low energy visible light waves. This is known as 'fluorescence'. When microorganisms coated with fluorescent dye are observed under UV microscope they appear brightly illuminated objects due to fluorescence. It is used for diagnosis of specific infections (e.g. Rabies in brain tissue).

g) **Inverted microscope:** This special kind of optical microscope is used in cell culture to observe the specimen in liquid medium. The light source and condenser are placed uppermost which directs the light on the stage. The front part of objective is set uppermost.

h) **Stereoscopic microscope:** It is a pair of microscope mounted side by side with a small angle between the optical axes. It is used in biological laboratories for dissection and microsurgical procedures. The magnification range of this microscope is 5-250×.

i) **Polarizing microscope:** It has additional feature to observe the specimen under polarized light. It is used to observe the effect of stress in biological samples and nature of crystals in geological samples.

j) **Reflecting microscope:** In this type of microscope two mirrors (primary and secondary) are used which uses reflection property for making images. Primary mirror is larger and concave, whereas, the secondary mirror is convex and small.

k) **Confocal microscope:** The specimen in focus appears with colour in the image whereas out of focus substances appear as black. Generally laser is used as a light source. This microscopy is often used to detect three-dimensional structures of biological samples.

Electron microscope: The electron microscope uses electron beam and magnetic field to create an image. The resolving power of electron microscope is more than 100 times than optical microscope. The highest resolution of electron microscope is 10 angstrom (0.001µm / 1 nm) and the magnification is up to 4,00000×. The samples are presented in the form of an enormously thin dry film. The film is placed between the magnetic objective and magnetic condenser. There are two types of electron microscopy i.e. scanning and transmission electron microscopy (SEM and TEM). The resolution is better in TEM but the SEM can produce a three dimensional picture ('micrograph') with a clear surface topography.

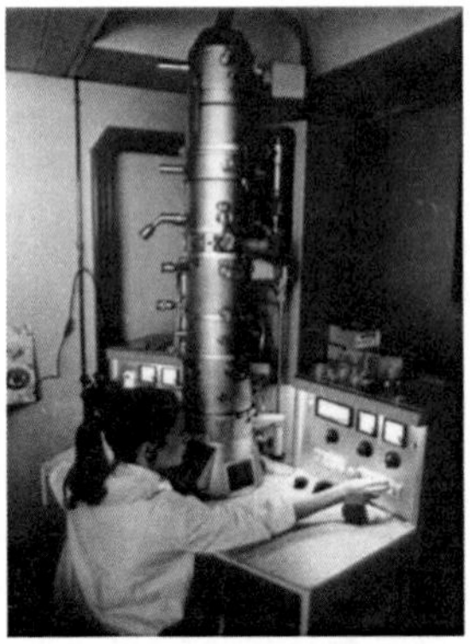

Fig. 4: Electron microscope (Courtesy of the National Library of Medicine)

There are several techniques used in electron microcopy for detection of cellular structure.

a) *Negative staining*: Detailed structure of viruses and bacterial flagella can be detected with the use of electron dense material such as phosphotungstic acid.

b) *Utrathin sectioning*: It is used for sectioning microbial cells. The bacterial cells are embedded in a plastic block and the block is cut into ultrathin sections (60 nm). The sections are used for microscopic examination with 'electron microscope stains' such as uranium and lanthanum salts.

c) *Freeze etching*: The specimen is sectioned in a frozen block without using chemical based fixation. The technique can avoid the formation of artifacts.

d) *Shadow casting*: Thin layer of platinum is deposited on the microbial cell in an oblique angle. The microbe produces a shadow on the uncoated side. The shadow gives a topographical representation of the microbial surface.

Cryo-electron tomography (cryo-ET) is a recent technique developed for three-dimensional study of macromolecules present in the cells. It is used for detection of bacterial cytoskeletal filaments, cell division, chemotaxis systems, motility machineries, invasion of bacteriophage etc. Most bacterial cells are considered large for this tomography. 'Minicells' are found suitable for cryo-ET. Minicells are produced by aberrant cell divisions of parent bacterial cells. It contains bacterial membranes, peptidoglycan, ribosomes, RNA, protein, plasmids but no chromosome. The minicells cannot divide or grow, but they have normal cellular functions. Other than cryo-ET, the minicells are current topic of discussion as a noble drug delivery system or a vaccine candidate.

Disadvantages of electron microscopy

i) High maintenance cost as the instrument is sensitive to vibration and magnetic field

ii) Trained manpower is required to operate the instrument and to prepare the samples efficiently

iii) Live cells cannot be examined

iv) Thin sectioning of the sample is required due to low penetration power of electron beam.

During drying for making the thin film the cell structures are sometimes altered.

Micrometry

Micrometry is the science of measurement of the object observed under microscope. It is performed with measuring device (micrometer) attached to the microscope. There are two types of micrometer i.e. stage and ocular micrometer.

a) *Stage micrometer*: This micrometer can be adjusted on a glass slide and it has a finely graduated scale. In the scale 1 mm is divided into 100 divisions which is equivalent to 10 μ (0.01 mm).

b) *Ocular micrometer*: It is adjusted inside the eyepiece. There are 50-100 divisions engraved into the scale.

Measurement of microbes

1. The stage micrometer is kept under low power of microscope and is observed through the eyepiece having ocular meter.
2. One division of ocular micrometer is calibrated with the following formula

   One division of ocular micrometer = Number of stage micrometer divisions / Number of ocular meter divisions × 10

   For example, 6 ocular divisions coincide with 8 divisions of stage micrometer.

   One division of ocular micrometer = 8/6 × 10 = 13.3 μ. Three readings are taken in a similar way and the mean value is considered.
3. The slide containing the stained bacterial cell is placed on the stage. If the length of a bacterial cell is 10 ocular divisions, measurement will be 10 × 13.3 μ = 133 μ.

Bacterial stains and techniques

The bacteria are colourless and have same refractive index to the aqueous solution present in the surrounding. It is difficult to observe the structural details until the diaphragm of the microscope is adjusted. It needs a lot of expertise. So the bacteria are coloured with stains to make them easily visible under microscope. The staining also allows study of internal structures of the bacterial cell, such as cell wall, nuclear material, mesosome etc.

Bacterial stains are organic compounds (dye) consist of 'chromophore' and 'auxochrome' group attached to a benzene ring. The chromophore group confers colour and the auxochrome group is responsible for electrolytic dissociation. On the basis of auxochrome group the stains can be classified into acidic, basic and neutral (cytological classification). The acidic stains (anionic / negative charged; e.g. eosin) are used to detect cell cytoplasm and basic dyes (cationic / positive charged; e.g. methylene blue, crystal violet, carbol fuchsin, gentian violet, methyl violet) can stain cellular constituents (nucleus, metachromatic granule). Neutral stains are complex salt of a dye acid and dye base (e.g. eosinate of methylene blue). Bacterial cell surface is mildly negative charged (in neutral pH) and attracts basic stains. The process of staining is an ion-exchange reaction. Eosin (acidic stain) cannot stain a bacterial cell as both are negative charged and electrostatically repeal each other.

Preparation of smear

The slides supplied from a manufacturer contain a greasy coat which hinders in making a proper smear. To remove the greasy coat the slide is rubbed with a clean soft cloth and it is flicked through the flame of a Bunsen burner. The cotton should not be used for rubbing as the fine threads present in cotton is attached with the slide and it will appear as artifact after staining.

a) During preparation of a direct smear from tissue samples, the tissue is held firmly with a sterile forcep and a sterile scalpel is inserted into the tissue. The material is scraped deep from the tissue and is placed over a clean, grease free slide. With the help of another slide held in an angle over the material, a thin smear is prepared.

b) From liquid specimens, the smear is prepared with a sterile swab.

c) For making smear from bacterial culture, a drop of sterile distilled water is placed over the slide. With the help of a bacteriological loop (standard diameter 4 mm) the culture is taken and the smear is prepared. It should be thin so that individual bacterial cell can be observed.

Fixation of smear

Fixation of smear is required to kill the vegetative bacteria (endospores are resistant), to adhere it to the slide due to coagulation of bacterial protoplasm and to make it permeable to the stains. Generally the fixation is done by air drying or flicking over the flame (smear is kept upside) of a Bunsen burner. Excess heat is avoided. For Giemsa staining the dried smear is fixed with methyl alcohol.

Types of staining

1. Simple staining

The staining of bacteria with a single stain (e.g. methylene blue) is known as simple staining. The dried smear is flooded with the stain and is kept for a specific period of time. It is washed with tap water; air dried and is observed under microscope. Simple staining is useful for detection of bacterial morphology (bacillus/coccus), special staining characteristics (bipolar staining) and presence of granules (higher colour intensity).

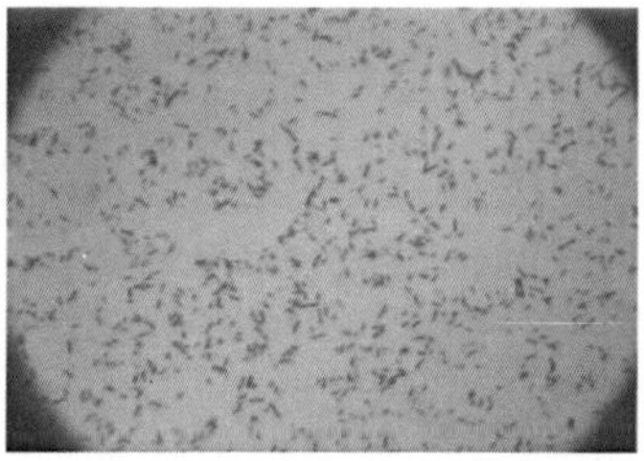

Fig. 5: Gram-positive mixed infection, 100X

2. **Differential staining**

a) *Gram's staining*: Christian Gram developed the technique in 1884 which is still considered as the fundamental technique for identification of bacteria. The four reagents used in the technique are primary stain (crystal violet / Gentian violet / methyl violet), mordant (Gram's iodine), decolourizer (95% ethyl alcohol / acetone / ether) and counter stain (carbol fuchsin / safranin). The bacteria which retain the primary stain are Gram-positive (violet / purple) and which are decolourized are Gram-negative bacteria (red / pink-red). There are several explanations of the fact as described under principle of Gram's staining.

Principle of Gram's staining

i) Earlier it was thought that Gram-positive bacteria contain magnesium-ribonucleoprotein which is absent in Gram-negative bacteria.

ii) Beveridge and Davies (1983) first explained the mechanism of Gram's staining. The mordant (negative charge) and primary stain (positive charge) makes a complex (crystal violet-iodine complex, CVI) which is retained in Gram-positive bacteria. The complex comes out during decolourization in Gram-negative bacteria so that the counter stain can enter the bacterial cell. Gram-negative bacterial cell wall contains more lipid than Gram-positive bacteria. During decolourization with ethanol the cell wall lipid in Gram-negative bacteria is extracted and porosity / permeability are increased. So the complex (CVI) comes out. The cell wall of Gram-positive bacteria become dehydrated in presence of ethanol and the permeability is reduced. The CVI complex cannot come out.

iii) Another explanation states that peptidoglycan content of Gram-negative cell wall is low and less cross-linked. So the cell wall is more porous even after ethanol treatment. The porous cell wall allows the easy exit of the complex (CVI).

b) Acid-fast staining

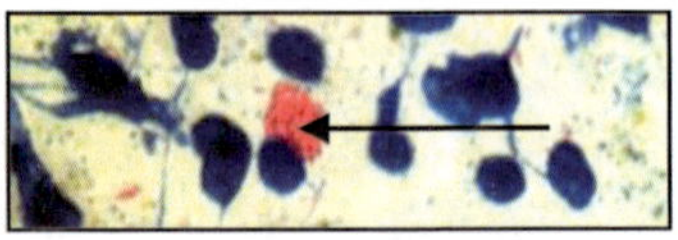

Fig. 6: Colour should be added so that red coloured ZN-positive rods can be seen (Courtesy of Premanshu Dandapat, ICAR-IVRI)

It is difficult to demonstrate gram staining nature of few bacteria (*Corynebacterium-Mycobacterium-Nocardia*, CMN group) due to high lipid content of the cell wall. The stains are relatively impermeable to these bacterial cells. With the help of heat (mordant) the strong carbol fuchsin can penetrate the lipid barrier. Once stained, decolourization of the bacteria is difficult even with acid-alcohol (20% sulfuric acid-95% ethyl alcohol). The staining technique is thus known as 'acid fast' staining (like 'colour fast cloth' which means colour is not lost during washing). The counter stain (methylene blue / malachite green) is applied to create the contrasting background. Paul Ehrlich (1882) first observed acid fast property of the bacteria and the staining technique. It was improved by Ziehl and Neelsen, so it is currently known as 'Ziehl and Neelsen' staining (ZN staining).

Later ZN staining was further modified for different purposes as enlisted below.

i) Instead of 20% sulfuric acid, 3% hydrochloric acid (HCl) is mixed with 95% ethyl alcohol. This modification is useful to differentiate *Mycobacterium tuberculosis* from saprophytic *Mycobacterium* spp.

ii) 0.5-1% sulfuric acid is used for demonstration of *Nocardia* and *Actinomyces*.

iii) < 5% sulfuric acid is used for demonstration of *Mycobacterium leprae*

c) ***Negative staining:*** The method of staining the background instead of the microbe is known as 'negative staining'. The bacteria will appear as stainless / transparent against a coloured background. India ink or nigrosine stains are used for it. The negative staining is useful for detection of spirochaetes, exact cell size and morphology of bacteria. As no heat is applied during the method morphology is not altered.

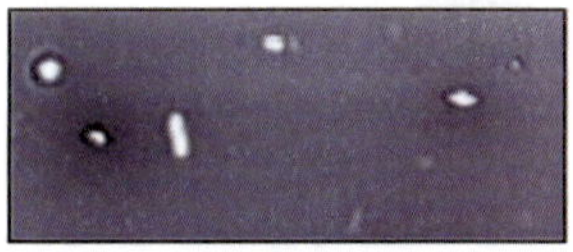

Fig. 7: Negatively stained bacteria with India ink

d) ***Special staining:*** The special staining is used for demonstration of bacterial parts such as capsule, endospore and flagella.

i) *Capsule staining:* For demonstration of bacterial capsule the background and the bacterial cells are stained with acidic (nigrosine) and basic dyes (crystal violet, safranin, methylene blue), respectively. The capsule appears as unstained halo surrounding the stained bacterial cells.

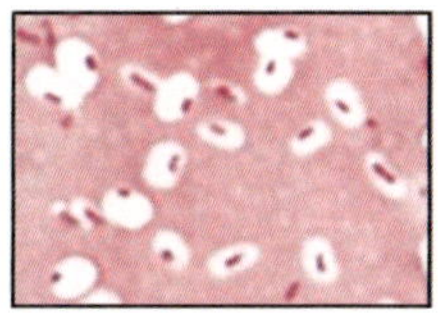

Fig. 8: Capsule staining of *Klebsiella* spp.

ii) *Endospore staining*: Bacterial endopsores (produced generally by Gram-positive bacteria with few exceptions) are heat and chemical resistant due to presence of spore coat or exosporium. Malachite green-Schaeffer and Fulton and Dorner methods are commonly used. The spores appear blue and the bacteria appear red in these staining methods.

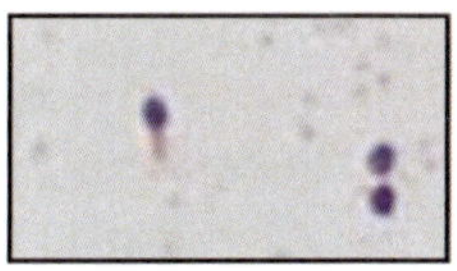

Fig. 9: Bacterial endospore staining with Malachite green-Schaeffer stain

iii) *Flagella staining:* Bacterial flagella are a thin and delicate structure which cannot hold much amount of stain. There are two types of flagella staining methods i.e. wet and dry methods. In wet method, a mordant (20% tannic acid-5% tartar emetic / phenol- aluminum potassium sulfate- tannic acid) is used which allows the stain (dilute silver sulphate / 'Ryu' stain) to be deposited on the flagella. The flagella become sufficiently thick to be visible under microscope. 'Ryu' stain is a saturated ethanolic solution of crystal violet.

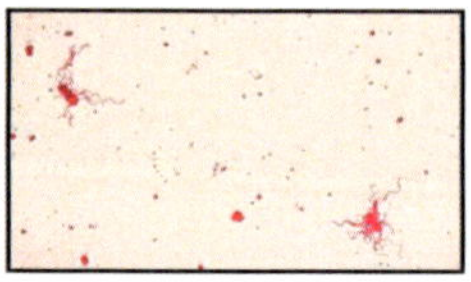

Fig. 10: Bacterial flagella (Leifson staining) (Courtesy of Public Health Library)

In dry method (Leifson staining) 1.2% basic fuchsin in 95% ethyl alcohol mixed with an equal volume of 0.75% NaCl and 1.5% tannic acid is used. Freshly prepared stain works better.

Observation of live bacteria by hanging drop method

Unstained live bacterial cells are observed by hanging drop method to detect cellular morphology (size, shape, arrangement of cells) and motility of the bacteria. A special kind of slide containing one/two depressions (wells) at the center is used. A loop full of bacterial suspension is placed over a cover slip. The vaseline is applied around the well of the slide. The slide is inverted and is put over the cover slip placing the depression exactly over the bacterial suspension. It is gently pressed and due to presence of vaseline the cover slip gets firmly attached with the slide. The slide is observed under low power objective of optical microscope.

4

Structure and Morphology of Bacteria

Bacteria can be defined as a group of diverse and ubiquitous prokaryotic single cell microorganisms. The size of bacteria varies with genera/species. In cocci the diameter varies between 0.5-1 µm. The measurement of bacillus / rod shaped bacteria is 4-8 µm × 1-1.25 µm. The surface area and volume ratio of bacteria is very high. The nutrients are absorbed through a large surface area and it is rapidly distributed into a small volume. So the growth rate and metabolism of bacteria is very high. The bacterial cell mass is packed near the surface and no circulatory system is required to distribute the nutrients. The growth and metabolism rate of bacilli are more than cocci because surface area and volume ratio of a sphere (cocci) is lowest among all the geometrical forms.

Shape of bacteria

The shape of bacteria is mostly regulated by the rigid cell wall covering the bacteria. Different shapes of bacteria are observed.

a) Spherical/oval: Coccus (cocci in pleural) e.g. *Staphylococcus*, *Streptococcus* (although *Staphylococcus* and *Streptococcus* are not a true sphere. The cocci cells have constrictions present in the sphere) 

b) Rod / cylindrical: Bacillus (bacilli in pleural) e.g. *Bacillus anthracis* 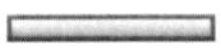

c) Rods with helical curve: Spirillum

   i) Rod with single curve (comma shaped) : e.g *Vibrio* 
   ii) Rod with multiple curves: e.g. *Spirilla* (rigid helical), *Spirochaetes* (flexible) 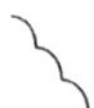

d) Coccobacilli (shorter than bacilli, appears stumpy): e.g. *Pasteurella multocida* 

e) Rectangular / triangular : e.g. *Haloarcula* (non-pathogenic halophile found in dead sea) 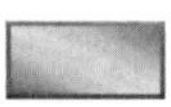

f) Star-shaped: e.g. *Stella humosa* (common in freshwater, soil and sewage)

g) Stalked bacteria (bacteria with external appendages): e.g. *Caulobacter crescentus* (common in lake, stream)

Arrangement of bacterial cells

Coccus shaped bacterial cells show following arrangement:

a) Diplococci: The cells divide in one plane and remain present in pair

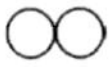

b) Streptococci: The cells divide in one plane and remain present in a chain

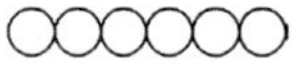

c) Tetrad: The cells divide in two planes and group of four cells is formed

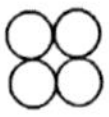

d) Staphylococci: The cells divide in three planes and irregular bunches of cocci cells is produced

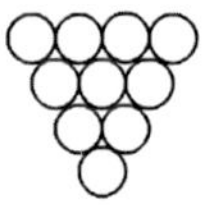

e) Sarcinae: The cells divide in three planes and regular cuboidal arrangement of cocci cells is produced 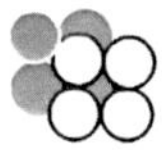

Bacillus / rod shaped bacterial cells show following arrangement:

a) Diplobacilli: Two bacilli cells are arranged in pair

b) Streptobacilli: The bacilli cells are arranged in chains (e.g. *Bacillus subtilis*)

c) Trichome: The bacilli cells are arranged in chains but the area of contact between the cells is larger between the adjacent cells (e.g. *Sapropspira*)

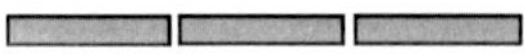

d) Palisade / 'Chinese letter' arrangement: The bacilli cells are arranged at an angle to each other. E.g. *Corynebacterium* spp. 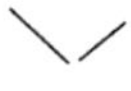

Bacterial cell structure

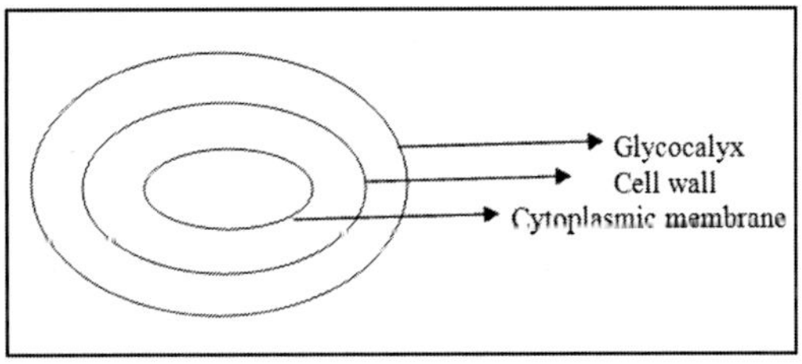

Bacteria are prokaryotic organisms. The cell is composed of nuclear material (not a true nucleolus) and cytoplasm. Many cell organelles present in eukaryotes are absent in bacteria (Table 1).

Glycocalyx: It is an additional polymeric covering present outside the cell wall in some bacteria. It has two types i.e. capsule and slime.

Capsule is a gelatinous, regular glycocalyx which forms a hydrophilic and amorphous envelope outside the bacterial cell. According to the thickness, the capsules are classified into 'microcapsule' (10-30 nm thick) and 'macrocapsule' (0.2-1 μm thick). Microcapsules cannot be observed by light microscopy. The bacterial capsule can be further classified into integral (e.g. *Klebsiella aerogenes*) and peripheral (e.g. *Pseudomonas aeruginosa*) types. The peripheral capsules are shed into the surrounding medium.

Bacterial capsule is composed of polysaccharide (neutral hexose, 6-deoxyhexose, polyol, uronic acid, amino sugar) except in *Bacillus anthracis*. In *Bacillus anthracis,* the capsule is composed of protein consisting D-glutamic acid. It is rare as L-isomers of amino acids are commonly found in nature. Single type of polysaccharide in the composition of capsule ('homopolysaccharide capsule') is observed in *Streptococcus mutans*. The capsule composed of different types of polysaccharides is known as 'heteropolysaccharide' capsule.

Due to hydrophilic nature capsules are difficult to stain. Most of the stains do not adhere to the capsule. So the capsules are stained by negative staining method with India ink or nigrosin. Several physiological factors such as high C : N ratio, ion concentration can influence the formation of capsule. The capsule production can be increased by sub-inhibitory dosage of antibiotics which converted the normal bacteria into hypervirulent in a mice model.

Function of bacterial capsule is described below.

i) Capsule prevents drying of bacterial cell by binding with water molecule (hydrophilic nature)

ii) Capsule protects the bacterial cell by preventing the attachment of bacteriophage

iii) It is antiphagocytic and plays a major role in virulence. The capsule covers C3b and prevents its binding with the C3b receptors present on the phagocytes.

iv) It helps bacteria to get attached with the host cell surface (teeth, hair) and environment (soil, rock). Extracellular glycocalyx plays a major role in biofilm formation. Biofilms are microbial communities adhered on biotic or abiotic surfaces and act as a major site for persistence and horizontal gene transfer. The biofilm producing organisms (80% of clinical isolates) are coated with an exopolysaccharide (EPS) matrix and become less susceptible to environmental stress, antibiotics, disinfectants and the host immune system. Bioflim forming uropathogenic *E. coli*, enterohaemorrhagic *E. coli*, *Salmonella*, cystic fibrosis associated *Pseudomonas* are global concern currently. The author elucidated healthy livestock, ducks and companion animals as a carrier of biofilm-producing *Enterobacteriaceae* in West Bengal, India.

v) Capsule can increase the stability of bacterial suspension in a liquid medium (broth). Capsule is composed of charged molecules (sugar) and in a suspension all the bacterial cells having same charge will repeal one another. Thus bacterial cells are prevented from aggregation and sedimentation.

vi) In nitrogen fixing bacteria (*Rhizobium trifolii*), the adhesin ('trifoliin', a lectin) for attachment with plant root gets adhered with bacterial capsule and mediates the adhesion. The adhesion is required for nodule formation in the plants and nitrogen fixation.

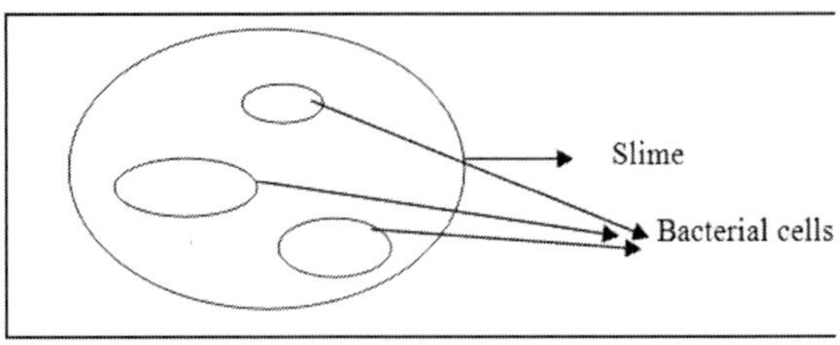

'Slime' is irregular diffused glycocalyx which can cover many bacterial cells together. Due to presence of slime layer the bacterial colonies in solid medium (agar media) become sticky (e.g. *Actinobacillus* spp.). The slime layer can also protect the bacterial cells from dehydration and loss of nutrients.

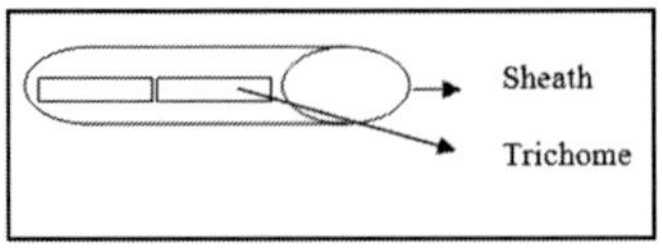

Sheath: The marine and freshwater bacteria with trichome arrangement are covered with a hollow tube, known as sheath. The sheath is composed of ferric or magnesium hydroxides.

Prosthecae: The marine and freshwater bacteria (*Caulobacter*, *Ancalomicrobium*, *Stella*) possess semi-rigid extension of cell wall, known as 'prosthecae'. The diameter of prosthecae is less than the bacterial cells. It increases the surface area for better nutrient absorption and it may help in adhesion with biotic or abiotic surfaces.

Stalk: Ribbon-like / tubular appendages found at the exterior of bacterial cells (*Gallionella, Plantomyces*). It helps in attachment of bacterial cell.

Cell wall: It is a rigid complex of membrane and associated macromolecules present between the glycocalyx (absent in majority of bacteria) and cytoplasmic membrane of bacterial cells. The cell wall constitutes 10-40% of dry weight of the bacterial cell depending upon the species and culture condition. Currently the word 'bacterial cell envelope' is introduced in place of 'cell wall'. The nomenclature 'cell wall' is not suitable to describe gram-negative membrane which additionally contains 'outer membrane' outside the peptidoglycan layer. Two unique molecules present only in prokaryotes, peptidoglycan and lipopolysaccharide are major constituents of the cell wall. The cell wall is absent in *Mycoplasma* and L-form of bacteria.

Function of cell wall

a) Maintenance of bacterial cell shape and rigidity

b) The cell wall provides protection against osmotic lysis. Most of the bacteria reside in hypotonic medium. The fluid can enter the bacterial cell to burst (osmotic shock) it

c) Maintenance of ionic balance between inside and outside of bacterial cells

d) Protection against antibacterial substances and host defence

e) It helps bacteria to sense the environment

f) It contains trans-envelope transport machineries

g) Adhesion to biotic or abiotic surfaces and invasion of eukaryotic cells

h) It supports flagellar motors and fimbriae

i) It acts as matrix for different biosynthesis

j) It is associated with cell division

Chemical composition of cell wall

Peptidoglycan ('murein') is the major constituent of bacterial cell wall and is responsible for the cell wall rigidity. The molecule is sensitive to lysozyme. The lysozyme is found in macrophages and polymorphonuclear leukocytes, secreations (tears, saliva, human milk, mucus) and egg white. The peptidoglycan has few unique properties.

i) It is an insoluble, porous and cross-linked amino sugar. Chemically it is a polymer of N-acetyl-glucosamine (NAG), N-acetyl-muramic acid (NAM) and amino acids. The schematic chemical structure of peptidoglycan is described below.

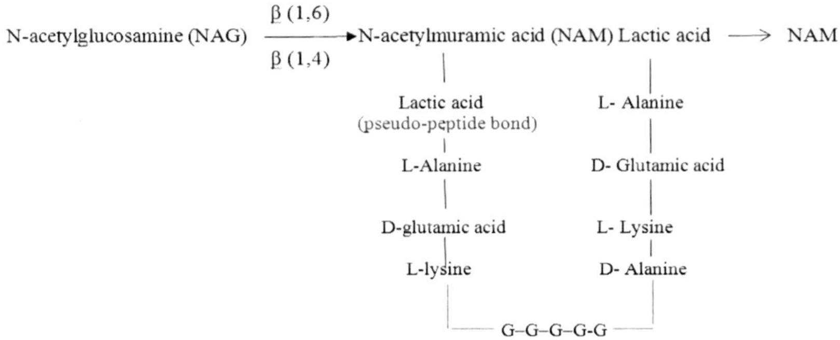

ii) Presence of D-amino acids is rare in nature and is only found in bacterial peptidoglycan

iii) L-lysine in peptidoglycan of vegetative bacteria is replaced with meso-diaminopimelic acid (meso-DAP) in peptidoglycan of bacterial spores. It is a rare symmetrical molecule with both optical activity (D and L) and hence is termed as 'meso'.

iv) The cross linkage of the polymer depends on penta-Glycine bridge between two amino-sugar strands. In Gram-negative bacteria (*E. coli*), most of the penta-Glycine bridges are unlinked and low (20%) cross linkage in the molecule is observed. Higher (90%) cross linkage is found in Gram-positive bacteria (*Staphylococcus*).

v) A peudo-peptide bond is detected between lactic acid and L-Alanine

vi) In *Mycobacterium* and *Nocardia*, N-glycosyl glucosamine are found in place of N-acetyl-glucosamine.

vii) Half of the muramic acids in *Staphylococcus* possess an acetyl group on 6th position (O-acetylation) which makes the molecules resistant to lysozyme. Unsubstituted glucosamine is found in few strains of *Bacillus cereus* making them resistant to lysozyme

viii) The bacterial cell wall also possess autolysins which can degrade own peptidoglycan so that extension of the chain can be done during cell division and growth

The cell wall of Archaeobacteria is composed of glycoproteins and polysaccharides, not peptidoglycan.

Cell wall of Gram-positive bacteria

Gram-positive cell wall is present between the glycocalyx (absent in majority of bacteria) and cytoplasmic membrane. It is composed of mostly peptidoglycan along with secondary / accessory carbohydrate and protein. The protein layer is the outermost layer and it is a fibrillar structure. The layer also contains accessory carbohydrate (teichoic acid) in most of the Gram-positive bacteria other than protein. In *Clostridium*, protein is the major macromolecule.

Teichoic acid is a poly-ribitol / poly-glycerol phosphate. The polymer is composed of alternating units of a polyhydroxy alkane (glycerol/ribitol) joined by phosphodiester linkage. On the basis of variations in the repeating structural units teichoic acids are classified into five types (I-V). Due to negative charge of the phosphate, the teichoic acid can bind with magnesium ions (positive charged). Magnesium ions provide thermal stability to the membrane. Teichoic acid also acts as receptor for bacteriophage and major antigen for bacterial typing scheme. In presence of phosphate, teichoic acid is converted into teichuronic acid. There are three types of teichoic acids i.e. intracellular teichoic acid, membrane teichoic acid and lipoteichoic acid (LTA, linked to glycolipid). The synthesis of lipoteichoic acid is essential for bacterial growth. It may also inhibit the activity of antibiotics and autolysin and thus it saves the membrane integrity. The bacterial autolysins regulate cell division and biofilm formation. So the bacteria with reduced LTA display pleiotropic phenotypes. Immunostimulatory role of type I-LTA is detected.

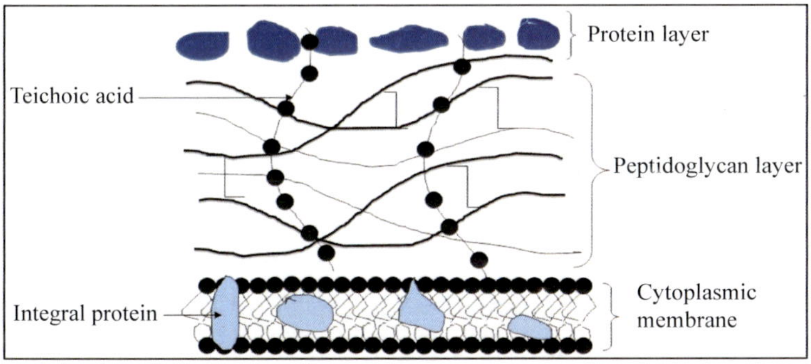

Peptidoglycan layer present beneath the protein layer is thicker (20-30 nm) than Gram-negative cell wall (3-5 nm). More than 50% (80-90% in *Micrococcus luteus*) dry weight of Gram-positive cell wall is due to peptidoglycan. However in Gram-positive bacterial cells having thick protein layer, the peptidoglycan layer in thinner (like Gram-negative bacteria).

Lipid content of Gram-positive cell wall is less except in *Corynebacterium*, *Mycobacterium* and *Nocardia* (CMN group of bacteria). In CMN group of bacteria lipid content is high due to presence of mycolic acid.

Cell wall of Gram-negative bacteria

Outer membrane: Gram-negative cell wall is more complex than Gram-positive cell wall due to presence of an additional layer outside the cell wall, known as 'outer membrane'. The outer membrane is a bilayer structure and is composed of lipopolysaccharide (LPS), phospholipid and proteins. The lipid constitutes 11-22% of dry weight of the cell wall. The outer membrane acts as impermeable barrier to prevent the entry of molecules which may damage the cell wall (e.g. lysozyme) and to prevent the exit of enzymes present in periplasmic space.

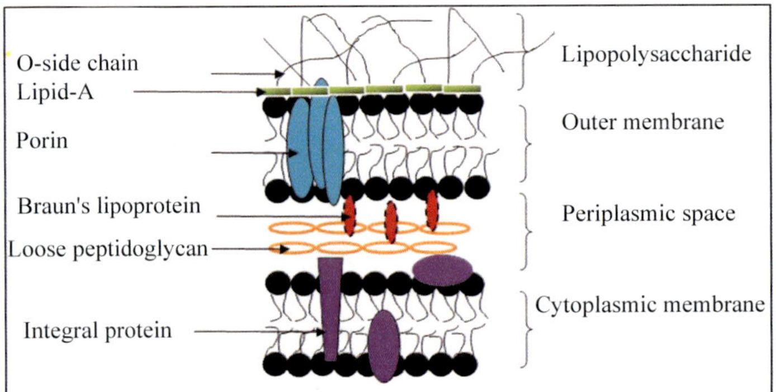

Gram-negative bacterial cell wall

Lipopolysaccharide (LPS) is also known as 'endotoxin' and is composed of three units i.e. lipid-A, core and O-antigen.

a) Lipid-A: It is phosphorylated glucosamine disaccharide along with fatty acids. The fatty acids help in anchoring the molecule in outer membrane. Lipid-A is responsible for 'toxicity' of the endotoxin (LPS). During lysis of Gram-negative bacterial cell by host immune system, the cell wall fragment containing LPS is released into the circulation. It causes fever, and diarrhoea followed by shock ('endotoxic shock')

b) Core: The core is the middle structure between lipid-A and O-antigen. It is composed of heptose and keto-deoxyoctulosonate (KDO)

c) O-antigen (somatic antigen / O-side chain): The somatic antigens are polysaccharide chains extending like whisker from outer membrane. The O-antigens are attached with core / lipid-A by WaaL ligase enzyme. The polysaccharide composition of O-antigen varies between the bacterial strains. E. coli is classified into 186 serogroups (O-serogroups) based on O-antigen structure variation.

O-antigen is not a permanent part of LPS. It is present in smooth-LPS found in virulent bacterial strains. It is absent in rough-LPS possessing bacterial strains which are easily penetrable by the antibiotics. In a group of bacteria (Haemophilus, Neisseria, Bordetella, Campylobacter), O- antigen is permanently absent in all strains due to absence of WaaL ligase enzyme. The strains instead possess lipo-oligosaccharide (LOS) composed of lipid-A and core. The LOS can also act as endotoxin and B-cell mitogen like LPS.

The proteins present in outer membrane are known as 'outer membrane protein' (OMP). There are three major groups of OMPs i.e. porin, transmembrane protein and peripheral proteins.

a) Porin: it is a trimeric protein of outer membrane which makes a pore (1 nm diameter) through which the molecules can diffuse. Porin protein is made of beta-sheets linked together by beta-turns at cytoplasmic side and amino acid loops on the other end. The beta-sheets are arranged in antiparallel fashion to form a cylindrical structure ('beta-barrel'). The porin channel is partially blocked with a loop, known as 'eyelet'. The eyelet projects into the cavity and controls the size of molecule which can pass through the porin channel. Diffusion of small hydrophilic metabolites such as sugar, ion, and amino acids is regulated by porin channel. Few antibiotics also use the channel to enter the bacterial cell. In *E. coli* several types of porins are observed such as maltoporin (maltose uptake), phosphoporin (phosphorus uptake), OmpF/OmpC (response to changes in osmolarity) etc.

b) Transmembrane protein: It helps in spanning outer membrane. It is associated with enzyme production and secreation, adhesion with biotic/abiotic surface and binding of antibiotic for structural modifications (e.g. penicillin-binding protein). DedA ('SNARE-associated family' based on homology to yeast Tvp38) is a highly conserved, integral membrane protein found in most of the sequenced genomes of eubacteria and archaea. DedA is associated with cell division, temperature sensitivity, membrane lipid synthesis, and generation of proton motive force.

c) Peripheral protein: It helps in transport of large molecules (e.g. iron) which cannot enter through the porin channel.

***Periplasmic space*:** It is the space between outer membrane and cytoplasmic membrane in Gram-negative bacteria. The space is occupied with 'periplasm' composed of enzymes required for cell wall growth, binding proteins which help in transport of molecules within the cell and beta-lactamase enzyme responsible for degradation of beta-lactam antibiotics. The oxidative protein folding takes place in the periplasmic space which can provide stability of many secreted proteins. The protein oxidation is regulated by a family of thioredoxin-like enzymes (DsbA-DsbG) specially in high-GC-content bacteria (e.g. *Actinomyces oris*, *Corynebacterium diphtheriae*). The DsbA and DsbB work together to catalyze disulfide bond formation in proteins to be secreated outside.

The space contains loose network of peptidoglycan. The 'loose peptidoglycan' is characterized with 50% cross linkage and absence of penta-Glycine bridge.

In Gram-positive bacteria, the space between cell wall and cytoplasmic membrane is considered as periplasmic space currently in few genera. It can be seen by electron microscopy. Although it is not exactly equivalent to the periplasmic space found in Gram-negative bacteria and no protein oxidation system is observed. Hence the misfolding is observed in proteins secreated by Gram-positive bacteria exposed to oxidative stress.

Cytoplasmic membrane (common in Gram-positive and Gram-negative bacteria)

The cytoplasmic membrane is present beneath the cell wall in both Gram-positive and Gram-negative bacteria. Together with cell wall it constitutes the bacterial 'cell envelope'. The membrane is 7.5 nm thick and damage to the membrane can cause death of the bacterial cell. It is a phospholipid bilayer in which proteins are held firmly (integral proteins). These proteins are removed only by the treatment of the membrane with detergent. Few other proteins are loosely attached to the membrane (peripheral proteins). The peripheral proteins can be removed by mild treatment. The phospholipid bilayer provides fluidity of the membrane which allows the components to move laterally. This kind of phospholipid bilayer arrangement with impregnated proteins is known as 'fluid mosaic model'. The sterol is absent in bacterial cytoplasmic membrane (except *Mycoplasma*) unlike eukaryotic plasma membrane.

Function

a) The membrane acts as hydrophobic barrier

b) The membrane contains several enzymes required for respiration and synthesis of capsular / cell wall components

c) It is the site for generation of 'proton motive force'. The force drives ATP synthesis, nutrient transport and flagellar motility. The proton gradients are used to generate chemiosmotic potential. Two protons are expelled to generate one ATP.

***Outer membrane vesicles* (OMV):** It is an outgrowth on the surface of a gram-negative bacterial cell ('bleb'). It plays major role in horizontal gene transfer, antibiotic resistance and virulence. In *Acinetobacter*, the OMVs help in transport of OmpA (major virulence factor) to the host cells. In few bacteria the OMV can generate protective immunity. So it is used as a vaccine candidate now a day.

***Mesosome*:** It is a membrane invagination in the form of a convoluted tubule commonly found in Gram-positive bacteria. It is the equivalent organ of mitochondria present in eukaryotes. Chapman and Hiller (1953) first observed mesosome and J.D. Robertson (1959) first named it. There are two types of mesosomes i.e. central (septal) and peripheral (lateral). The central mesosome is situated near the nuclear material and is associated with DNA replication and cell division. The peripheral mesosome is associated with export of extracellular enzymes.

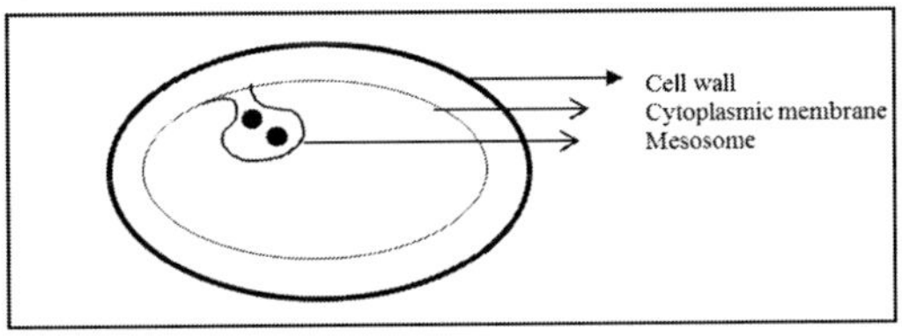

***Cytoplasm*:** Bacterial cell material surrounded by cytoplasmic membrane is divided into cytoplasm and nuclear material. The cytoplasm is granular in appearance due to presence of free ribosomes (no endoplasmic reticulum). The synthesis of secreatory proteins takes place in the ribosomes adhered with inner surface of cytoplasmic membrane. The bacterial ribosome is 70S composed of two subunits i.e. 50S and 30S. Following cytoplasmic granules and vacuoles are detected.

a) Metachromatic granule (Volutin granule/Babes Ernst body): It acts as phosphate reserve and is common in *Corynebacterium* sp. It can be stained by Albert / Neisser's stains.

b) Polyhydroxy-butyrate granule (PHB): It acts as carbon and energy reserve and it is common in aerobic bacteria. It can be stained by Nile blue (fat soluble dye).

c) Sulphur granule: It is found in saprophytic bacteria grown in hydrogen sulphide rich environment.

d) Gas vacuole: It is common in aquatic and cyanobacteria. The membrane of vacuole is impermeable to water but the gases can enter and fill it, when required. The vacuole is required for maintaining the buoyancy of aquatic bacteria.

***Nuclear material*:** The bacterial cells do not have a typical membrane bound nucleus (except *Planctomycetes*). The genetic material (deoxyribose nucleic acid, DNA) is confined at the centre of the cell in a specific area, known as 'nuclear material' / 'nucleoid'/ 'chromatin body' / 'bacterial chromosome'. The genes are arranged in chains like 'beads on a string' in the bacterial chromosome. The chromosome length is *more* than the bacterial cell diameter. So it is compacted in rosettes of radial loops. The chromosome (eubacteria and archae) is always circular. If the chromosome is made linear with hairpin telomeres, it remains stable and functional. Single chromosome is found in eubacteria and archae except in *Vibrio*, *Brucella*, *Haloarcula* (two chromosomes). The reason for single chromosome in bacteria is presence of only one replicon driven by the *oriC*/DnaA pair. There is no histone protein ('naked' DNA) and the nucleoids are present like a 'wire loop' held together loosely by a proteinaceous core. In true sense bacterial DNA is not 'naked' and is surrounded with nucleoid-associated proteins and transcription factors. The ratio of protein to DNA in a bacterial genome is 0.02. Introduction of DNA superhelicity provides stability of the wire loop structure. Mesophilic bacteria use DNA gyrase to introduce negative-supercoil and thermophilic bacteria use reverse gyrase to introduce positive supercoils.

The bacterial genome is highly compact with minimal intragenic regions and almost no repeats. Few introns are present which mostly encode selfish elements. Large uninterrupted foreign DNA sequences are found in bacterial genome resulting from horizontal gene transfer. The foreign DNA may enter the bacterial cells through nutrients or with the help of extrachromosomal 'mobilome' (plasmid, phages). It later becomes integrated into the bacterial chromosome. The horizontal gene transfer from neighbouring bacteria helps in survival of recipient bacteria in a new habitat or hostile environment or with the exposure to antibiotics. Few bacterial plasmids possess niche-specific essential genes and chromosome-like GC content. They are known as 'chromids'.

Appendages

Flagella

Flagella ('flagellum' in singular) are hair like helical appendages protruding out from the eubacterial cells. It is the organ of motility. The diameter of flagella is 0.01-0.02 µm. In archae, the flagellum is known as 'archaellum'. With the help of flagella the motile bacteria can swim in liquid medium. The speed is detected up to 135 µm/s. The bacterial flagella can be seen by light microscopy with special staining (Leifson staining)

Flagella are not considered as sole locomotory organs of bacteria. Few bacterial species (*Neisseria gonorrhoeae*, *Pseudomonas aeruginosa*) show 'twitching and social gliding motility' with the help of type IV fibrils at a slow speed (0.1 µm/s). Spirochaetes (*Leptospira*) can show twitching motility in viscous medium (e.g. connective tissues) with the help of periplasmic flagella residing within the cells ('endoflagella' / 'axial filament'). 'Swarming motility' is detected mostly in *Proteus* spp. and also in *Pseudomonas aeruginosa* and *Clostridium tetani*.

Based on the position of flagella the bacteria can be classified into following types.

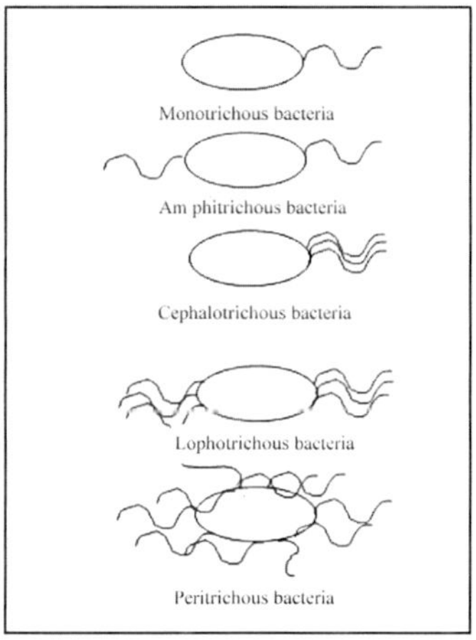

a) Monotrichous : Bacteria with one flagellum at one end (e.g. *Pseudomonas aeruginosa*)
b) Amphitrichous : Bacteria with one flagellum at both end (e.g. *Aquaspirillum* sp.)
c) Cephalotrichous : Bacteria with cluster of flagella at one end
d) Lophotrichous : Bacteria with cluster of flagella at both ends (e.g. *Pseudomonas* sp.)
e) Peritrichous: Bacterial cell surrounded with flagella (e.g. *Salmonella* Typhi)

Mechanism of bacterial motility: The movement of bacteria towards a favourable stimulus (sugar, amino acids) is known as 'positive chemotaxis'. When the bacteria can sense the unfavourable environment they can move away from the place ('negative chemotaxis'). Before moving away from the place or changing the direction of swimming there is a phase called 'tumbling'. In 'tumbling' phase the bacteria stop movement. Bacteria with polar flagella swim in a backward and forward way. Change in flagellar rotational direction can alter the direction of movement. The peritrichous bacteria during movement create a bundle of flagella. The bundle rotates anticlockwise and the bacteria move in opposite direction (A). The average rotational frequency of flagellar bundles in *E. coli* is 80 Hz (revolutions per second). During tumbling phase, all the flagella become free from the bundle and rotate individually (B). As a result there is no movement of bacterial cell. The flagellar motor is powered with proton motive force (PMF) or sodium ion motive force (NaMF). The force is created with the movement of a proton or sodium ion from external environment into the bacterial cell. The force can activate F0F1-ATPase (ATP synthetase) to generate ATP. The ATP helps in rotation of flagella. The flagellar motor is known as 'smallest rotary device in nature'.

Brownian movement: It is the vibration of bacterial cells *in same direction* due to collision with water molecules. Kinetic energy present in all molecules causes

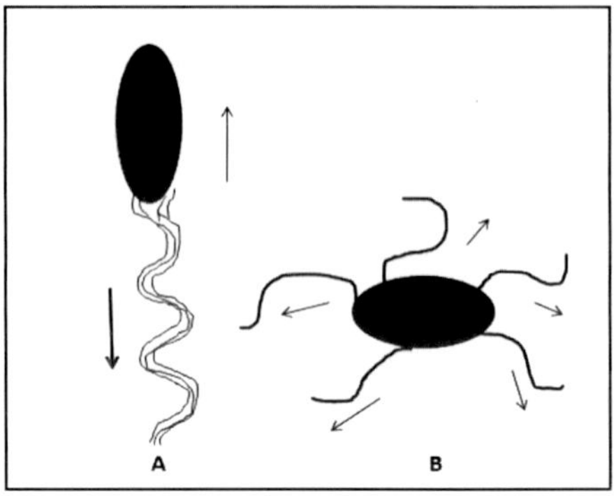

this kind of movement. Sometimes it is confused with true bacterial motility. In true bacterial motility the bacteria shows movement in *different directions*. Some bacteria will 'move' forward / backward and some bacteria will 'tumble' in the same position.

Structure of flagella: Flagellum is a helical structure. It is made of 'flagellin' protein. Theoretically three types of helixes are possible. Left handed, right handed and zero-handed. The helix is left handed in most of the bacteria. In few exceptions such as in *Caulobacter cresentus* and *Rhizobium melilotti* the right handed helix (curly flagella) is detected. In *Rhodobacter* the helix is left handed but is converted into right handed during rotation on a bacterial cell. This conversion of helix handedness is known as 'polymorphism'. If a mixture of left handed and right handed helix are allowed to polymerize the result depends on the larger proportion of the helix present in parents.

A flagellum consists of three structural parts i.e. filament, hook and basal body.

Filament: The filament is composed of flagellin protein. The protein is encoded by *Hag* (H-antigen) or *FliC* gene. Current nomenclature supports the name *FliC*. There are six genes in the eubacterial genome known as *FliC1-FliC6*. The flagellin protein has four structural regions (two terminal and two central regions). The central region amino acid sequence is highly variable between the bacterial species and *Salmonella* serovars. On the basis of the variation H-typing is conducted. Toll-like receptor (TLR 5) present within the body of the host can recognize the variable domain of flagellin (H-antigen) and produce antibodies. The variable domain is absent in environmental bacteria and they cannot produce anti H-antigen antibodies.

Hook: It acts as universal joint between the filament and basal body of the flagella. The hook acts as both flexible and rigid joint. During cessation of movement no rotation of filament is detected. However, the hook rotates around the filament axis and along the tubular axis of itself. The hook is composed of protein (FlgE). Three minor proteins (HAP1, HAP2, HAP3) are also present in the hook-filament region. HAP 1 and HAP 3 are present at the junction of hook and filament. HAP 2 is present at the tip of the filament and it is known as 'filament cap protein'. HAP 2 helps in polymerization of flagellin to make the filament. HAP 3 helps in assembly of filament. The mutant cells which do not possess HAP 3 show impaired movement when attached with a solid surface.

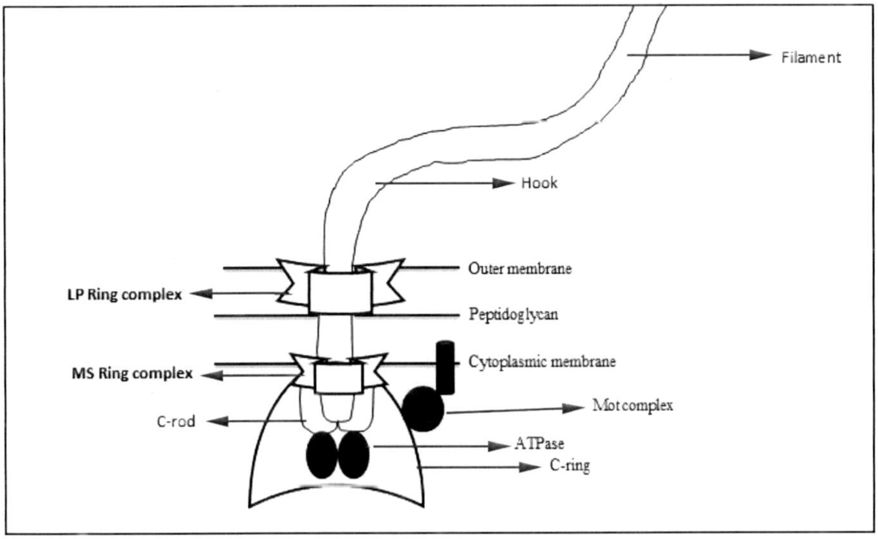

Basal Body: The basal body consists of rings with a rod passing through the rings. It is the motor of flagella. In Gram-negative bacteria, there are five parts of basal body i.e. LP ring complex, MS ring complex, periplasmic rod, C ring and C rod.

The LP ring complex is attached with outer membrane of Gram-negative cell wall. Due to absence of outer membrane the LP complex is not found in Gram-positive bacteria. The LP ring acts as a bushing around the rod. It is composed of two flagellar proteins i.e. FlgH (L ring) and FlgI (P ring). In few Gram-negative bacteria such as in *Wolinella succinogenes* (basal disk) and *Vibrio alginolyticus* (T/H ring) additional rings are found in LP complex. The additional rings help in stable flagellation and stable rotation of the motor.

MS ring is the base on which other parts of flagella are made. It is associated with cytoplasmic membrane of both Gram-negative and Gram-positive bacteria. The lower part of M-ring is hidden into the membrane and the other parts are exposed to the periplasmic space. Both the rings are composed of FliF protein.

Periplasmic Rod is the tubular polymer around which the rings are constructed. The rod has two parts i.e. proximal and distal. The rod is composed of four proteins (FlgB, FlgC, FlgF and FlgG).

The cytoplasmic (C) ring is a cup-shaped structure attached to the cytoplasmic surface of the M ring. It is composed of three proteins (FliG, FliM and FliN). It acts as switch which can change the direction of flagellar rotation.

C-rod is composed of six proteins (FlhA, FlhB, FliO, FliP, FliQ and FliR). It acts as export apparatus of the flagella.

Fimbriae: Fimbriae (fimbria in singular) are non-helical (straight) filamentous appendages generally found in Gram-negative bacteria (except *Streptococcus*, *Staphylococcus*, *Corynebacterium*). They are thinner (3-10 µm in diameter), shorter and more in numbers than flagella. The fimbriae do not possess basal body and are originated from outer membrane of Gram-negative cell wall. They help in adherence of bacteria with other bacteria, biotic and abiotic surfaces and twitching motility (type IV fimbriae). Fimbriae are found to be essential for virulence in *E. coli* (P-fimbriae in uropathogenic *E. coli*), *Vibrio, Dichelobacter* (type IV fimbriae) and *Streptococcus*. Fimbria is composed of a protein ('pilin'). There are five types of fimbriae (type I-V). Among them type I and type V fimbriae are mannose sensitive. Mannose can prevent the attachment of sensitive fimbriae with the surfaces. The fimbriae are visible only with electron microscopy.

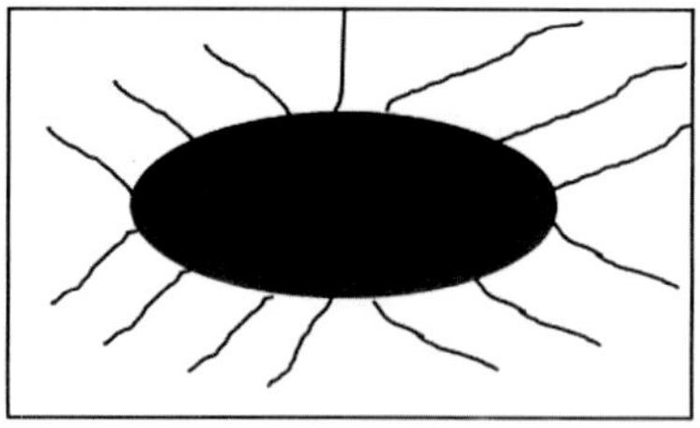

Pili: Pili (pilus in singular) are a kind of fimbriae used as appendage in bacterial conjugation. Many microbiologists use both the terms interchangeably although few differences between fimbriae and pili are described. Pili are less in numbers, longer and wider than fimbriae. Few pili possess an axial hole and a terminal knob. Pili are essential for virulence in certain bacteria such as in *Acinetobacter* spp., chaperone/usher pili ('Csu pili') are associated with biofilm formation.

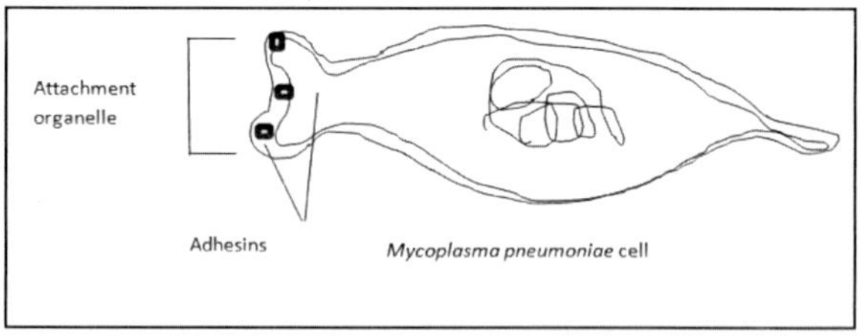

Attachment organelle: It is a polar extension of bacterial cell (*Mycoplasma*) and is associated with adherence, gliding motility and cell division. The proteinaceous 'core' is present at the center of the organelle. P1 and P30 are major cytoskeletal proteins associated with attachment organelle in *Mycoplasma pneumoniae*. The motor of gliding motility is present in attachment organelle. The gliding motility is required for penetration of mucus layer by *Mycoplasma*.

Bacterial spore

The spores are dormant form (little or no metabolic activity) produced by bacteria for survival under unfavourable condition. After spore formation metabolic activity is detected for few minutes which ceases with time. In suitable conditions and in presence of germinants the spores are able to produce vegetative cells. The bacterial spores do not act as reproductive unit. The spores are produced either within the bacterial cell (endospore) or outside the cell (exospore). Spores were first observed by Kohn (1875). Robert Koch (1876) first made detailed study of bacterial spores. The spores are highly resistant to heat, desiccation, chemical disinfectants and radiation. The spores can resist the boiling for one hour or more.

Importance of bacterial spores

a) Bacterial spores are unique system which can remain dormant for many years but can germinate within a few minutes

b) The spores of *Bacillus anthracis* are potent bio-terrorism threat

c) The spores of few bacteria such as *Bacillus* spp., *Clostridium difficile* may act as public health threat with the production of gas gangrene, tetanus, botulism, anthrax, pseudomembranous colitis

d) The spores of few bacteria such as *Bacillus* spp. may cause spoilage of foods

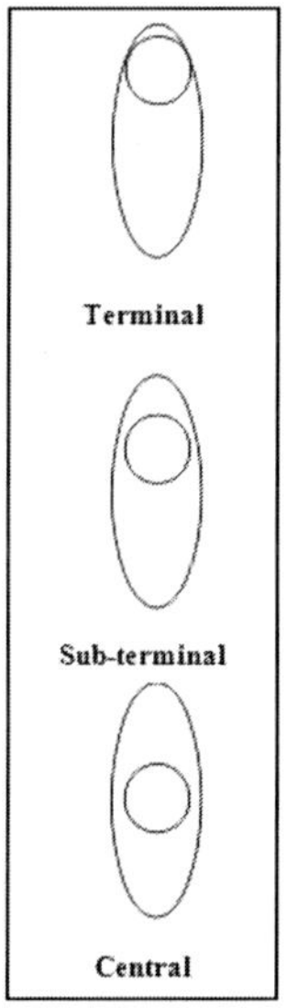

Location of endospore

Location of endospores varies between the bacterial species.

a) Terminal: Endospore is present at one end of bacterial cell (e.g. *Clostridium tetani*)

b) Sub-terminal: Endospore is present at near the end of bacterial cell (e.g. *Bacillus subtilis*)

c) Central: Endospore is present at centre of bacterial cell (e.g. *Bacillus cereus*)

Structure of spores

Core or protoplast: The core is composed of chromosome (DNA), small-acid soluble- spore proteins (SASP), dipicolinic acid (pyridine-2, 6-dicarboxylic acid) chelated with Ca^{++} (CaDPA) and low water content (25-50% of wet weight). Ribosomes and few enzymes are also present in the core but no metabolic activity is detected. The SASP can protect the DNA from heat and radiation. The calcium-dipicolinate can remove water molecule by contraction of spore membrane (calcium-contractile theory). Low water content of spore is responsible for minimum metabolism and heat resistance.

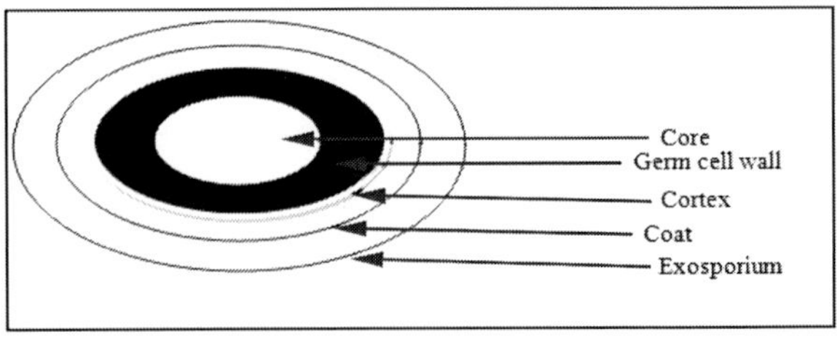

Germ cell wall: It provides osmotic stability in germinating spores.

Cortex: Cortex is composed of peptidoglycan which is different from vegetative cell peptidoglycan. The spore cortex peptidoglycan contains unsubstituted muramic acid, low cross linkage and incomplete peptide chain of L-alanine. It also contains meso-diaminopimelic acid (DAP) in place of L-lysine of vegetative peptidoglycan. The meso-DAP is converted into dipicolinic acid which is found in the core in chelated form.

Coat: The coat prevents entry of toxic materials into the spore and contains several enzymes required for germination.

Exosporium: It is the outermost lipid-protein membrane of the spore. It can produce protective antibodies in the host.

Germination of spore: The germination of spore occurs in presence of a stimulus, known as 'germinant'. The germination is followed by 'outgrowth' which converts the spore into a vegetative bacterial cell. The amino acids (L-alanine, L-valine, L-asparagine), high pressure, temperature and cationic surfactants (dodecylamine) may act as spore germinants. The germinants can bind with specific receptors (germinant receptor, GR) present in spore membrane. After binding a short lag period is observed before the commitment. The 'commitment' is the change of spore membrane permeability or strength so that dipicolinic acid (CaDPA) is released from the spores. The binding of germinants with their receptors may produce a channel in the spore membrane. The monovalent cations are released through the channel.

Sometimes the germinant receptors provide signal to the germinants such as SpoVA channel protein or GerD protein. The SpoVA channel protein helps in release of CaDPA. The normal function of germinant receptors is dependent on GerD protein. The GerD protein also helps in formation of germinant receptor cluster in the spore membrane. The cluster of germinant receptor is known as 'germinosome'.

After release of CaDPA the cortex lytic enzyme (CLE, e.g. CwlJ in *Bacillus*) degrades cortex peptidoglycan layer of the spore. The core can absorb water molecule (hydration) and it is expanded.

Protoplast: It is the bacterial cell without cell wall. It is surrounded by only cytoplasmic membrane. The protoplast can be prepared by treating Gram-positive bacterial cell with lysozyme or cell wall destroying antibiotics (e.g. penicillin). Protoplast has respiratory and biosynthetic capabilities and it can grow in size but it cannot divide like a true bacterium. In absence of inducers (lysozyme, penicillin) the protoplasts can revert back into parent bacterial cell. The protoplasts are maintained in isotonic medium because osmotic shock can lyse the cell in absence of cell wall. *Mycoplasma* and L-form of bacteria are considered as 'natural protoplast'. In the laboratory artificial protoplasts are used for preparation of genetically modified organisms. In absence of cell wall the protoplasts can uptake foreign DNA easily.

Spheroplast: It is partial cell wall deficient bacteria prepared from Gram-negative bacteria. The peptidoglycan layer is absent in spheroplasts and it is surrounded by cytoplasmic membrane and outer membrane. Due to membrane tension of two membranes present in spheroplasts it takes a spherical shape, hence it is known as spheroplast. In laboratory, spheroplasts are used as a vehicle of modified DNA to transfect the eukaryotic cells. It is also used to study bacterial ion channel through a technique known as 'patch clamp'.

Table 1: Differences between prokaryote and eukaryote cells

Characteristics	Prokaryote cell	Eukaryote cell
Size	4-8 µm × 1-1.25 µm	More than 5 µm
Nucleus	True nucleus absent. Nuclear material is not covered with nuclear membrane (except Planctomycetes)	True nucleus with nuclear membrane is present
Genome	i) The genes are arranged in a chain in the circular chromosome. Single chromosome is found in prokaryotes except Vibrio, Brucella (two chromosomes)	i) More than one chromosomes in eukaryote (human-46, cattle-60)
	ii) No centromere in the prokaryote chromosome (except 'plasmid centromeres' in Caulobacter)	ii)Centromere present
	iii) Prokaryotic genomes are jam-packed with genes with almost no repeats	iii)More numbers of repeats
	iv) Very less numbers of introns	iv) More numbers of introns (3.7 introns / kbp protein coding region)
	v) More numbers of foreign elements are present due to horizontal gene transfer	v)Less foreign elements
	vi) Due to low numbers of promoters (-10 promoter,-35 promoter, upstream elements), many genes are controlled by a single promoter present within an operon	vi)Promoter numbers and types is high (TATA box, initiator elements, GC box, CAAT box etc.)
	vii) No histone proteins in the chromosome	vii) Histone present
	viii) No mitotic division of the chromosome	viii) Mitotic division of chromosome occurs
	ix) The chromosomes have a single, unique replication origin; 1/2 polymerase enzymes are involved	ix)Multiple replication origin; more than 4 polymerase enzymes are associated
	x) Self-replicating, extra chromosomal plasmids are present. Few essential genes are carried by the plasmids such as genes required for environmental adaptation, antimicrobial resistance etc.	x) No plasmids
	xi) G+C content of DNA is 28-73 mol%	xi) about 40 mol%

Characteristics	Prokaryote cell	Eukaryote cell
Sexuality	Merozygote (partial diploid)	diploid
Cytoplasmic membrane	No sterol; respiratory and photosynthesis enzymes are present	Sterols present; not associated with respiration / photosynthesis
Cell wall	Peptidoglycan and lipopolysaccharide present	Peptidoglycan and lipopolysaccharide absent
Gas vaculoes	present	absent
Mesosome	present	absent
Ribosome	70S ('S'=Svedberg unit) , distributed freely in cytoplasm	80S, present in endoplasmic reticulum membrane
Mitochondria, chloroplast, endoplasmic reticulum,		
Golgi apparatus	Absent	Present
Pinocytosis	Absent	Present

Table 2: Differences between Gram-positive and Gram-negative bacteria

Gram-positive bacteria	Gram-negative bacteria
Peptidoglycan layer is thicker (20-30 nm)	It is thinner (3-5 nm)
Peptidoglycan comprises 50% dry weight of the cell wall	Peptidoglycan comprises 10% dry weight of the cell wall
Teichoic acid present	Teichoic acid absent
Outer membrane absent	Outer membrane present which is composed of phospholipid, proteins (OMPs), and LPS
Lipid content of cell wall is less	Lipid content of cell wall is more (11-22%)

5

Growth and Nutritional Requirements of Aerobic and Anaerobic Bacteria

Growth of bacteria can be defined as change of total population mass, not individual increase in size or mass. Macroscopically visible growth of bacteria on the solid medium is known as 'colony'. It is estimated that if *Escherichia coli* are allowed to grow, a single bacterial cell can produce a daughter population with the mass of the whole earth within 2 days! In the environment the bacteria are not actively growing all the time. The mechanisms behind the growth-arrested states of environmental bacteria are not well understood.

Bacterial reproduction

Bacterial reproduction is an asexual process which occurs by binary fission, budding, fragmentation and condiospore or sporangiospore formation. There is no possibility of genetic exchange (reassortment) as it is originated from a single parent cell. Bacterial gene transfer occurs by transformation, transduction and conjugation methods (discussed later in details). These are one-directional DNA transfer methods and are not associated with reproduction. The donor bacteria can give the genetic material to the recipient and the *vice-versa* does not occur.

Binary fission: In binary fission, bacterial DNA is replicated first and then the parent cell separates. Each daughter cell receives a complete genome, identical to the parent cell. Bacterial DNA replication begins when the cells reach a specific mass. If the cell diameter is constant, longer cells will begin DNA replication earlier than the shorter cells. The shorter cells need time to reach a critical mass required for the initiation of DNA replication. The ugtP proteins were identified to be associated with shorter cells and delayed DNA replication in Gram-positive bacteria (*Bacillus subtilis*). It was confirmed later that the ugtP act as inhibitor for Z-ring formation.

Bacterial DNA replication: The bacterial DNA replication is a rapid method (1000 nucleotides / minute) but it occurs with few errors. It starts from a single origin of replication and it is a bi-directional method. There are three types of

DNA polymerase enzymes in bacteria known as DNA polymerase-I, II and III. DNA polymerase III is the enzyme for replication which adds deoxyribose nucleotides at the 3'-OH group of growing DNA chain. The required energy for addition of deoxyribose nucleotides is present within the bond of three phosphate groups attached to each nucleotide (triphosphate). Initiation of replication occurs at a specific sequence of the genome known as 'Ori-C'. In bacteria generally single copy of 'Ori-C' is found. In *E. coli*, 'Ori-C' is approximately 245 bp long and is rich in adenine-thymine (AT) sequences. For initiation of DNA replication supercoiled DNA should be relaxed (negative supercoiling) with DNA gyrase (topoisomerase-II) present in mesophilic bacteria. Helicase enzyme separates DNA strands. The 'Y' shaped replication fork is formed at the origin of replication. The formation of fork makes the single stranded DNA available for replication. DNA-polymerase III can add new nucleotides at 5'-3' direction by making a covalent phosphodiester bond between the free 3′-OH end and the 5′ phosphate of the new nucleotide. A short RNA sequence (known as 'primer', 5-10 nucleotides long) can provide the free 3'-OH group where the new nucleotides are added which are complementary to the parent strand. This kind of continuous nucleotide synthesis occurs in 'leading strand'. The leading strand always grows towards the replication fork. Another strand grows away from the replication fork. Then DNA polymerase III moves back towards the replication fork and starts synthesis of new nucleotides again in the direction away from the replication fork. These steps will generate small DNA fragments, known as 'Okazaki fragments' (discovered by Reiji and Tsuneko Okazaki, Japan, 1966). Every Okazaki fragment is added with a RNA primer. The strand with Okazaki fragments is known as lagging strand. The synthesis of lagging strand is discontinuous. With the progress of replication, RNA primers are removed by DNA polymerase-I. The gap ('nick') created after removal of primer is sealed by the enzyme DNA ligase. The ligase can catalyze the formation of a covalent phosphodiester linkage between the 3′-OH end of one DNA fragment and the 5′ end of the other fragment. Termination of DNA replication occurs through interlocking of circular chromosome and separation from each other. It is done by bacterial topoisomerase IV enzyme. Both DNA gyrase and topoisomerase IV are unique enzymes present in prokaryotes. They are used as target for antibiotics (e.g. quinolone).

> Why bacteria replicate very fast?
> a) The chromosome is circular so that two replication forks always terminate simultaneously
> b) Fastest replisomes are employed by bacteria
> c) Transcription and replication occurs simultaneously
> d) Reduction in number of sites where RNA polymerases become idle
> E.g. For *E. coli*, standard chromosome doubling time is 45 minutes

Cell separation (cytokinesis): The cell separation begins after completion of bacterial DNA replication. A septum is produced at the center of the parent cell with an inward growth of cytoplasmic membrane first, followed by inward growth of cell wall. Formation of septum divides the parent cell into two daughter cells. The septum formation takes place beneath an equatorial ridge present in the cell wall of bacteria. Current finding indicates the role of FtsZ, a bacterial cytoskeleton protein (tubulin homolog) that initiates and directs cytokinesis. The polymerization of FtsZ takes place just before the cell division near the center of a cell as a ring ('Z-ring'). FtsZ is attached with the cell membrane by specific FtsZ-interacting proteins (e.g. EzrA). During the first step of cytokinesis, early proteins that directly bind FtsZ stabilize the Z-ring. In the second step the Z-ring matures with the recruitment of downstream proteins into the site of cell separation. It is followed by depolymerization and constriction of Z-ring which separates the parent cell into two daughter cells. The protein complex which accumulates in response to FtsZ and is associated with cytokinesis is known as 'divisome'.

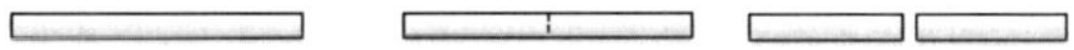

Cytokinesis in rod shaped bacteria

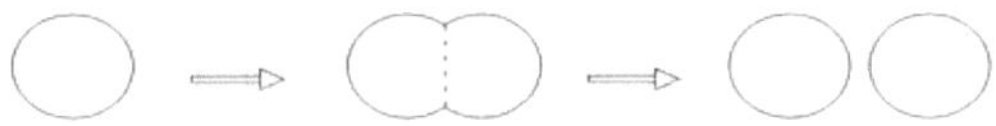

Cytokinesis in coccus bacteria

In Gram-negative bacteria (*E. coli*) FtsZ activity is regulated by 'Min'-system. MinD and MinE proteins make the gradient of FtsZ-inhibitor (MinC) highest at the cell poles and lowest at the center of the cell. MinC concentration at the center of the cell drops below the critical level when the cell is sufficiently long. Then FtsZ is activated to form the Z-ring and cytokinesis proceeds.

During septum formation old cell wall is broken and is replaced with a newly synthesized peptidoglycan. This newly synthesized peptidoglycan partly forms (15%) the wall of daughter cells also.

Elongation: The separation of daughter cells is followed by elongation of cells in case of rod shaped bacteria (e.g. *Bacillus* spp.). The elongation is regulated by an actin homologue cytoskeleton protein of bacteria (MreB). MreB forms long fibrils around the cylindrical portion of rod shaped cells. MreB acts jointly with FtsZ to produce the 'rod' shape of the Gram-negative bacteria. In Gram-positive bacteria, few homologues of MreB protein take part in cell elongation.

Variation in cell diameter (5-7 %) is observed between bacterial strains growing under different growth phases. Bacterial cells (*E. coli*) in logarithmic growth phase are longer and wider than the same bacterial strains present in stationary phase. The cells also become larger in a rich growth medium. Sometimes variations in cellular length (1-4% variations in *E. coli*) are observed between the bacterial strains of same species growing under same conditions. Faster growing bacteria are larger in size. Molecular regulatory mechanism for variation in cell size is poorly known. It is observed that in Gram-negative bacteria (*E. coli*), FtsA can stimulate FtsZ activity and overproduction of both FtsA and FtsZ is associated with reduced cell size (30% reduction). In Gram-positive bacteria teichoic acid mutant (bacteria without techoic acid in cell wall) are longer in size probably due to decreased assembly of Z- rings.

Budding: A small bud (protuberance) is developed at one pole of the bacterial cell. The bud enlarges and separates from the parent cell to become an individual cell. Budding is found in *Rhodoblastus acidophilus* (formerly known as *Rhodopseudomonas acidophila*), a gram-negative purple non-sulfur bacterium.

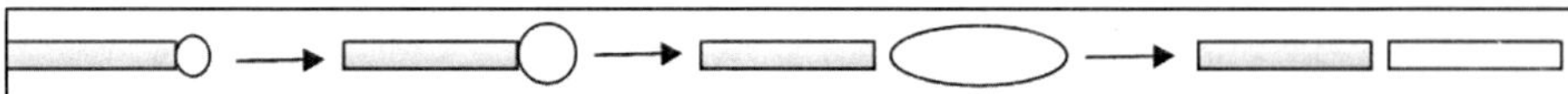

Budding

Fragmentation: Filamentous bacteria (*Nocardia*) can reproduce by fragmentation of filaments to produce coccus or short rods. Each of the cells grows to become filamentous bacteria.

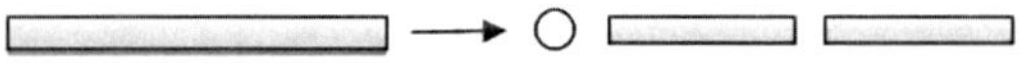

Fragmentation

Conidiospore / Sporangiospore: *Streptomyces* are unique bacteria with properties of eukaryotic fungi such as production of spores for reproduction. The vegetative mycelial form of the bacteria is converted into aerial reproductive hyphae. Formation of septum in hyphal tips can generate different types of spores such as condiospores, sporangiospores like fungi. Each of the spores can produce a daughter bacterium.

Growth cycle (growth curve) of bacteria

The growth curve of bacteria is a curve plotted with the data reagrding numbers of bacteria at various time intervals. The growth curve has four phases i.e. lag phase, log phase, stationary phase and phase of decline. There is a preparatory period between each of the phases, known as 'transitional period'. This preparatory period is demarcated with a 'bend' between the phases in the curve.

Lag phase: This is the preparatory phase of bacterial cells after inoculation into the fresh medium. The bacterial cells are metabolically active. The cells increase in size but do not multiply. Different enzymes, co-enzymes and vitamins are synthesized in this phase required for the cellular growth. The period of lag phase is variable depending upon the nutrient concentration. The period is lengthy in a nutritionally poor medium.

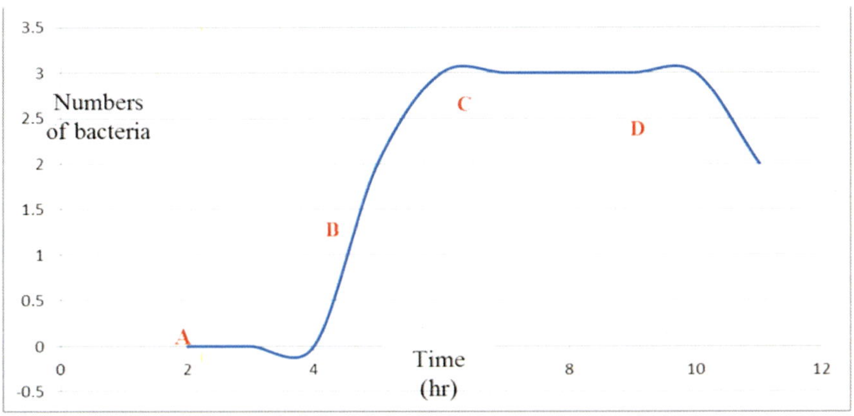

Standard bacterial growth curve plotted with numbers of bacteria (Y-axis) against time (X-axis). A, Lag phase; B, Log phase; C, Stationary phase; D, Phase of decline

Logarithmic phase or exponential phase: In this period the cells reproduce (DNA replication and binary fission) in a constant rate until the substrate concentration becomes sufficiently low. The numbers of bacteria when plotted against time produces a straight line (B). The cells are uniform in their chemical composition and metabolic activity. Log phase cells are commonly used for bacterial metabolism studies. The time taken by bacterial population to become double is known as 'generation time'. It depends on nutrients and physical conditions of the medium. It is calculated by t / n formula ('t' = time interval, 'n' = numbers of generation). The generation time for *Clostridium perfringens* is 10 minutes, *E. coli* is 15-20 minutes and *Staphylococcus aureus* is 30 minutes. The numbers of generations in a specific time interval (per hour) is known as 'growth rate'. It is the reciprocal of generation time (n / t).

Stationary phase: The logarithmic phase is followed by a bend and another straight line (C) in the growth curve. The population mass remains constant in the stationary phase. The growth is stopped or the growth rate is same with the death rate of the cells. Cessation of growth occurs due to lack of nutrients, accumulation of toxic metabolites or antibiotics in the medium. If a bacterial cell is transferred from stationary phase into a fresh medium the cell starts to multiply.

Phase of decline: In this phase the growth is completely stopped. Individual cells start to die and numbers of dead cells crosses the numbers of live cells. So the downward trend in the numbers of bacteria is detected in the growth curve (D). The death rate also varies between the bacterial species like the growth rate. Gram negative cocci shows faster death rate than other bacteria.

Measurement of bacterial growth

Measurement of bacterial growth actually determines bacterial mass, not individual cell growth. Bacterial cultures are highly heterogeneous. The growth estimates are based on averages of population which might be varying in length, diameter, age and cell wall composition. The following methods are employed to measure bacterial growth directly or indirectly.

a) *Direct microscopic count*: The unstained bacterial suspension can be counted accurately in Petroff-Hausser counting chamber (or Neubauer chamber) using a microscope. Dense bacterial population should be diluted before counting. A drop of suspension is poured over Petroff-Hausser counting slide. Most counting chambers consist of 400 small squares each with an area of 0.0025 mm^2, 25 large squares with areas of 0.04 mm^2 and the suspension depth (height of the coverslip) is 0.02 mm. The investigator makes several counts of the number of bacteria found within one or more of the larger squares. These numbers are recorded and mean value is calculated. The total number of cells in a milliliter of the original suspension can then be calculated. The number of bacteria is expressed as numbers of bacteria / ml. This method is useful for enumeration of bacteria in vaccines and cultures.

b) *Electronic counter*: The bacterial suspension is placed into an electronic particle counter through narrow orifices. The orifices are attached with compartments containing electrically conducive medium. When the bacteria pass through the orifices it generates electrical resistance. The resistance is converted into a signal which can be counted. The technique requires sophisticated instrument and it cannot differentiate live and dead bacterial cells.

c) *Flow cytometry*: Flow cytometry can accurately enumerate the number of bacteria present in a suspension. The high-affinity nucleic acid stain which can penetrate both Gram-positive and Gram-negative cell wall is used. The stain after binding with bacterial nucleic acid produces a strong fluorescence. A calibrated suspension of polystyrene microsphere is present in the suspension which produces forward light scatter. A plot of fluorescence and forward scatter is prepared (cytogram). The bacterial population can be calculated from the ratio of fluorescence and forward scatter. The technique can process large numbers of samples accurately in less time. However flow cytometry is suitable for pure culture or less contaminated samples because inorganic particles can strongly interfere with bacterial counts. Processing of environmental samples such as soil, sediments require detachment of bacterial cells before flow cytometry. The detachment of bacterial cells can be performed with chemicals (ionic and non-ionic detergents), mechanical force (ultrasonication), and treatment with enzymes.

d) *Pour plate method*: The method is used to enumerate colony-forming bacteria in liquid specimens. The method detects only live bacterial count. The inoculum of test sample is serially diluted (10-fold dilution). A particular dilution is selected on the basis of prediction of bacterial number present in the sample. The inoculum (1 ml) from the selected dilution is placed at the center of sterile Petri dish. Molten cooled agar (15ml) is poured into the Petri dish containing the inoculum and it is mixed well. After the solidification of the agar, the plate is inverted and incubated at 37°C for 24-48 hours. The bacteria will grow as 'colony' both on the surface and within the agar. The colonies within the agar are small and confluent. All the colonies are counted either manually or by a colony counter. The number of bacteria present in the test sample is detected using the following formula and is expressed as colony forming unit (cfu) / ml.

Number of bacteria (cfu / ml) = Number of colonies × dilution factor

The method has the advantage that no ready-made media is required. Microaerophilic bacteria grow better at the sub-surface.

Dis-advantages:

- The pour plate method is not suitable for heat sensitive bacteria as most of them are lysed after coming in contact with hot molten agar
- Reduced growth of obligate aerobes are observed at the depth of the agar
- Media preparation is time-consuming

e) *Spread plate method*: In this method the serially diluted sample is used. Similar to pour plate method, an inoculum (10 μl) from a selected dilution (10^{-3}) is spread over the already prepared agar plate with L-spreader. The plate is inverted and incubated at 37°C for 24-48 hours.

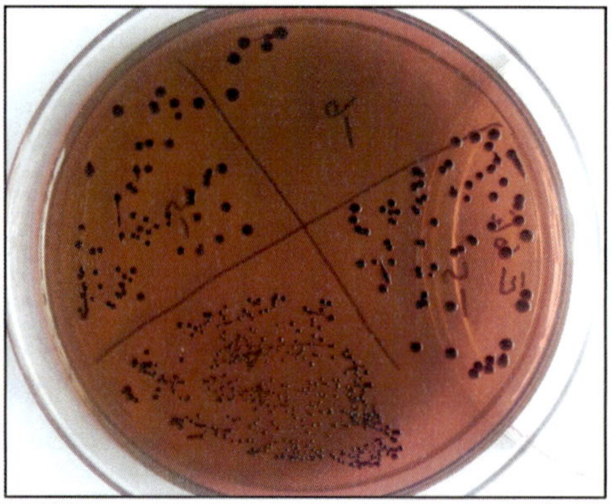

Colonies appeared in different dilutions in spread plate method

The bacteria will grow as 'colony' on the surface of the agar. All the colonies are counted either manually or by a colony counter. The number of bacteria present in the test sample is detected using the following formula and is expressed as colony forming unit (cfu) / ml. The culture plates with more than 250-300 colonies cannot be counted and are known as 'too many to count (TMTC)'. Plates with less than 30 colonies are designated as 'too few to count (TFTC)'.

$$\text{Number of bacteria (cfu / ml)} = \frac{\text{Number of colonies} \times \text{dilution factor } (10^3) \times 10^3}{10 \text{ (inoculum size)}}$$

Advantage of this method is heat-sensitive bacteria can be enumerated accurately. However, the method is not suitable for enumeration of microaerophilic bacteria which does not grow properly in this method.

f) *Automated colony counting platform*: In traditional methods of plate counting more time is required for full appearance of bacterial colonies on the solid media. Possibility of human error is also there in manual colony counting. The automated colony counting platform consists of an incubator, robotic moving parts for sample processing and digital imaging system. The imaging system can measure cellular autofluorescence and accurately enumerate the microcolonies. The microcolonies are not fully grown bacterial colonies and their appearance on the solid media requires less time. The automated platform is costly and is restricted in food and pharmaceutical industries.

g) *Membrane filter count*: The technique is useful for counting bacteria in air and water samples. The known volume of sample is passed through the membrane filter. The filter containing the trapped bacteria is placed over plates containing pads with special medium. The bacteria produce colonies over the membrane filter which is counted. The numbers of bacteria are expressed as colony forming unit (cfu) / ml.

h) *Turbidimetric method*: Bacterial population (> 10^7-10^8 cfu / ml) present in liquid medium can produce turbidity. The turbidity can be expressed as measurement of bacterial cell mass present in the solution by spectrophotometer or colorimeter. The optical density (OD) measures the amount of light scattered (deflection) by bacterial cells. It is not absorption of light by the bacterial cells (except pigmented phototrophic bacteria). The small glass tube (cuvette) is used to keep the bacterial suspension within the instrument. The cuvette with uninoculated broth is used to set the instrument at optical density zero. It is followed by measurement of optical density of the test cultures. In ultraviolet (UV) spectrophotometry, the light belong to 550-700 nm wavelength can be used. The UV light of 600 nm (OD 600) is generally preferred for bacterial population as the cells are not lysed at this wavelength. UV can also cause mutation of bacterial population. The OD values of test bacteria can be plotted in a standard graph (time as the X-axis and OD as the Y-axis) to calculate the bacterial concentration. The turbidimetric method can calculate both live and dead bacterial cells. Miniaturized charge-coupled device (CCD) based spectrophotometers with 3D printing are used currently for enumeration of pathogenic and anaerobic bacteria.

In absence of spectrophotometer or colorimeter, McFarland standard tubes are used to calculate approximate concentration of bacterial cells. The tubes contain mixture of barium chloride and sulphuric acid (barium sulphate) or latex particles. The tubers with various turbidity are represented with McFarland standard number 0.5, 1, 2, 3, 4 representing approximately 1.5×10^8 cfu / ml, 3.0×10^8 cfu / ml, 6.0×10^8 cfu / ml, 9.0×10^8 cfu / ml, 12.0×10^8 cfu / ml bacterial concentration, respectively. The bacterial concentration equivalent to McFarland standard number 0.5 is recommended for antibiotic sensitivity test.

i) *Dry weight estimation*: Dry weight estimation of bacterial cells is an indirect way for measurement of bacterial growth. Polyhydroxy butyrate can accumulate in the bacterial cells during log phase of the growth. More amount of polyhydroxy butyrate is accumulated into the bacterial cells in subsequent growth phases and it also increases the dry weight of bacterial cells. The dry weight is expressed as mg / ml.

j) *Nitrogen estimation*: Nitrogen is the integral part of bacterial proteins. Rise in nitrogen concentration indicates bacterial growth. Nitrogen can be estimated by Kjeldahl method. Nitrogen is converted into ammonia and the ammonia is measured either by volumetric titration or colorimetrically with Nessler's reagent. The nitrogen concentration is expressed as mg / ml.

k) *Real time PCR*: Real-time polymerase chain reaction (RT-PCR/ Q-PCR) can be used for accurate enumeration of bacterial population

l) *Adenosine triphosphate (ATP) bioluminescence*: This assay measures ATP concentration in a sample which indicates the concentration of organic matter or microbes. The instrument contains luciferase enzyme which catalyzes the conversion of ATP into adenosine monophosphate (AMP). The conversion results emission of light which is detected by the bioluminometer and quantified in relative light unit (RLU). This technology is used for microbial quantification in food industry and health care settings.

Nutritional requirements of bacteria

The chemicals and environmental elements that are utilized for bacterial growth, biosynthesis and energy production are known as nutrients or nutritional requirements. The nutrients are broadly classified as macronutrients and micronutrients.

Macronutrients: Carbon, oxygen, hydrogen, nitrogen, sulphur, phosphorous, potassium, calcium, magnesium and iron are macronutrients for bacteria and it constitutes more than 95% dry weight of the cell. Carbon, oxygen, hydrogen, nitrogen, sulphur and phosphorous are building blocks of four major macromolecules of life i.e. carbohydrate, lipid, protein and nucleic acid. Nitrogen constitutes amino acids, purine, pyrimidine, carbohydrate, lipid, enzymes and co-factors. Few bacteria (*Azotobacter*, *Rhizobium*) can assimilate atmospheric nitrogen by nitrogenase. This group of bacteria is known as 'nitrogen fixing bacteria'. Other bacteria use inorganic (nitrate, nitrite, ammonium salts) or organic compounds (amino acids) as nitrogen source. Phosphorus makes nucleic acids, phospholipids, ATP, teichoic acid, enzyme cofactors. Most of the bacteria use inorganic phosphorus. However, *E. coli* can use both inorganic and organic phosphorus (hexose 6- phosphate). The sulphur can make amino acids (cysteine and methionine), carbohydrates, and vitamins (biotin and thiamine).

Other macro elements (potassium, calcium, magnesium and iron) exist in bacterial cells as cations and act as cofactors for enzymes (K^{+}, Mg^{++}, Fe^{++}), helps in heat resistance of bacterial spores (Ca^{++}), stabilization of ribosome and cell membrane (Mg^{++}) and electron transfer (Fe^{++}).

Different indigestible carbon containing molecules such as amyl alcohol, paraffin, rubber, pesticides can also be used by bacteria as carbon source. During degradation of indigestible compounds the bacterial nutrients are also metabolized at the same time by a process known as 'co-metabolism'. The digested products can be utilized as nutrients by other groups of bacteria.

Micronutrients: Manganese, zinc, cobalt, molybdenum, nickel and copper acts as micronutrients for bacteria. Manganese (Mn^{++}) supports enzymes to catalyze transfer of phosphate groups. Zinc (Zn^{++}) is present in active sites of the enzymes. Cobalt (Co^{++}) constitutes vitamin B12. Molybdenum is required for nitrogen fixation by the bacteria. Sodium (Na^{+}) is required for growth of halophiles such as marine bacteria, cyanobacteria and photosynthetic groups of bacteria.

Growth factors: Other than macro and micronutrients the bacteria also require few organic macromolecules for survival and growth, known as 'growth factors'. The growth factors are essential cell components or precursors of such components and cannot be synthesized by the bacteria. The growth factors include amino acids (for protein synthesis), pyrimidines and purines (nucleic acid synthesis), and vitamins (Table 2).

Water: The water plays following role in survival and growth of bacteria.

a) In food industry it is observed that bacterial growth is dependent on 'water activity (Aw)' of food items. The water activity is the ratio of the vapour (water) pressure detected in food items to the vapour pressure of pure water at a specific temperature. The Aw (0.7-0.85) is considered as indicator for effective sterilization of food items. Drying, salting and freezing can reduce water activity of food items and subsequently reduce the available water to the bacteria in usable form. As a result bacterial growth is reduced.

b) All the nutrients must be dissolved in water to enter the bacterial cells

c) The water provides a suitable environment for all metabolisms within the bacterial cell

d) Water is required for many hydrolytic reactions

e) Due to high specific heat the water provides resistance to sudden change of environmental temperature

Types of bacteria based on nutritional requirements are described in Table 1. There are four major nutritional groups of bacteria. Most of the pathogenic bacteria, fungi and protozoa belong to chemoorganoheterotroph. Other three groups are photolithoautotrophs (algae, purple and green sulphur bacteria, cyanobacteria), photoorganoheterotrophs (purple and green non-sulphur bacteria), chemolithoautotroph (sulphur-oxidizing bacteria, hydrogen bacteria, nitrifying bacteria, iron-oxidizing bacteria). Few groups of bacteria (e.g. *Beggiatoa, Desulfovibrio*) utilize inorganic energy or electron sources and organic carbon sources. These groups are known as 'mixotrophs'.

Cultivation of bacteria

The artificial cultivation of aerobic or anaerobic bacteria is known as 'bacterial culture'. The aim of bacterial culture in the laboratory is to obtain pure culture. 'Pure culture' is the bacterial growth consists of single bacterial species. In 1881 Robert Koch developed solid plate technique for isolation of bacterial pure culture.

A growth medium or culture medium is a solid, liquid or semi-solid combination of nutrients to support the growth of bacteria. The culture medium is used for general cultivation and maintenance of bacteria in the laboratory. Liquid artificial medium which can support the bacterial growth is known as 'broth'. Agar (jelly-like substance extracted from red algae) is composed of linear polysaccharide agarose and agaropectin. Agar is added (@1.5-2%) in the artificial medium as solidifying agent to convert the liquid medium into solid. Silica gel is preferred as solidifying agent for growth of autotrophs.

Types of medium

a) *Chemically defined medium (synthetic medium)*: The artificial medium for growth of autotrophs (or few heterotrophs) in which the exact chemical composition is known. The researcher should know about the exact nutritional requirements of a specific bacterium to use this medium. For example, ammonium chloride (nitrogen source), potassium di-hydrogen phosphate (phosphorus and potassium source), magnesium sulphate (magnesium source), calcium chloride (calcium source), sulphur, CO_2 (carbon source) and sterile distilled water are added in a suitable proportion to make a defined medium.

b) *Complex medium*: It is the undefined medium for cultivation of bacteria where the exact chemical constitution is not known. It is composed of complex materials of biological origin such as meat extract, yeast extract, peptone and agar. Meat extract and peptone are the source of carbohydrates, amino acids, water soluble vitamins and salt. Yeast extract is the source of vitamin B-complex. Agar is added to solidify the medium. Complex medium is the most common medium used in the bacteriology laboratory for cultivation of unknown pathogens which require a numbers of growth factors either known or unknown. For example, nutrient agar composed of 1% peptone, 1% meat extract, 0.5% salt and 2% agar.

c) *Selective medium:* The medium with ingredients enhancing the growth of a particular group of bacteria and does not enhance or inhibits the growth of others present as contaminant or saprophyte in the clinical samples. E.g. azide blood agar is selective medium for isolation of *Streptococcus* and few strains of *Staphylococcus*. Sodium azide has a bacteriostatic effect on most Gram-negative bacteria.

d) *Differential medium*: A culture medium containing certain reagents or supplements which allows differentiation of various kinds of bacteria. E.g. MacConkey lactose agar can differentiate lactose fermenting (*E. coli*) and non-fermenting groups of bacteria (*Salmonella*).

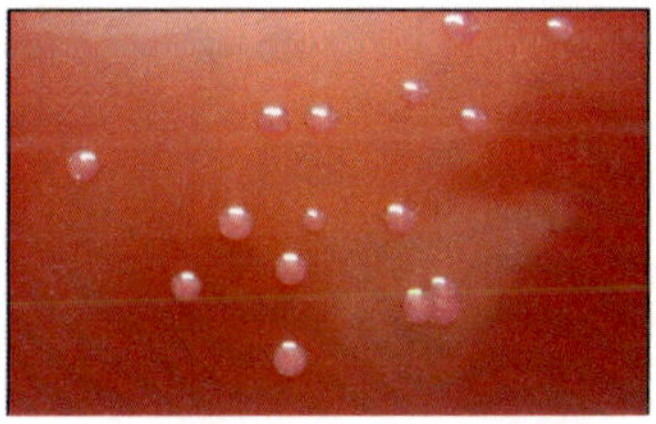

Lactose fermenting colonies in MacConkey agar

e) *Maintenance medium*: It is the artificial culture medium which maintains viability and physiological characteristics of bacterial culture. E.g. medium without glucose. The glucose enhances bacterial growth and produces acid as end product. The end product shifts the pH towards acidic site which kills the bacteria. So, the medium without glucose can maintain the viability.

f) *Enriched medium*: It is the artificial culture medium which contains enrichment for growth of fastidious bacteria (bacteria with complex or particular nutritional requirements). E.g. Blood agar, chocolate agar, serum agar, egg yolk agar

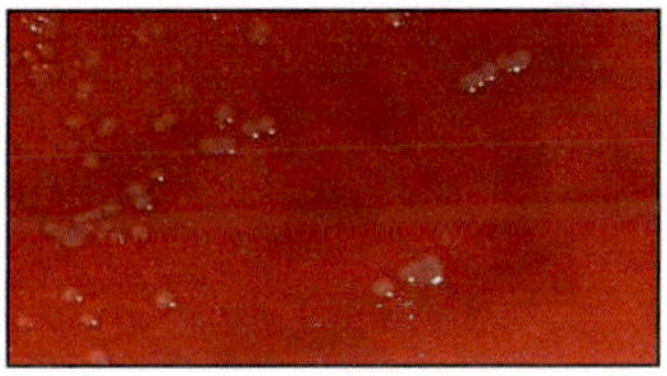

Non-Haemolytic colonies in blood agar

g) *Enrichment broth*: It is the liquid culture medium which selectively supports a specific group of bacteria. E.g. tetrathionate broth and selenite F broth for isolation of *Salmonella*

h) *Semisolid medium*: It is the culture medium with 0.5% or less agar. It is used for detection of bacterial motility and growth of microaerophiles.

i) *Transport medium*: It is used for transport of clinical specimens suspected for bacteria from the site of collection to the laboratory. Transport medium prevents drying of specimens and inhibits overgrowth of contaminants. E.g. Cary Blair transport medium (*Vibrio cholerae*), Sach's buffered glycerol saline (bacillary dysentery), alkaline peptone water etc.

Conditions for bacterial growth

a) *Temperature*: The growth of bacteria is effected by temperature as all the chemical synthesis and reactions within the cell are temperature dependent. Optimum growth temperature is the temperature which allows most rapid bacterial growth within a short period of time. Based on temperature requirement for growth the bacteria can be classified into following types.

   i) Psychrophile: The group of bacteria which can grow at -20°C to +10°C. Optimum growth temperature for psychrophiles is 15°C or lower. Examples are *Pseudomonas, Vibrio, Bacteroides, Flavobacterium, Arthrobacter, Micrococcus* etc. Psychrotrophs (facultative psychrophiles) are able to grow at 0°C but prefer to grow at 20°C-30°C. The cytoplasmic membrane lipid of psychrophiles contains more *cis*-unsaturated fatty acids or methyl-branched fatty acids which reduces the bacterial melting point and maintains membrane fluidity at low temperature. The cold-adapted enzymes are also detected in psychrophiles which have activities at low temperatures. Many cold-shock proteins (GroEL, DnaK), antifreeze proteins (AFP) and cold-acclimation proteins (Caps) are detected in psychrophiles which helps in adaptation to extreme low temperature. Trehalose and exopolysaccharides (EPSs) have important role in cryoprotection in psychrophilic bacteria.

   ii) Mesophile: The group of bacteria which can grow at 25°C to 40°C. Optimum growth temperature for human and animal pathogens is body temperature (37°C) of the host.

   iii) Thermophile: The group of bacteria which can grow at above 45°C. Optimum growth temperature for thermophiles is 60°C-80°C. It can be classified into two types i.e. extreme thermophiles (T_{opt} > 65°C) and hyperthermophiles (T_{opt} > 80°C). Thermophiles are found in hot springs, deep sea hydrothermal vents, and decaying plant matters such as peat bogs and compost. Thermophiles can survive in high temperature due to possession of thermostable enzymes, high GC content, and adaptation of all key synthesis and metabolisms to high temperature. Examples include *Thermus aquaticus*, *Pyrococcus furiosus* which are used in production of thermostable enzymes. The thermostable enzymes (Taq DNA polymerase, Pfu polymerase) are commonly used in polymerase chain reaction (PCR) in the laboratories.

b) *Oxygen and carbon-di-oxide requirements*: On the basis of free oxygen requirement the bacteria can be classified into following types.

I) *Aerobic bacteria*: The aerobic bacteria require oxygen for growth. The aerobes can tolerate up to 21% oxygen.

II) *Anaerobic bacteria*: The anaerobic bacteria do not require oxygen for growth. Instead oxygen is toxic to anaerobic bacterial cells. In anaerobic respiration (energy production), NO_3^-, $SO_4^=$, fumerate, trimethylamine oxide act as terminal electron acceptor in place of oxygen. Anaerobes can be further classified into three following sub-types.

i) Obligate anaerobes: These bacteria cannot survive in the presence of oxygen [partial O_2 pressure (pO_2) of>0.5%) due to 'oxygen toxicity'. The oxygen is beneficial to aerobes because they have protective mechanisms. During cellular synthesis of chemicals a single electron is added with oxygen molecule and the superoxide radical is generated. The superoxide radical can produce toxic hydrogen peroxide or hydroxyl radicals by reacting with hydrogen ions. Hydrogen peroxide can oxidize various molecules of bacterial cells. The hydroxyl ions are most reactive free radicals which can damage bacterial cells. Aerobic bacteria have superoxide dismutase, catalase and peroxidase enzymes as a protective mechanism. Superoxide dismutase can destroy superoxide radical. Catalase and peroxidase can break hydrogen peroxide to generate water and oxygen. So, aerobic bacteria can tolerate oxygen. True anaerobes lack superoxide dismutase, catalase, and peroxidase. True anaerobes can get their energy only through glycolysis. Examples are *Peptostreptococcus*, *Clostridium tetani*, *Propionibacterium,* sulfate-reducing bacteria and methanogenic *Archaea.*

ii) Facultative anaerobes: These anaerobic bacteria can survive both with and without oxygen. They do not require oxygen for their survival but they can survive in presence of oxygen.

iii) Aerotolerant anaerobes: These anaerobic bacteria cannot grow or carry out the metabolism but they can survive in presence of oxygen (2-8%) due to possession of superoxide dismutase and peroxidase enzymes. They use fermentation for energy generation during presence or absence of oxygen. Examples are *Streptococcus*, *Clostridium perfringens* etc.

III) *Microaerophilic bacteria*: This group of bacteria requires low level of oxygen (2-10%) for survival but they cannot tolerate the oxygen level (21%) normally present in the atmosphere. Examples are *Vibrio cholerae*, *Campylobacter*, *Neisseria*, *Legionella*, *Helicobacter* etc.

IV) *Capnophilic bacteria*: This group of bacteria requires carbon-di-oxide (5-10%) for survival. E.g. *Campylobacter*, *Brucella* (few strains) etc.

c) *pH*: The optimum pH for bacterial growth is 6.5-7.5. These neutrophilic bacteria can grow well in host body as most of the human tissue has pH 7.0-7.2. In artificial medium buffers are used to adjust the pH. Phosphate buffer (pH 6.8) is most commonly used in the medium for bacterial growth.

d) *Special requirements*: The phototrophic bacteria requires illumination, deep sea bacteria requires high hydrostatic pressure for growth.

Anaerobic bacteria cultivation

Cultivation of anaerobes requires special precautions to avoid the oxygen exposure.

a) *Candle jar method*: It is the simplest technique for cultivation of facultative or aerotolerant anaerobes. The culture plates with inoculum are placed in a sealed desiccator or glass jar. A candle is lighted within the desiccator or jar. The whole jar is placed into the incubator. The free oxygen is consumed by the burning candle and carbon-di-oxide (3%) is produced. The method can be made more effective with addition of chopped potatoes / vegetables at the bottom of the jar. Respiring plant tissues will also help to absorb the free oxygen. In place of candle a piece of yellow phosphorus was used earlier. On drying the phosphorus ignited spontaneously. It continued burning till the availability of free oxygen. Due to possibility of explosion the technique was later modified with a candle.

b) *Anaerobic jar*: The jar was first made by McIntosh and Fildes (1916). In the jar hot platinum or palladium was used as catalyst for the chemical reaction of oxygen with hydrogen to produce water. The hydrogen was supplied from a Kipp's apparatus in which zinc was allowed to act with hydrochloric acid to generate hydrogen. Alkaline solution of pyrogallol was also used in the jar to absorb oxygen. Currently 'GasPak system' is used which contains dried powder of sodium borohydride and sodium bicarbonate. The chemicals react with water to generate hydrogen and carbon-di-oxide (10%). The hydrogen then reacts with oxygen present within the jar in presence of palladium catalyst. A methylene blue capsule is placed within the jar as an indicator for anaerobic condition. In absence of oxygen the coloured capsule becomes colourless due to production of reduced leuco compound from oxidized methylene blue.

Earlier a culture plate with inoculum of *Clostridium tetani* was placed within the jar as an indicator. In true anaerobic condition *C. tetani* grows.

c) *Roll tube method*: This technique is recommended for isolation of obligate anaerobes such as methanogens and archaea. It is a complex technique to be used in clinical laboratories. The roll tubes (Hungate tubes) are filled with medium. The medium is prepared by boiling in an oxygen-free nitrogen atmosphere. The roll tubes (Hungate tubes) are placed in an anaerobic glove box. Resazurin is used as an indicator for oxygen-free condition. The bacterial colonies are detected on the walls of the tubes after incubation.

d) *Anaerobic chamber*: The chamber was first developed by Dick Coy, an engineer under the supervision of Rolf Freter, Professor of Microbiology in University of Michigan. The chamber was equipped with instrument for generation of hydrogen gas to keep the oxygen level at 0-5 ppm and temperature control unit. Later Coy's anaerobic chamber was modified as per the necessity.

e) *Use of aerobic bacteria*: It is an old technique which was described first by Fortner in 1928. Two culture plates of same diameter are selected with suitable media. One plate is inoculated with known aerobic bacteria (*Serratia*, coliform bacillus) and the other one is with inoculum of suspected anaerobic bacteria. Two plates are fitted at their rims and sealed with petri seal. The system is incubated. The growth of aerobes will consume the free oxygen of the system and anaerobic condition will be developed after a certain period. The method is not suitable for obligate anaerobes.

f) *Brewer's anaerobic lid*: It was invented by Brewer in 1942. It can be used for isolation of facultative anaerobes and microaerophiles as an alternative to anaerobic jar. The solid medium is poured over a sterile Petri dish with 0.2% sodium thioglycolate. After solidification of media it is inoculated with the suspected anaerobic bacteria. The Petri dish is covered with Brewer's anaerobic lid. The lid touches periphery and traps some air in the center. Sodium thioglycolate removes the oxygen from the trapped air. Moist air present at the junction of lid and rim of the Petri dish prevents the entry of air further. An anaerobic condition is thus created at the center of the plate.

Anaerobic culture medium: The anaerobic culture medium should contain suitable terminal electron acceptor for anaerobic respiration (oxygen acts as terminal electron acceptor in aerobic respiration), donor elements and carbon sources. The bacteria should grow in a reducing environment where the energy is generated by fermentation or anaerobic respiration. Sodium thioglycolate

(0.01-0.2%), glucose (1%), cysteine hydrochloride (> 0.05%), glutathione, sodium sulphide, sodium carbonate-oxalic acid, ascorbic acid (0.1%), metallic iron (wires, nails, steel wool), fresh sterile animal tissues (guinea pig kidney) can be used as reducing agents in the media. The growth factors such as yeast extract, pyrimidines, peptone, casitone, casamino acid (rumen fluid) are added. The growth factors act as a source of volatile fatty acid and heme.

Cooked meat medium first prepared by Robertson (1915-16) is the most common fluid medium for the cultivation and maintenance of anaerobic bacteria in the laboratory. The medium contains cooked sterile muscle tissues which acts as the source of glutathione and cysteine (reducing agent). Unsaturated fatty acids present in meat also utilize oxygen for auto-oxidation. The auto-oxidation is catalyzed by haematin present in the meat. The cooked meat, glucose and peptone also provide nutrients to the growing bacteria. Currently it is modified as 'cooked M-medium' which is approved by FDA for cultivation of *Clostridium perfringens* from food items.

Table 1: Types of bacteria based on nutritional requirements

Nutritional requirements	Types of bacteria
Carbon: It acts as backbone of all organic molecules and carbon containing molecules also act as source of hydrogen and oxygen	Autotroph- Bacteria which uses CO_2 as sole or major source of carbon Heterotroph- Bacteria which uses reduced, preformed organic matters as source of carbon
Energy	Phototroph- Bacteria which utilize light as a source of energy Chemotroph- Bacteria which utilize chemical compounds (organic / inorganic) as a source of energy
Electron	Lithotroph- Bacteria which utilize inorganic compounds as a source of electron Organotroph- Bacteria which utilize organic compounds as a source of electron

Table 2: Vitamin as growth factors for bacteria

Vitamin	Growth stimulation
Thiamine (B1)	*Bacillus anthracis*
Riboflavin (B2)	*Clostridium tetani*
Niacin (B3)	*Brucella abortus*
Pyridoxine (B6)	*Lactobacillus*
Cyanocobalamin (B12)	*Lactobacillus*
Vitamin K	*Bacteroides*

6

Normal, Opportunistic and Saprophytic Bacterial Flora

Normal bacterial flora is the bacteria which live on another living being (human or animals) or inanimate object without causing infection

Opportunistic bacteria are part of normal bacterial flora which can produce infection during lowered immunity (immunosuppression) of host or when transferred into other parts of the body

Saprophytic bacteria live on dead or decaying organic matter

Infection

Infection can be defined as a pathological condition occurred due to multiplication of microbes.

Intoxication can be defined as pathological condition due to ingestion of microbial toxin (e.g. aflatoxin produced by *Aspergillus* fungus).

Mycetism is the pathological condition due to ingestion of fungus (e.g. toxic mushroom) which produces toxicity within the body of the host

Types of infection

Following types of infections are common in animals and human.

a) Acute infection: The infection is short duration type but with severe outcome. E.g. anthrax or black quarter in animals, strangles in horses, Glasser's disease in pigs etc.

b) Chronic infection: The infection of long duration type is known as chronic infection. E.g. tuberculosis in cattle, paratuberculosis in cattle, actinomycosis (lumpy jaw) in cattle, actinobacillosis (wooden tongue) in cattle etc.

c) Primary infection: A localized infection caused by specific microorganism which can lowers the body immunity and opens the door for other microorganisms or same microbe. E.g. chicken infectious anaemia in poultry

d) Secondary infection: The infection established after the occurrence of primary infection due to lowered body defense. E.g. *Escherichia coli* infection in poultry followed by chicken infectious anaemia

e) Local infection: It is restricted in a specific part of the body. E.g. infectious keratoconjunctivitis (pink eye) in cattle, urinary tract infection by *E. coli* etc.

f) General infection: It can spread throughout the body via blood, lymph and can infect all the vital organs. E.g. miliary tuberculosis in deer, typhoid in human etc.

g) Fulminating infection: It happens suddenly with severe intensity. E.g. fowl cholera in poultry, Ebola and Lassa fever in human

h) Mixed infection: More than one type of microorganisms is associated with the infection. E.g. shipping fever in cattle, foot rot in sheep etc.

i) Exogenous infection: The infection is caused by the bacteria transmitted from external sources of infection such as contaminated food, drinking water, air, coitus etc. e.g. cholera in human, tuberculosis in animals etc.

j) Endogenous infection: The infection is caused by the bacteria residing on the skin and in the nose, mouth, throat, gastrointestinal tract and genital tract. Due to lowered body defense the bacteria multiply and enter the deeper tissues to produce the infection. E.g. wooden tongue in cattle.

k) The types of infection can also be categorized according to the causative agents such as bacteria (bacterial infection), virus (viral infection), fungi (fungal infection), protozoa (protozoal infection) etc.

Sources of infection

The sources of microbial infection may be human, animals and the environment where the organisms are residing as pathogen, commensal and saprophytes. The animals or human acts as source of infection during incubation period, clinical phase showing symptoms, convalescence (recovery phase), and carrier stage.

Transmission of infection

Transmission of infection takes place into animals and human through different portals (entry points) such as alimentary, respiratory, urogenital, and integumentary systems, and the ear and eye. Types of transmissions based on portals are described in Table 1. After entry through the preferred portals the bacteria will reach to the 'site of predilection' for multiplication with the help of their 'virulence factors'. The site of predilection consists of cells and products which can help in bacterial survival and stimulate multiplication.

a) Ingestion (alimentary tract): Through ingestion the pathogens (bacteria) adhere to the mucosa present in tonsil, villus, crypts, Peyer's patches etc. The bacteria are trapped in the mucus layer present over the surfaces except M-cells (microfold cell). The mucus is produced by goblet cells present in the epithelial layer. The mucosal layer acts as one of the primary protective layer of the host which prevents the entry of pathogens. The layer is a physical barrier to the entry of bacteria due to its thickness and high viscosity. The mucus layer is thickest in colon (850 µm) and thinnest in jejunum (130 µm) depending on the concentration of goblet cells. It is the source of lysozyme and immunoglobulin (Ig-A) which can also neutralize the invading bacteria. The beneficial bacteria (*Lactobacillus*, *Bifidobacterium* etc.) can adhere with the mucosal layer by attaching with the receptors. Due to absence of empty receptors the pathogens cannot adhere with the mucosal layer. It is also a kind of host defense mechanism known as 'competitive exclusion' ('Nurmi concept'). These beneficial commensal also compete for nutrients with the pathogen, secrete antimicrobials and stimulate cross-protective immune factors of the host to lyse the pathogens. These beneficial bacteria are known as 'probiotics' and feeding of probiotics in poultry is a part of national program in European countries (e.g. Sweden) to control pathogens (*Salmonella*). The M-cells are present over the Peyer's patches in the small intestine. M-cells are commonly used by the bacteria for penetration of intestine as the cells are not covered with mucus layer. Few bacteria can cross the mucus layer with the help of antigen presenting cells such as dendritic cells.

b) Inhalation (respiratory tract): The pathogens can enter through the nostrils and deposit on nasal turbinates, pharynx, trachea, and bronchioles depending on shape, size, weight, and electrostatic charge of the pathogens. The pathogens are inhaled with inanimate objects such as dust, soil, sputum or other body fluids, known as 'fomite'. The larger fomites (> 1 µm) containing bacteria and fungi are trapped into the nasal turbinates. Whereas the smaller fomites (< 1 µm) containing virus and few bacteria can enter into the alveoli and bronchioles. After inhalation all the fomites are lodged into the mucociliary

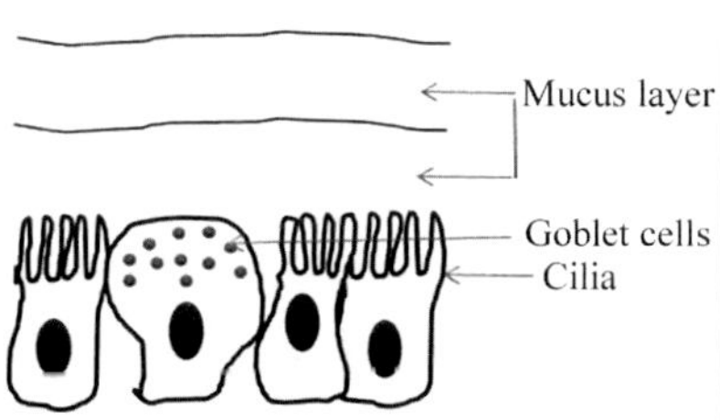

Muco-clilary apparatus

layer present in the nasal turbinates. The mucociliary apparatus is unique defense system of the respiratory tract. The upper part of the apparatus is composed of biphasic mucus layer consists of a gel like substance where the fomites are trapped. The lower part of the apparatus contains epithelial cells fitted with cilia. The continuous beating of cilia can move the gel and trapped fomites. In nasal cavity the movement of cilia always tries to pass the fomites towards pharynx so that it can be swallowed for easy passage through the digestive tract where the pathogen can be lysed with gastric acid. The cilia cannot beat when the mucociliary apparatus is damaged by respiratory viruses (Influenza virus, infectious bovine rhinotracheitis virus etc.). In absence of ciliary clearance the secondary bacterial infections with the fomites are lodged into the lungs directly due to the gravitational force. Thus secondary bacterial pneumonia can take place. Sometimes the passage of air through nasal turbinates produces a centrifugal violent air movement (turbulence) which dislodges the fomites from the mucosa. Depending on the size the fomites can enter into the deeper part of the alveoli and bronchioles.

c) Ascending infection (urogenital system): The pathogens can enter urinary and genital system through the damaged mucosa following coitus with infected animals or use of contaminated straws / semen in artificial insemination.

d) Cutaneous penetration (skin): The skin is the external barrier which protects the host from microbial invasion through its dryness, acidic pH, sebum (oils) and normal bacterial flora. The normal flora competes with invading pathogens for nutrients and receptors. The bacteria can adhere with the skin via direct contact. The bacteria can penetrate the skin if it is damaged due to abrasions, trauma, scratches and bite. The insects such as mosquitoes and blood sucking flies help in bacterial entry into muscle, blood, lymph during bite.

e) Direct contact (eye and ear): The microbes can adhere with the cornea, conjunctiva and lacrimal duct of eye and external acoustic meatus of ear by direct contact.

Pathogenicity, virulence, determinants of virulence

'Pathogenicity' can be defined as the capacity of the bacteria to cause any disease or harm in a host. It depends on host immunity, type of bacterial strains, and numbers of bacteria in exposure. 'Non-pathogenic' is a relative terminology for microbes, as apparently non-pathogenic bacteria may become pathogenic during decreased host resistance. The 'non-pathogenic' nomenclature is applied to those bacteria which are not yet confirmed to have pathogenic potential. Although purely beneficial bacteria such as *Lactobacillus*, *Bifidobacterium* exists as commensals in the body. Few beneficial bacteria present in the environment help in mineralization.

'Virulence' refers to the degree of pathology caused by the bacteria. Virulence is the quantitative measure of the pathogenicity. It can be expressed as the ratio of numbers of animals showing clinical symptoms to the numbers of animals exposed to the causative bacteria.

Determinants of virulence

The clinical infection is the outcome of war between the bacterial virulence determinants and immunity of the animals. Bacterial determinants of virulence consist of 'virulence factors' and 'toxins'. **Virulence factors** are glycoproteins or glycolipids expressed by bacteria which help in bacterial adherence with host cell membrane, invasion of skin or mucosa, endocytosis or phagocytosis, replication and dissemination locally, regionally and systematically, evasion and suppression of host immune response, and acquisition of nutrients. According to Koch's postulate the presence of virulence factors can differentiate pathogenic strains from the non-pathogenic strains of the bacteria. Currently it is considered that genes encoding virulence factors present in pathogenic strains can differentiate them from non-pathogenic strains (molecular Koch's postulate). The expression of virulence genes depends on several factors including host immunity. Examples and functions of bacterial virulence factors are enlisted in Table 2. The major functions conducted by bacterial virulence factors include adhesion, colonization and invasiveness. **Adhesion** is the process of bacterial attachment to host cells, tissue and biologic substances. **Colonization** is the bacterial adherence, multiplication, and establishment of infection. **Invasiveness** is the ability of bacteria to invade tissues. Adhesion and colonization of the bacteria is primary requirement of pathogenesis. Due to peristalsis, mucociliary undulations (beating of cilia) and micturition there is always a possibility of bacterial passage if not colonized. After colonization the bacteria start to express invasins required for spreading.

Bacterial secreation system

The virulence factors are transported from the bacterial cytoplasm to other cellular compartments, eukaryotic cells (host) and environment by a co-ordinated process known as protein secreation. In the body of the host secreation of virulence factors is required to establish the infection and in the environment it is required to compete with other environmental bacteria. There are several secreation systems used by bacteria such as general secreation (Sec), twin arginine translocation (Tat), type 1 secreation system (T1SS), type 2 secreation system (T2SS), type 3 secreation system (T3SS), type 4 secreation system (T4SS), type 5 secreation system (T5SS), type 6 secreation system (T6SS), type 7 secreation system (T7SS), SecA2, Sortase and injectosome. The type secreation systems (T1SS-T6SS) are common in Gram-negative bacteria, SecA2, Sortase, injectosome and T7SS in Gram-positive bacteria, and Sec/Tat are common in both types of bacteria. Sec and Tat secreation systems are highly conserved and are detected in bacteria, archae and eukaryotes. Sec system secreates unfolded proteins but Tat system secreates folded proteins. Different types of virulence factors secreated by various secreation systems are enlisted in Table 3.

Pathogenicity island (PAI)

Jo¨rg Hacker and colleagues (1980) first noticed that genes encoding virulence factors are located in a mobile genetic element in bacterial chromosome. Later, Hacker (1994) coined the term 'pathogenicity island' to describe the 70 kbp region of uropathogenic *E. coli* chromosome which can encode haemolysin and the region is absent in non-pathogenic strains. The PAIs can encode several virulence factors such as adhesins, invasins, and secreation systems. The size of PAI is 10 to 200 kbp and is generally located near tRNA genes. The borders of PAI contain insertion sequences which help in their transfer to other bacterial strains. The GC content and codon usage pattern of the PAIs is different from the rest of the bacterial genome. These findings indicate about acquisition of this genetic element from external sources into the bacterial chromosome. It is supposed that *E. coli* O157:H7 (food borne pathogen) is originated from acquisition of such pathogenicity island which can encode shiga toxins, intimin and T3SS. The PAIs are common in most of the Gram-negative and few Gram-positive (e.g. *Listeria*) bacteria.

Bacterial toxin

Bacterial toxin is the poison produced by the bacteria to cause lysis of the host cells. There are three kinds of bacterial toxins known as exotoxin, endotoxin (lipopolysaccharide) and lipoteichoic acids. Exotoxin is released by live Gram-positive bacteria. Endotoxin and lipoteichoic acids are released by dead Gram-negative and Gram-positive bacteria, respectively during lysis of bacteria by antibiotics or bactericidals. The potency of toxins is expressed with LD50 / MLD (lethal dose 50 / minimum lethal dose). LD50 is the dose of toxin which kills 50% of the test animals. MLD is the dose of toxin which kills 100% of the test animals. LD50 is calculated by Reed and Muench method.

Exotoxin: They are potent biological toxins secreated by live Gram-positive bacteria. They act by direct lysis of cells (pore formation), apoptosis, and activation of inflammation. The exotoxins are named as per their target cells or tissues such as haemolysin (lysis of red blood cells), leukotoxin (lysis of leukocytes), enterotoxin (acting on intestine by dysfunction of ion pumps, e.g. cholera toxin, *E. coli* enterotoxins), cytotoxin (pore formation, e.g. *Staphylococcus aureus* α-toxin), and neurotoxins (acting on nerve tissues e.g. botulinum toxin and tetanospasmin act by cleavage of SNARE proteins). Majority of the exotoxins belong to A-B toxin system in which the toxin gets attached with the host cells via B-subunit and then the toxic part (A) enters the host cells. Cholera toxin, botulinum toxin, diptheria toxin, tetanus toxin etc. are the examples of A-B toxin system.

Endotoxin: The endotoxins are lipopolysaccharide (LPS) present in Gram-negative bacterial cell wall. It is released into the host body after death of the bacteria. The lipid-A part of LPS is responsible for the toxicity of the endotoxin. The endotoxins act on endothelial cells, platelets, macrophages and few organs. The endotoxins can release pyrogens (causing fever) from leukocytes and damage platelets causing intravascular clotting (disseminated intravascular coagulation, DIC). It becomes lethal if released in large amount into the circulation which causes excess release of proinflammatory cytokines and nitric oxide from macrophages and endothelial cells, respectively. It further causes activation of the complement system and coagulation cascades followed by 'endotoxic shock'. It is characterized by fever, hypoglycaemia, thrombosis, hypovolemic shock and death. Differences between bacterial exotoxin and endotoxin are described in Table 4.

Lipoteichoic acid (LTA): It is a kind of toxin secreated by dead Gram-positive bacteria. It binds to endothelial cells, activates complement pathway and helps in release of reactive oxygen and nitrogen species, acid hydrolases, proteinases and cytokines toxic to host cells from neutrophils and macrophages. Lipoteichoic acid acts as a 'Gram-positive endotoxin' in *Staphylococcus*.

Toxoid and antitoxin

Toxoids are chemically modified bacterial exotoxins which retain their antigenic property but are not toxic in nature. Generally the toxins are treated with formaldehyde to produce toxoids. The toxoids can generate antibodies which neutralize the toxin. The toxin neutralizing antibodies are known as *antitoxins*.

Tetanus toxoids are used as prophylactic measure (vaccine) in animals and human which offers long term protection against tetanus. Ant-tetanus serum or tetanus immunoglobulin (ATS / TIG, antitoxin) can be used as both prophylactic and curative measure against tetanus in animals and human. The prophylaxis with ATS (1500 IU) is done during surgical injury, castration, docking, deep wound soiled with dust and mud in animals with no history of tetanus toxoid immunization or unknown immune status. The curative ATS (10,000-50,000 IU in cattle and horses; 3000-15,000 IU in sheep and pigs) is applied to the animals with symptoms of tetanus. The horses are injected with tetanus toxin and the equine plasma is collected to purify the antibodies which can neutralize *Clostridium tetani* toxins. ATS can produce protection for 1-2 weeks only.

Epizootic, enzootic and panzootic diseases

Epizootic (Greek *epi-* upon + *zoon* animal) is a disease which appears as new cases in a certain time period, in a certain animal population, at a higher incidence rate than expected. E.g. African swine fever in China (2019), rinderpest in India (1869-70) etc. The analogous term of 'epizootic' in human population is 'epidemic'. When the epizootic is restricted to a locality it is known as 'outbreak'.

When the epizootic disease spreads worldwide it is known as '**panzootic**' ('pandemic' in human). Examples are highly pathogenic avian influenza (H5N1), Newcastle disease in racing pigeons (1980) etc. There are three conditions to be satisfied for the disease to become 'panzootic' i.e. the disease should be infectious, new to the population and it spreads easily and continuously among the animal population.

Common diseases that occur at a constant but relatively high rate in the animal population are called '**enzootic**' diseases. E.g. Low pathogenic avian influenza in poultry etc.

Bacteremia, septicaemia and toxaemia

Septicaemia is the clinical condition caused by invasion and multiplication of pathogens in the bloodstream.

Bacteremia is the condition in which bacteria are present in the bloodstream. It may be originated from infections (pneumonia, urinary tract infection) or ordinary dental surgeries.

Toxaemia is the condition in which toxins are present in the bloodstream. It may be originated from a local bacterial infection.

Table 1: Routes of transmission

Portal	Route of transmission
Alimentary system	Ingestion
Respiratory system	Inhalation
Urogenital system	Ascending infection
Integumentary system (skin)	Cutaneous penetration
Ear and eye	Direct contact

Table 2: Bacterial virulence factors and function

Virulence factors	Function
Capsule	Antiphagocytic, role in adherence with the host cell membrane
Flagella	Bacterial motility, H-antigen also helps in adherence and is antiphagocytic
Fimbriae	Adherence with the host cell membrane
O-antigen	Antiphagocytic
Adhesin	Helps in bacterial adhesion with cell membrane by attachment with mucus, mucins, extracellular matrix (ECM) proteins
Invasin	Helps in bacterial invasion of cell membrane through ligand-receptor interaction or breakdown of extracellular matrix
a) Hyaluronidase	It lyses hyaluronan (hyaluronic acid) present in ECM of skin, mucosa, connective tissue, nervous tissue. Thus it helps in spreading of bacteria through the tissues ('spreading factor'). Few bacteria use hyaluronan as a carbon source for growth
b) Collagenase	It breaks down collagen present in ECM of muscle tissues
c) Neuraminidase	It breaks down neuraminic acid (sialic acid) present in host cell membrane
d) Haemagglutinin	It helps in binding with host cell membrane
e) Kinase	It lyses fibrin and prevents blood clotting which is required for separation of bacteria
f) Lecithinase	Lysis of host cell membrane
g) Phospholipase	Lysis of host cell membrane
Immunoglobulin protease	It degrades immunoglobulins required for adaptive immunity
Lipase	Destroys lipids present in host cell membranes and disrupts lipid metabolism
DNase	Degrades cellular DNA
Haemolysin	Lysis of red blood cells
Siderophores	Acquisition of iron for bacterial growth

Table 3: Bacterial secreation systems and secreated virulence factors

Secreation system	Secreated virulence factor
'Tat' system	Phopholipase C (e.g. Mycobacterium tuberculosis, Pseudomonas)
T1SS	Export of antibiotics and toxins outside the bacterial cell (e.g. MARTX toxin of Vibrio cholerae)
T2SS	Proteases, lipases, phosphatases, carbohydrate processing enzymes
T3SS ['needle and syringe' like structure, known as 'injectisome' (note the spelling difference with 'injectosome' of Gram-positive bacteria)]	It can inject the virulence factors directly into eukaryotic host cells by crossing three membranes i.e. bacterial cytoplasmic membrane, bacterial cell wall and eukaryotic cell membrane. It is essential for secreation of virulence factors in Yersinia, Salmonella, and Shigella
T4SS	It can transfer the proteins into other bacteria or eukaryotic cells. It can transfer DNA (bacterial conjugation), DNA-protein complexes in Brucella suis, Neisseria gonorrhoeae etc.

Secreation system	Secreated virulence factor
T5SS	Toxins and receptor binding proteins secreated by Neisseria gonorrhoeae, Yersinia enterocolitica, Shigella etc.
T6SS	It transfers proteins into another bacteria and host cells (e.g. Pseudomonas, Vibrio cholerae)
T7SS	Common in transport of virulence factors (e.g. ESX-1) through mycolic acid containing cell wall ('mycomembrane' present in Mycobacterium, Corynebacterium, Nocardia)
SecA2	Secretes proteins associated with stress responses, cell wall repair and metabolism (e.g. Staphylococcus, Streptococcus)
Sortase	In Gram-positive bacteria, sortase enzyme attaches the proteins (e.g. pilin of pili) secreated via cytoplasmic membrane to the cell wall (e.g. Staphylococcus, Streptococcus)
Injectosome	Like T3SS it can inject virulence factor (NAD glycohydrolase) of Gram-positive bacteria (Streptococcus pyogenes) into eukaryotic cells (keratinocyte)

Table 4: Differences between bacterial exotoxin and endotoxin

Exotoxin	Endotoxin
Secreated by live bacteria	Secreated by dead Gram-negative bacteria
Protein in nature	Lipopolysaccharide in nature
Heat sensitive	Heat stable (resistant to autoclaving)
Lethal dose is small	Lethal dose is large
Toxoid can be produced with exotoxin	Toxoid cannot be produced with endotoxin
Neutralization is easily possible with antitoxin	Neutralization is not easily possible with antitoxin
Each toxin has separate mechanism of action	All endotoxins act in a similar way

7

Bacterial Genetics

The genetics is the study of inheritance and variability of organisms. Bacterial genetics is a sub-field which specifically studies transmission of genetic information from one bacterium to its progeny or between the interbreeding bacteria and the expression of genetic information.

Mutation

Hugo de Vries (1848-1935, Dutch botanist) coined the term 'mutation'. It is originated from a Latin word which means 'to change'. The heritable change in bacterial DNA sequences is known as bacterial mutation. The mutation will generate a new type of bacteria with altered genotypical and phenotypical characteristics, known as 'mutant'. The parent bacterial cell from which the mutants are generated is known as 'wild type'. In nature bacterial mutation is a rare incidence. The spontaneous mutation occurs at a rate of 1 in 10^5 to 10^8. The phenotypical expression of mutation occurs quickly as the bacteria are haploid with shorter generation time.

Types of mutation

a) Point mutation: It occurs due to substitution of a single nucleotide with another in a DNA sequence. The substitution may occur with similar types of nucleotides [purine (A/G) / pyrimidine (C/T) replaced with another purine/pyrimidine] or different types of nucleotides (purine with pyrimidine or *vice-versa*). The substitution with similar types of nucleotides is known as *transition* and the substitution with different types of nucleotides is called *transversion*. The nucleotide substitution results following types of mutations.

   i) *Missense mutation:* Production of an altered amino acid in a protein sequence due to change in codon (sequence of three DNA or RNA nucleotides that produces a specific amino acid) is known as missense mutation.

   ii) *Nonsense mutation:* Production of a stop codon (UAG, UAA, and UGA) is called missense mutation. It will result premature termination of protein synthesis with incomplete protein products.

iii) *Silent (neutral) mutation*: Generation of same amino acid by the altered codon is called silent / neutral mutation as there is no change in the product. The same amino acid can be specified by different codons.

b) Frameshift mutation: Change in the reading frame of a gene due to addition or deletion of base pairs is called frameshift mutation. The total amino acids and their sequences are changed after frameshift mutation.

c) Lethal mutation: The mutation affecting vital function of bacterial cells and causing death is known as lethal mutation. Sometimes the mutant can survive in a specific environmental condition which is known as 'conditional lethal mutant'. For example, a temperature sensitive mutant can survive at 35°C, but not at 40°C.

d) Suppressor mutation: It is the reversal of mutant to wild-type bacteria by another mutation at a position different from the original mutation.

Different types of bacterial mutations result 'auxotrophs' (a mutant which requires a particular nutrient for the growth not required by the parent cells), antibiotic resistance, regulatory mutants (disruptions on regulatory sequences), constitutive mutants (continuous expression of genes) etc.

Mechanism of mutation

The spontaneous mutation (without exposure to mutants) occurs in the course of DNA replication. The nucleotide may be inserted, mispaired or deleted during synthesis of a new DNA strand by DNA Polymerase III. The bacterial DNA can exist in different forms known as tautomers. The tautomers are isomers in the positions of their atoms and in the bonds between the atoms. The nucleotides mostly exist in keto (C-O) and amino (C-NH2) forms and rarely in imino (C≡NH) and enol (C-OH) forms. The alteration in nucleotide base pair formation during DNA replication is known as 'tautomerization'. For example, A (adenine) in amino form can pair with T (thymine) in keto form, whereas, A in its imino form pairs with C. The T in enol form pairs with G.

The possibility of spontaneous mutation is more in lagging strand than the leading strand. The mutation may be carried forward to the progeny of the parent bacteria. The mispairing in DNA strands ('slip-strand mispairing') can generate addition or deletion mutations because some nucleotides replicate twice while the others cannot replicate. If the repeats are not in a multiple of three the frameshift mutation is generated.

The physical, chemical or biological agent which produces artificial mutation is known as mutagen. Different types of mutagens and their mechanism of action are enlisted in Table 1.

Techniques for detection of mutant bacteria

Replica plating

Joshua and Esther Lederberg (1952) first developed the replica plating technique for isolation of nutritional mutant bacteria. The bacterial colonies grown in a complete solid medium (nutrient agar) are exposed to a mutagen (e.g. UV radiation). The colonies are replicated on a sterile velvet pad with gentle pressure. The velvet pad is pressed over the agar plate consisting of a minimal medium, deficient for a nutrient (e.g. histidine amino acid). The histidine auxotrophs cannot produce any colony on the minimal agar plate although the colonies are present in the original plate from which the colonies are replicated.

Ames test

Bruce Ames (USA, 1970) first described the test procedure for isolation of nutritional mutants (auxotrophs). The test is conducted with mutant strains (mutation in histidine synthesis gene) of *Salmonella* Typhimurium. The strains require histidine for growth but cannot synthesize it. The bacteria are spread on an agar plate with a small amount of histidine. The histidine allows the bacteria to grow for an initial time. The histidine is exhausted soon. The medium will allow the growth of those bacterial strains that have mutated to gain the ability to synthesize their own histidine. The plate is incubated for 48 hours. The mutagenicity of a substance is proportional to the number of colonies observed.

Chromogenic substrate

The chromogenic substances are used to isolate mutant bacteria that cannot use carbon source (e.g. lactose, glucose etc.). The bacteria which can use carbon source possess β-galactosidase enzyme which hydrolyses lactose into glucose and galactose. The chromogenic substrate for β-galactosidase is 5-bromo-4-chloro-3-indolyl-β-D-galactoside (X-gal).The colonies are blue in X-gal containing medium if the bacteria are able to use carbon source. The mutants produce white coloured colonies in X-gal containing medium.

Polymerase chain reaction (PCR) and nucleotide sequencing

The nucleotides flanking the region of interest can be amplified with specific oligonucleotide primers in PCR. The PCR product is sequenced by Sanger dideoxy method to detect the mutational changes.

DNA microarray

The chromosomal gain and losses can be detected by DNA microarray method.

Bacterial gene transfer

In bacteria there are three methods of gene transfer from one bacterium to another which is known as transformation, conjugation and transduction.

Transformation

Transfer of 'cell-free' or 'naked' DNA from one bacterium to another is called transformation. It is the most common method of bacterial gene transfer in nature. In 1928, Griffith in his experiment observed that mixing of heat-killed and virulent (capsulated/ smooth strains) pneumococci with live and non-pathogenic (non-capsulated, rough strains) cultures can convert all non-pathogenic bacteria into virulent. Avery, MacLeod and McCarthy later showed that transfer of genetic material (DNA) from the killed bacteria was responsible for the conversion of non-pathogenic live bacteria into virulent. Thus the concept of transformation was established.

The capacity to uptake the naked DNA is known as bacterial 'competence'. It is regulated by quorum sensing and nutritional requirements of the bacteria. The competent bacteria use structures similar to type IV pili and type 2 secreation system (T2SS) for uptake of DNA. Till date at least 40 bacterial species is confirmed to be competent for transformation.

Free DNA is available in the environment originated mostly from dead bacterial cells and few live bacteria (e.g. *Neisseria* spp.). Transformation of foreign DNA is required for several purposes such as source of carbon, nitrogen and phosphorous, repair of damaged DNA in recipient bacteria and production of genetic diversity. The DNA of related environmental bacteria may serve as template for damage repair in recipient bacteria. The genetic diversity is associated with acquisition of new genetic information related to virulence, metabolism and antimicrobial resistance.

The major constraint in transformation is bacterial DNAase enzyme which can lyse the foreign DNA. The 'uptake' of DNA can be defined as conversion of foreign DNase-sensitive DNA into a 'DNase-protected' state within the bacterial cell. The DNase-protected state is observed when foreign DNA crosses the outer membrane in Gram-negative bacteria and cytoplasmic membrane in Gram-positive bacteria. The single strand of the foreign DNA can enter bacterial cytoplasm whereas the other strand is degraded into the environment (Gram-positive) or periplasmic space (Gram-negative bacteria). The bacteria use a group of proteins which partially spans the cell envelope required for foreign DNA entry.

Binding of DNA

Binding of foreign DNA is the first step of 'uptake' during transformation. In Gram-positive bacteria (*Bacillus subtilis*) ComEA protein acts as the major DNA-binding receptor. After binding, the surface endonuclease (NucA) cleaves the double stranded foreign DNA to generate single stranded DNA. In few Gram-positive bacteria (*Streptococcus pneumoniae*) a nick is produced first before separation of the double strands. In Gram-negative bacteria (*Haemophilus, Neisseria, Actinobacillus*) a specific sequence ['DNA uptake sequences (DUS)' or 'uptake signal sequences (USS)'] should be present in foreign DNA as a marker for efficient uptake. The DUS-mediated uptake is dependent on pilus.

The role of pili (pilus) in transformation is still not established although expression of pilin protein is required for effective transformation. The 'competence pseudopilus' generated in competent bacteria (both Gram-negative and Gram-positive) helps to bring the foreign DNA closer to the transport machinery. In Gram-positive bacteria the pseudopilus can span the thick cell wall. In Gram-negative bacteria it connects the outer membrane with the cytoplasmic membrane. The pseudopilus can retract and pull the foreign DNA from the bacterial surface to the transport machinery to cross the membranes as described below.

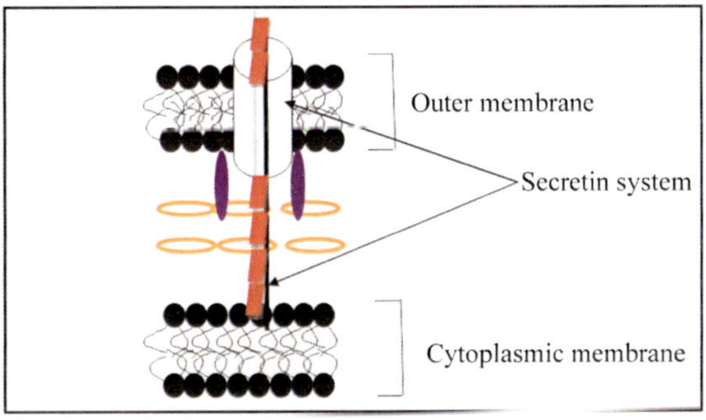

Gram-negative bacterial' 'secretin' system

Crossing the membrane (membrane translocation)

In Gram-positive bacteria (*B. subtilis*) ComEC (permease/channel protein) and ComFA (ATP binding protein) play major role in crossing cytoplasmic membrane of foreign DNA. ATP-binding cassette transporters (ABC transporters) use the energy derived from ATP hydrolysis for transfer of foreign DNA through the cytoplasmic membrane.

In Gram-negative bacteria the protein complex 'secretin' (12-14 subunits) helps in translocation of foreign DNA through the outer membrane. It is a 'doughnut' shaped structure (6-8.8 nm diameter) produced in outer membrane during translocation. The secretin forms aqueous channel through which the DNA can pass in. The best characterized secretin is PilQ of *N. gonorrhoeae* which also takes part in pilus biogenesis.

Fate of foreign DNA

Interaction with bacterial cytoplasmic protein protects the foreign DNA from lysis. The single stranded DNA can be integrated into the bacterial chromosome (recA dependent) or plasmid if sequence homology is present.

Transduction

In 1952, Norton Zinder and Joshua Lederberg discovered a new method of bacterial gene transfer in *Salmonella* Typhimurium which they called 'transduction'. It can be defined as transfer of the genetic component between two bacterial strains (donor and recipient) with the help of a bacteriophage.

There are two types of bacteriophages i.e. virulent / lytic and temperate phages. The lytic phages cause fragmentation of the bacterial chromosome into small pieces and lysis of the bacterial cells. Incidentally the phages can pick up a bacterial chromosome segment in place of phage DNA into their head. Now the transducing phage can inject the bacterial chromosome segment into freshly attacked bacteria. The temperate phages during attack generally do not lyse the bacteria. Instead the phage DNA is integrated into the bacterial chromosome. The integrated phage DNA is known as 'prophage' and the bacteria carrying the prophage is called 'lysogenic bacteria'. André Lwoff (1940) first observed lysogeny in *Bacillus megaterium.* The attachment of prophage takes place through 'reciprocal crossover' between the circular chromosomes of the phage and bacteria. The crossover point is known as 'λ attachment site' ('λ' phage). The attachment site is located between the genes *gal* and *bio* (*E. coli*) in bacterial chromosome. The lysogenic bacteria are resistant to infections with free phages and the prophages are carried into the daughter bacterial cells after divisions. In presence of 'inducers' (ultraviolet light) the prophages are activated. The activated prophages cause lysis of bacteria and release of new phage particles which may carry part of bacterial chromosome along with the phage DNA. When the new phages attack fresh bacteria they may insert the bacterial gene into the freshly attacked bacterial chromosome.

There are two types of transduction i.e. generalized and specialized. In generalized transduction the phages (P1, P22) can carry any part of the bacterial chromosome but in specialized transduction the phages carry only restricted part of the bacterial chromosome. In generalized transduction more number of genes is transferred than the specialized transduction. The generalized transduction was first noticed by K. Ikeda and J. Tomizawa (1965) during their experiments with temperate phage (P1) in *E. coli.*

The generalized transduction is used to calculate linkage value between the bacterial genes. The simultaneous transduction of multiple bacterial genes with a single phage particle is called 'cotransduction'. The bacterial strain receiving multiple transduced genes due to their close linkage is known as cotransductant. The linkage values are expressed as 'cotransduction frequencies'. More cotransduction frequency indicates the presence of higher linkage between the genes.

Conjugation

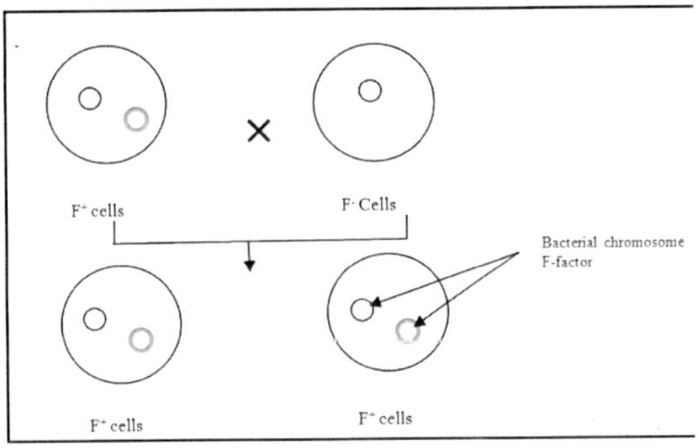

Gene transfer between F^+ and F^- cells

Joshua Lederberg and Edward Tatum (1946) discovered the conjugation method of bacterial gene transfer during their experiment with *E. coli*. Conjugation can be defined as transfer of self-replicating genetic factor and sometimes chromosomal DNA from a donor bacterial cell to a recipient through a conjugation pilus or sex pilus. In true sense it is not a sexual reproduction because in sexual reproduction both the partners donate equal genetic information to generate the offspring. In bacterial conjugation unidirectional transfer of genes occur from donor bacteria ('male') to the recipient ('female'). William Hayes (1952) identified that the 'maleness' of bacteria depends on possession of self-replicating genetic factor ['fertility factor' (F-factor)] which is transmitted during conjugation. The strains possessing 'F-factor' are known as F^+ / donor /male and the strains devoid of F-factor are F^- /recipient/female cells.

The pilus associated with conjugation (sex-pilus) brings two compatible bacteria (F^+ and F^-) together. A bridge with a pore is formed between the bacteria. The double strands of F-factor present freely in the cytoplasm of F^+ cells become separated into single strand. One strand of F-factor enters the recipient bacterium (F^-) through the pore. Each of the single strands in the F^+ and F^- cells replicates to produce the double stranded F-factors again. The F^- cell is thus converted into an F^+ cell. The possibility of F-factor transfer is very high (100%) during the cross between F^+ and F^- cells but transfer of chromosomal genes with F-factor has low possibility (one recombinant per 10^4 to 10^5 cells).

Gene transfer between Hfr and F⁻ cells

Luca Cavalli-Sforza (1949) discovered a subset of F^+ cells which contains F-factor integrated with the bacterial chromosome. Jacob and Wollman (1958) coined the term 'episome' for genetic elements which have alternate states of existence either as a cytoplasmic autonomous particle (plasmid) or integrated into the bacterial chromosome. The subset can produce recombinants with higher frequency (1000 times more) than normal F^+ cells. So the cells became known as high frequency of recombination (Hfr) cells. During crosses between Hfr and F^- cells the part of bacterial chromosome is transferred. The circular chromosome in Hfr cells unwinds first and begins to be transferred from a specific start point (origin or 'O'). The increasing distance of the genes present in the chromosome from 'O' start point reduces the probability to be transferred into the F^- cells. The transfer procedure is stopped before all the genes are transferred. The transfer process is a kind of rolling circle type of replication. During the transfer of one strand of the chromosome another strand is replicated. The Hfr cells again possess a whole chromosome after transfer. The transferred part of the chromosome in the recipient cells is either integrated into the recipient chromosome or is lost during subsequent cell divisions. The mating between Hfr and F^- cells does not generate F^+ cells (although frequency of recombination is high) because generally before the transfer of integrated F-factor the chromosomal strand (which is transferred) breaks and the transfer is stopped. The breakage can occur at any time during the transfer and the farthest genes from 'O' site have the least chance to be transferred ('gradient of transfer').

Sexduction or 'F-duction'

Jacob and Adelberg (1959) coined the term 'sexduction'. Sometimes the integrated F-factor is detached from Hfr chromosome with part of the bacterial chromosome. The F-factor containing the part of bacterial chromosome is known as 'F-prime (F')'. The bacterial cells with F' are called F' cells. During the mating of F' and F^- cells F-factor is transferred with the part of primary bacterial chromosome and the method is known as 'sexduction' or 'F-duction'. The recipient cells become secondary F' cells.

Plasmids and antibiotic resistance

Plasmids are circular or linear (N15 prophage of *E. coli*) self-replicating extrachromosomal double stranded DNA (replicon) which is common in eubacteria, archaea, and few eukaryotes. They are transmitted between the bacteria by conjugation. The average size of plasmid is 80 kbp (744 bp-2.5 Mbp) and the average GC content is 44 mol % (19.3-75.6 mol %). The size of plasmid is 10% of the host chromosome and it can accommodate minimum

400 genes. The GC content of plasmid is important in selection of bacterial hosts. Generally the GC content of the plasmid is similar with the host bacterial chromosome because replication of plasmid requires host bacterial respiratory enzymes. In few bacteria the GC content of plasmid and chromosome differs because the bacteria cannot afford higher energy to maintain G and C bonds (G and C is connected with 3 H-bonds than A and T connected with 2 bonds). More than 4600 plasmids of bacteria, archaea and eukaryotes are fully sequenced and 14% of the sequenced plasmids are conjugative type. The conjugative plasmids are not only transferred easily between the bacteria but also promote transfer of other plasmids. The plasmids carry genes for survival of bacteria in adverse environment in presence of antibiotics, heavy metals (mercury, cadmium, silver), survival of bacteria in hosts (virulence genes) and the genes encoding the enzymes for DNA repair.

Replication of plasmid

The plasmid DNA contains an origin of vegetative replication (*oriV*), genes for antibiotic/heavy metal resistance/virulence, promoter sequence and restriction digestion site. The plasmids which can be transferred have origin of transfer (*oriT*), relaxase and type IV pili coupling protein (T4CP). The replication takes place at *oriV*. The plasmids use different replication strategies such as theta-type replication, rolling-circle replication, and strand displacement-type replication. Repeated DNA sequences ('iteron') should be present in the plasmid to use theta-type replication strategy. The small multi-copy plasmids (pT181/Inc14, pC194/ Inc8, pMV158/ Inc11, pUB110/ Inc13) use rolling-circle replication strategy.

Classification of plasmid

A. The most common strategy for classification of plasmids is based on incompatibility (Inc). The 'incompatibility' is defined as inability of the plasmids with similar replication and partition systems to be propagated into the same host. The Inc groups are established in three types of bacteria such as *Enterobacteriaceae* (27 Inc groups), *Pseudomonas* (14 Inc groups) and *Staphylococcus* (18 Inc groups) based on amino acid sequences of replication initiation protein (Rep). Classification of plasmids on Rep protein varieties is known as 'replicon typing'. This kind of plasmid typing can recognize unidentified Inc groups also.

B. Another classification system of plasmids is based on amino acid sequences of relaxase enzyme which can classify the plasmids into six mobility (MOB) types (MOB_C, MOB_F, MOB_H, MOB_P, MOB_Q, MOB_V).

C. According to the type 4 secreation system (T4SS) amino acid sequence the plasmids can be grouped into four mating pair formation (MPF) classes such as MPF_F, MPF_G, MPF_I, and MPF_T.

D. Functional classification of plasmids consists of five types i.e. fertility/ F-plasmids, resistance plasmids / R-factors, Col-plasmids, virulence and degradative plasmids. Fertility plasmids are transferred by conjugation through sex pilus. Resistance plasmids consist genes for resistance against antibiotics and heavy metals. Before the development of plasmid concept they were known as 'R-factors'. Col-plasmids consist genes for bacteriocins. The virulence plasmids contain the genes associated with bacterial virulence. Degradative plasmids help in digestion of toluene and salicylic acid.

Transfer of plasmid

After conjugation of two compatible bacteria (donor and recipient) the plasmid double stranded DNA is cleaved at origin of transfer (*oriT*) site with the relaxase enzyme. The relaxase protein binds covalently with the single strand of plasmid DNA and the complex is transferred to the recipient cells with the help of type 4 secreation system (T4SS) and type IV pili coupling protein (T4CP). The FtsK-homologous protein was identified to help in transfer of *Actinomycetales* plasmids. In archaea the transfer of plasmid was detected only in *Sulfolobales* with an unknown mechanism.

Antibiotic resistance

Antimicrobials can be defined as any substance of natural, semisynthetic or synthetic origin that kills or inhibits the growth of a microorganism but causes little or no damage to the host. It is a broader term and it can be classified into several groups according to the type of microbes on which it acts such as antibiotics (bacteria), antivirals (virus), antifungals (mould and yeast), and antiparasitic (malaria agent). On the basis of mode of action antimicrobials are either microbicidal (lysis of microbes) or microbistatic (growth inhibition). Antibiotics can be defined as low molecular weight substance produced by a microbe that at little concentrations inhibits or kills other bacteria. First evidence of chemotherapy was noticed in 1899 when Emmerich and Löw prepared extract from *Pseudomonas aeruginosa* (pyocyanase). Paul Ehrlich (1854-1915, Germany) during his work with dyes noticed that specific aniline dyes can kill a specific group of microbes, not the others. Based on the idea of specificity Ehrlich began his quest for 'magic bullet' during 1904 to treat syphilis. Paul Ehrlich and Alfred Bertheim identified the chemical structure of atoxyl, a less toxic arsenical drug used to treat African sleeping sickness. They started to synthesize numerous derivatives of atoxyl and the arsphenamine derivative (compound 606, salvarsan) was found effective against syphilis in experimental rabbits, followed by limited human trials.

Alexander Fleming (1881-1955, United Kingdom) discovered the first antibiotic 'penicillin' in 1928. He observed that growth of *Staphylococcus aureus* was inhibited by a contaminant blue mould (*Penicillium*) in culture dishes. The observation was converted to the concept that certain microbes produce diffusible substances that can inhibit the growth of other microorganisms. Penicillin was introduced into the clinical practice during 1940 and as a wonder drug it saved several lives during Second World War. Identification of core structure (6-aminopenicillanic acid) paved the way for development of numerous derivatives such as penicillinase-resistant penicillins (methicillin, oxacillin, nafcillin), aminopenicillins (ampicillin, amoxicillin, bacampicillin), carboxypenicillins (carbenicillin, ticarcillin), and ureidopenicillins (mezlocillin, azlocillin, piperacillin).

'Antimicrobial resistance' (AMR) is the capacity of microbes to resist the lytic effects of antimicrobials. The term 'antibiotic resistance' is a subset of AMR which is applied to antibiotic only. It is the capacity of bacteria to resist the lytic effects of antibiotics. Alexander Fleming, the discoverer of first antibiotic also introduced the concept of AMR. It is a multi-factorial complex issue which can cause more death than cancer in coming decades. The antibiotics acted successfully against several deadly bacteria are useless now. The AMR increases the mortality, morbidity, prolonged hospital stay, man-day loss and increased treatment costs.

Mobile genetic element mediated antibiotic resistance

Plasmid mediated antibiotic resistance

The antibiotic resistance depends on transfer of resistance genes between the bacteria through mobile genetic elements (MGE) such as plasmids, transposon, integron etc. Resistance plasmids play major role in generation of antibiotic resistance. The plasmids encoded resistance includes against the common antibiotics such as cephalosporins, fluoroquinolones and aminoglycosides. Resistance plasmids are mostly 'conjugative' type (transferred easily between the bacteria, 30-100 kbp in size). The conjugative plasmids also promote transfer of 'mobilizable' plasmids (10 kbp) between the bacteria. The 'mobilizable' plasmids have own relaxasome but do not possess the genes required for mating pore formation. These deficient genes (compatible mating-pore genes) are provided by comparatively large conjugative plasmids. The plasmids are transferred along with the resistance genes though conjugation as described above. Sometimes mobilizable and conjugative plasmids are present in two separate bacterial cells and the method of plasmid transfer is known as 'retrotransfer'.

The conjugative plasmids have both broad and narrow host range depending on the distribution of receptors in the recipient bacterial cells. The receptors are required for effective conjugation of the plasmid. The example of broad host range plasmid is resistance plasmid RP1 (RP4 and RK4) which was first identified in *Pseudomonas aeruginosa*. It can transfer resistance gene into almost all Gram-negative bacteria.

The plasmids in natural bacterial isolates are persistent with antibiotic resistance genes even in absence of antibiotics. So the bacteria remain antibiotic resistant even in absence of selection pressure (antibiotics).

Transposon mediated antibiotic resistance

Transposons can move both intra and inter-molecularly i.e. it may jump within a DNA molecule or from one DNA molecule to another. There are two classes of transposons i.e. composite (class I; Tn5, Tn9, Tn10, Tn903, Tn1525, Tn2350, Tn4001, Tn4003) and complex transposons (class II; Tn3, Tn21, Tn2501). The most well studied transposon is Tn21 which possesses resistance determinants OXA and PSE (*Pseudomonas* specific enzyme) against aminoglycoside antibiotics. The transposons can move from chromosomal DNA to plasmid DNA or *vice-versa* with resistance genes.

Integron mediated antibiotic resistance

Stokes and Hall (1989) coined the term 'integron'. Integrons are mobile genetic elements which contains the genes required for excision and insertion of genetic materials from plasmids or chromosomes along with antibiotic resistance genes. There are several categories of integron based on amino acid sequences of integrase enzyme it possesses. For example, class 1 integrons possess class I integrase (IntI1), class 2 integrons possess class II integrase (IntI2) etc. Class 1 integrons are associated with resistance against streptomycin-spectinomycin (*aadA*) and sulfonamide-trimethoprim. It is common in both Gram-positive and Gram-negative bacteria such as *Enterococcus, Corynebacterium, Streptococcus, Escherichia, Klebsiella, Aeromonas, Enterobacter, Providencia* and *Mycobacterium*. The resistance genes such as streptothricin acetyltransferase (*sat1*), adenyl transferase (*aadA1*), dihydrofolate reductase (*dfrA1*) are present in class 2 integrons, common in *Enterobacteriaceae*, *Acinetobacter*, and *Psuedomonas*. The class 3 integrons contain beta-lactamase (IMP-1) encoding genes and are detected in *Acinetobacter, Alcaligenes, Citrobacter, Escherichia, Klebsiella, Pseudomonas, Salmonella* and *Serratia*.

Integrative and conjugative elements (ICE) mediated antibiotic resistance

Integrative and conjugative elements (ICEs) are common in both Gram-positive and Gram-negative bacteria. It can integrate with the bacterial chromosome with integration and excision module, conjugation module and regulation module. It can transmit the genes associated with resistance against antibiotics and heavy metals, virulence and biofilm formation. The information about ICEs is updated in the database ICEberg (http://db-mml.sjtu.edu.cn/ICEberg/).

Table 1: Classification of mutagens and their mechanism of action

Classification of mutagens	Mechanism of action
Physical mutagen	
Ultraviolet (UV) light	UV light (250 nm) makes a bond between adjacent pyrimidine bases (rarely purine bases) to produce a dimer. The dimers are covalently linked and do not fit within the helix structure. It prevents DNA conformation, replication and transcription. The dimer formation ultimately results a deletion mutation.
Chemical mutagens	
Base analog	5-bromouracil can act as analog of thymine. It acts as a wrong substrate during DNA replication and causes point mutations. It can pair with guanine in place of adenine
Deaminating agents (e.g. nitrous acid)	These agents can convert amino groups of the nucleotides into keto groups. Nitrous acid can convert cytosine into uracil which cannot pair with guanine. Deamination of adenine creates hypoxanthines which will base-pair with cytosine.
Alkylating agents (e.g. ethyl methanesulfonate, dimethyl nitrosoguanidine)	It adds alkyl group along with oxygen at the 6 position of guanine to create an O-6-alkyl-guanine. This addition leads to direct mispairing with thymine and results in GC → AT transitions
Interchalating agents (e.g. proflavin, acridine orange, ethidium bromide)	The agents can mimic base pairs and slip themselves in between stacked nitrogen bases ('interchalation') at DNA helix. The interchalation unwinds the helix slightly and increases the distance between adjacent base pairs. Thus the agent can disrupt the reading frame during translation and produces insertions or deletions
Reactive oxygen species (e.g. peroxide, superoxide, hydroxyl radical, singlet oxygen)	Hydroxyl radicals can convert guanine into 8-hydroxy-deoxyguanosine (8-OhdG) which mispairs with adenine instead of cytosine
Biological mutagen	
Transposons	Transposon is a DNA sequence that can change its position within a genome. Insertion of transposons into exons, introns and into flanking DNA can destroy or alter the gene activity. The faulty repair of the 'gap' created by the transposon at the old site form where it had moved can cause mutation.

8

Staphylococcus

Sir Alexander Ogston, a physician from Scotland, first elucidated the role of *Micrococcus* in formation of pus. He proposed the name '*Staphylococcus*' (In Greek 'staphyle' means bunch of grapes and 'kokkos' means berry). Anton J. Rosenbach isolated two different species of *Staphylococcus* and named them according to the pigmented appearance of colonies i.e. *Staphylococcus aureus* (in Latin 'aurum' means gold) and *Staphylococcus albus* (in Latin 'albus' means white). The studies of Bumm (1885) established the relationship of *Staphylococcus* with human infections. Nocard (1887) and Guillebeau (1890) isolated *Staphylococcus* from mastitis in sheep and cattle, respectively and established its pathogenic role in animals.

Properties of genus

1. *Morphology*: Staphylococci are gram positive cocci, capsulated, non-sporing and non-motile. Each coccus cell is 1μm in diameter. They are arranged in a group or grape like cluster as cell division occurs in more than one plane. During preparation of smear and staining the cluster is sometimes broken and cocci are seen in pair or single. Staphylococcal capsule is polysaccharide in nature. The capsule can inhibit phagocytosis and helps in virulence. The capsulation is variable among the species and strains. *S. aureus* is mostly capsulated whereas *S. hyicus* is non-capsulated. Staphylococcal cell wall contains three major components i.e. peptidoglycan (PG), teichoic acid (TA) and surface proteins (Figure 1).

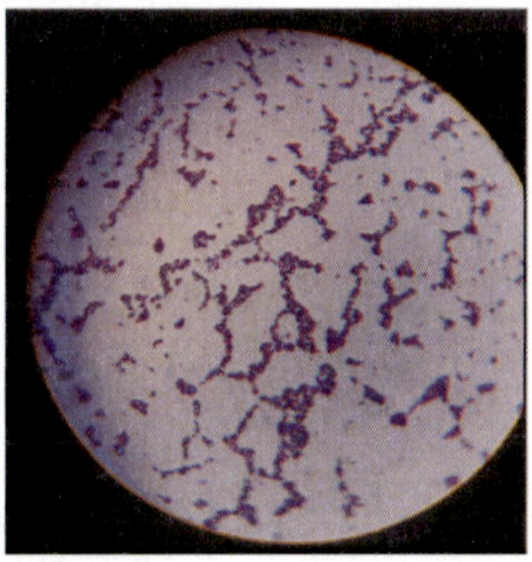

Fig. 1: Gram stained smear of *Staphylococcus aureus* isolated from mastitic milk (*Courtesy*: Achintya Mahanti, Department of Veterinary Microbiology, WBUAFS, Kolkata, India)

   a) Peptidoglycan (PG): PG is a polymer of glucosamine and muramic acid cross linked by pentaglycine (L-glycine) bridge. In other gram positive bacteria these glucosamine and muramic acids are N-acetylated. In *Staphylococcus* they are O-acetylated making them resistant to lysozyme.

b) Teichoic acids (TA): They are found in the cell wall of staphylococci like other gram positive bacteria. TA is either peptidoglycan associated or sometimes present outside the cell. TA contains ribitol in *S. aureus* cell wall whereas glycerol in *S. epidermidis* and *S. intermedius.*

c) Surface proteins: The surface proteins are known as 'microbial surface components recognizing adhesive matrix molecules'(MSCRAMMs) that mediate attachment of the bacteria to the host tissues and initiate colonization prior to an infection. The protein group includes fibronectin binding protein, clumping factors, collagen binding proteins etc. A kind of immunoglobulin binding protein is found on the surface of *S. aureus* known as 'Protein-A'. Carotenoid pigments present in the bacterial cell membrane produce golden coloured colonies of *S. aureus* in agar plates.

2. Staphylococci are aerobe or facultative anaerobe. They can produce energy by respiratory or facultative way.
3. Staphylococci are generally extracellular in nature. Certain types of host cells (fibroblasts, osteoblasts, keratinocytes and endothelial cells) can uptake staphylococci *in vitro*.
4. *Classification*: *Staphylococcus* belongs to *Micrococcaceae* family and the genus contains 32 recognized species among them 13 are restricted to human and rest to the animals. Major pathogenic species are *Staphylococcus aureus*, *S. intermedius, S. pseudintermedius, S. hyicus, S. epidermidis, S. schleiferi* subsp. *coagulans, S. haemolyticus, S. delphini.*

   S. aureus strains are further classified into several clonal complexes based on multilocus sequence typing (MLST) of housekeeping genes. The strains having identical sequences at all loci of the housekeeping genes are considered as a 'clone' and designated with a unique sequence type (ST). The sequence types which vary in sequences at more than three loci are grouped into clonal complexes (CC). Assignment of ST / CC of the sequences can be done by eBURST algorithm (http://eburst.mlst.net).
5. *Resistance:* Staphylococci are heat-sensitive (60°C temperature for 60 minutes). The bacteria can withstand drying for several weeks specially within pus or within the medium containing 7.5% salt concentration. Staphylococci are sensitive to common disinfectants like phenol, mercuric chloride. They are also sensitive to bacteriostatic dye like crystal violet (1: 500000) and bile salts. Resistance to beta-lactam antibiotics (e.g. penicillin) occurs through the production of penicillinase enzyme.

Methicillin resistant Staphylococcus aureus (MRSA)

S. aureus was effectively treated with penicillin group of antibiotic during its discovery. Later the bacteria evolved to produce the plasmid encoded enzyme penicillinase, responsible for lysis of penicillin. Methicillin (a type of penicillin) was developed to combat penicillin-resistant bacteria. However *S. aureus* became resistant to it also through a different mechanism. These resistant strains are called MRSA. Methicillin can block the penicillin binding proteins (PBPs) of the bacteria required for their cell wall synthesis. MRSA can synthesize a new form of PBP known as PBP2a, resistant to methicillin. The PBP2a is encoded by *mecA* gene found on the bacterial chromosome within a large mobile genetic element called staphylococcal chromosome cassette *mec* (SCC*mec*). MRSA are not only resistant to methicillin but also to all β-lactam antibiotics, including synthetic penicillins, cephalosporins and carbapenems as well as other groups of antibiotics like aminoglycosides, macrolides, lincosamides, streptogramins and tetracyclines. Major human originated MRSA clones are CC1, CC5, CC8, CC22, CC30 and CC45 which are prevalent throughout the world. Seventeen epidemic strains of human MRSA (EMRSA1-17) were described with frequent detection of EMRSA-15 and EMRSA-16 associated with clinical infection. The most widely prevalent livestock associated MRSA (LA MRSA) belonged to CC 398 lineage and was described in pigs and other food animals in different parts of the world. In South-East Asia, ST 9 clonal complex is widely prevalent among farmed pigs.

6. *Natural habitat:* Staphylococci are ubiquitously present in the environment such as in soil, water and air. The bacteria have the inherent ability to form biofilms on biotic and abiotic surfaces. All warm blooded animals and human can act as the reservoir. The bacteria reside in the external nares, nasal passage, saliva, skin, perineum, external genitalia, respiratory and intestinal tract of human and animals. Bovine udder is another important site of bacterial residence.

7. *Genome: S. aureus* genome is circular in shape and is 2.8-2.9 Mbp in size with 33 mol% GC content. The genome is composed of core genome, accessory component and foreign genes, assimilated by intra-species gene transfer. The core genome occupies 75% of the genome and is responsible for metabolism and housekeeping. Rest 25% of the genome consists of mobile genetic elements such as transposons and staphylococcal cassette chromosome (SCC). The genome also contains several genomic islands (GI) harbouring the foreign genes, and the genes associated with virulence (toxic shock syndrome toxin and enterotoxin) and antibiotic resistance. *S. aureus* GIs are composed of integrated prophage, *oriC* environ, *ν*Sa (*ν* = island). The *ν*Sa has two classes i.e.

*v*Sa*n* ('*n*' denotes location of the attachment site in the chromosome) and *v*Saα-*v*Saε. The *v*Sa*n* is associated with pathogenicity and resistance genes whereas, *v*Saα-*v*Saε contains genes encoding staphylococcal superantigens, exfoliative toxin, virulence gene regulators (T and U).

The plasmids of *S. aureus* belong to three classes. Class I plasmids are 1-5 kbp and occur in high copy numbers (15-50 per cell). They usually encode a single antibiotic resistance determinant. Class II plasmids are of intermediate size and occur in intermediate copy numbers, and they usually encode β-lactamase only. Class III consists of large conjugative plasmids (40-60 kb). It can carry multiple resistance determinants against trimethoprim, gentamicin and ethidium bromide.

8. Staphylococci can be used for detection of other bacterial antigens like *Brucella, E. coli* and viral antigens like foot and mouth disease (FMD). Staphylococcal cells are sequentially treated with formalin (2% v/v, overnight at 4°C) and heat (80°C for 5 minutes). The cells are coated with monoclonal antibodies against specific bacterial or viral antigen. Equal amount of the staphylococcal cells with antibodies and test bacterial suspension is mixed and observed for agglutination in positive case. The technique is called 'co-agglutination'.

Isolation, growth and colony characteristics

Staphylococci can be isolated in routinely used bacteriological media like nutrient agar, blood agar or specific media like mannitol salt agar (MSA), lipovitellin salt mannitol agar (LSM), Vogel-Johnson agar (VJ), Baird Parker agar, potassium thiocyanate-actidione-sodium azide-egg yolk-pyruvate agar (KRANEP), *Staphylococcus* medium number 110. The bacteria can tolerate 5-10% sodium chloride. The salt tolerance capacity is used in the selective medium to inhibit the growth of other bacteria (MSA, LSM). Potassium tellurite and lithium chloride are also used as selective agents to inhibit the growth of contaminants as found in Vogel-Johnson and Baird Parker agar. Fermentation of mannitol will shift pH of the medium which is detected by phenol red indicator.

If the bacteria are present in low number in the samples, initially they are inoculated into enrichment broths like tryptone soya broth with sodium chloride and pyruvate, Giolitti and Cantoni Broth and liquid Baird-Parker medium. All enrichment broths or media plates are incubated at 37°C. Sometimes reduced oxygen tension with increased CO_2 concentration favours the growth. It has a wide pH range for growth but the optimum is 7.2. Colony characteristics of *S. aureus* in different isolation media are described in Table 1. The typical large, creamy white, beta hemolytic colonies of *S. aureus* is described in Figure 2.

Small colony variants (SCV)

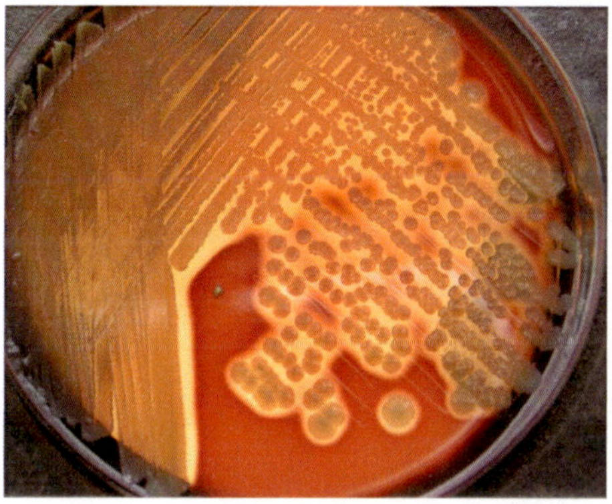

Fig. 2. Large, creamy white, beta hemolytic colonies of *Staphylococcus aureus* (*Courtesy*: Rebecca Buxton, American Society for Microbiology)

Small colony variants of *S. aureus* are a type of slow growing subpopulation producing non-pigmented, tiny colonies on the agar. They may persist within lung, udder for a long time and cause chronic fibrosed lungs in human and persistent mastitis in cattle, respectively. They exhibit reduced rate of metabolism and are less virulent, but due to their slow growth and reduced cell wall synthesis, they are more tolerant of β-lactam antibiotics than their wild-type parents. Induction of SCV acts as a protective mechanism for survival of *S. aureus* during competition with other pathogens.

Table 1: Colony characteristics of *S. aureus* in different media

Media	Colony characteristics
Nutrient agar	Round, smooth, convex, glistening with entire edge. *S. aureus* from cattle, human and other Domestic animals produces golden yellow coloured colonies in nutrient agar. The canine *S. aureus* isolates, *S. intermedius* and *S. hyicus* produce non-pigmented colonies
Blood agar	Haemolytic
Mannitol salt agar	Colonies are surrounded by bright yellow zone. Phenol red indicator produces yellow colour in acidic pH due to fermentation of mannitol
Lipovitellin salt mannitol agar	Colonies are found with opaque zone against yellow background
Vogel-Johnson agar	Black, convex and shiny surrounded by yellow zone
Baird Parker agar	Black, shiny and convex with narrow white entire margin and surrounded by a clear zone
Potassium thiocyanate-actidione-Sodium azide-egg yolk-pyruvate agar (KRANEP)	*S. aureus* produces golden yellow colonies with a precipitation zone of egg yolk after 48 hours of incubation. The medium remains opaque
Oxacillin Resistant Screening Agar Base (ORSAB)	MRSA produce intense blue coloured colonies
CHROM agar	MRSA produce rose to mauve coloured colonies
MRSA ID	Green coloured colonies

Biochemical characteristics

Table 2: *S. aureus* produces following biochemical reactions that can be used for detection of the organism.

Biochemical test	Expected result
Catalase	(+ve)
Oxidase	(-ve) (except *Staphylococcus sciuri*)
Indole	(-ve)
Methyl red	(+ve)
Voges- Proskauer	(+ve)
Urease	(+ve)
H_2S production	(-ve) or slight production
Nitrate reduction	(+ve)
Carbohydrate fermentation:	
Glucose	acid without gas
sucrose	acid without gas
Maltose	acid without gas
Mannitol	acid without gas
Lactose	acid without gas
Glycerol	acid without gas
Gelatin hydrolysis	(+ve)
Methylene blue reduction	(+ve)

Antigenic Characteristics

Serotyping of the Staphylococcal isolates is possible using the capsular antigen. The capsule is polysaccharide in nature. It can be subdivided into 12 types. Most mastitic and human clinical isolates of *S. aureus* produce thin microcapsule of 5 or 8 type.

Toxins and virulence factors produced

Extotoxins

Staphylococci produce several exotoxins which help in establishment of infection. The activity of the toxins is described below.

a) *Alpha-toxin (α-haemolysin)*: This is the best characterized exotoxin produced by animal and human strains of Staphylococci. The strains (20-50%) associated with bovine mastitis produce α-toxin. It is encoded by *hla* gene. It causes lysis of red blood cells collected from several species such as rabbit, sheep and ox at 37°C by formation of pores in the cellular membrane. Through the pores cellular contents come out causing osmotic cytolysis. The toxin causes local tissue damage by disruption of macrophage function. It can act as a dermonecrotic toxin after injection into the skin of the rabbit and lethal to the rabbit if injected intravenously. It also causes lysis of leukocytes (leukocidal).

b) *Beta-toxin (β-haemolysin)*: It is a type of sphingomyelinase (phopholipase C) causing lysis of cellular membrane having higher content of sphingomyelin. It is encoded by *hlb* gene. It is produced by animal strains of staphylococci specially those associated with bovine mastitis (75-100%). The toxin enhances bacterial growth in the udder. It is also known as *hot cold lysin*. It produces a zone of incomplete haemolysis at 37°C in a blood agar plate prepared with red blood cells of cattle, sheep and goat. This haemolysis becomes clear and complete at 4°C. This type of haemolytic activity is referred as *hot cold lysis*. The toxin has no lethal, dermonecrotising and leukocidal activities.

c) *Gamma-toxin (γ-haemolysin)*: It can act on rabbit, sheep and human red blood cells but not on horse RBC. It is a bi-compartmental toxin and the 'protease' part helps in unmasking the second part. The second compartment is associated with cell membrane binding. It is encoded by *hlgA,B,C* gene.

d) *Delta-toxin (δ-haemolysin)*: It produces narrow zone of complete haemolysis with red blood cells of different species. It has a detergent like cell damaging activity. It is encoded by *hld* gene. Serum and skin lipids can neutralize the toxin.

e) *Leukocidin (Panton-Valentine Leukocidin)*: MRSA strains produce leukocidin responsible for lysis of leukocytes (human, cattle, and rabbit) by formation of a pore in cellular membrane. The toxin is associated with severe skin infections. The toxin has two components known as F (fast) and S (slow) based on electrophoretic mobility of the components. This is encoded by *lukF,M* gene. This is the first bacterial leukocidin discovered. It may cause immunomodulation in animals which has a specific role in mastitis.

f) *Toxic shock syndrome toxin (TSST-1)*: The toxin (22 Kda) is also known as superantigen. It can form a trimolecular complex with MHC class II present on the surface of antigen presenting cells and T-cell receptor (V_β domain). The complex can stimulate T-cell proliferation in absence of antigen (mitogenic stimulation) to produce excessive cytokines such as tumour necrosis factor (TNFα) and interleukin (IL-1). It causes capillary leak, epithelial damage, hypotension and cardiovascular shock. The cells to which the toxin binds are also destroyed by cytotoxic T cells. The toxin decreases cellular and humoral immunity to allow the bacteria to propagate. It is encoded by *tst* gene. The toxin is resistant to heat and protease.

g) *Enterotoxin*: It is a heat stable protein and like TSST-1 acts as mitogen to stimulate lymphocytes to produce more IL-1 (superantigen). It is the most potent protein mitogen. It is resistant to pepsin and trypsin. There are nine antigenic types described (A, B, C, D, E, G, H, I, R) and two staphylococcal like proteins (SEL J, SEL P). The toxin is produced by 30% of *S. aureus* strains and *S. intermedius* strains associated with food poisoning in human. When the preformed toxin is ingested along with the food it causes nausea, vomition and diarrhoea in human. The symptoms appear within 1-6 hours of ingestion. Most of the animals are found resistant to this toxin (except kitten and monkeys). The toxins are encoded by *SE (s)* gene.

h) *Exfoliative toxin (epidermolytic toxin):* This is a 30Kda protein and like TSST-1 acts as superantigen. It is produced by few strains of *S. aureus* and *S. hyicus*. It has two types ETA (encoded by chromosomal gene *eta*) and ETB (encoded by plasmid gene *etb*). It causes separation of cells from one another in stratum granulosum (skin layer) and blisters in infants or adults. In infants the condition is known as 'staphylococcal scalded skin syndrome'. In animals, it is associated with 'exudative dermatitis' in pigs.

Virulence factors

In addition to the exotoxins, Staphylococci produce several virulence factors like exoenzymes, cell surface structures, adhesins encoded by more than 50 virulence associated genes known as 'virulons'.

Exoenzymes

i) *Coagulase*: The production of heat stable coagulase enzyme can sub divide staphylococci into two major groups i.e. coagulase positive staphylococci (CPS) and coagulase negative staphylococci (CNS). *S. aureus, S. intermedius, S. schleiferi* subsp. *coagulans* are eaxmples of CPS. Whereas *S. lugdunensis, S. epidermidis, S. hyicus, S. haemolyticus* belong to the CNS group. Coagulase positive staphylococci can produce two major types of coagulase i.e. cell bound coagulase and extracellular free coagulase. The free coagulase can convert fibrinogen into fibrin that forms a layer surrounding the bacterial cells *in vivo* and protects the bacteria from phagocytosis. It can coagulate plasma *in vitro*. However its role in pathogenesis is uncertain as few strains of CNS are also found equally pathogenic like coagulase producers.

ii) *Lipid degrading enzymes*: *S. aureus* can produce lipases, esterases and fatty acid modifying enzymes (FAME). First two enzymes degrade skin lipids and help in bacterial multiplication. Lipid degradation can generate antibacterial fatty acids, modified by FAME. The skin abscess producing strains of *S. aureus* can generate FAME to neutralize the antibacterial effects of the fatty acids.

iii) Catalase: All staphylococci produce catalase enzyme to survive in presence of oxygen. As the oxygen can produce superoxide radicals that generate hydrogen peroxide in a sequential chemical reaction. Catalase can neutralize this hydrogen peroxide which is otherwise toxic to the bacterial cells.

iv) *Protease*: *S. aureus* produces a variety of proteases like hyaluronidase, nuclease, staphylokinase, serine proteases, cysteine proteases, zinc metalloproteinase (aureolysin). They are encoded by *hysA, nuc, sak, htrA, sspBC, aur*, respectively. Hyaluronidase acts as 'spreading factor' and helps in tissue invasion of the bacteria and diffusion of the toxins produced. Hyaluronidase along with nuclease can degrade the pus materials to generate nutrients for the growing bacteria within a lesion.

Table 3: Major virulence factors produced by staphylococci

Virulence factors	Function
Capsule	Antiphagocytic as it prevents opsonization.
Peptidoglycan	PG can stimulate the production of endogenous pyrogen and act as chemoattractant for the leukocytes. So more amount of PG is found in the local infections such as skin abscess and joint infections.
Teichoic acid	Extracellular TA can prevent opsonization by reducing the availability of complement components to the bacteria and helps in bacterial virulence.
Protein A (It is found in 98% surface of *S. aureus* animal and human strains. It is encoded by *spa* gene.)	a) It can bind with Fc portion of IgG1, IgG2 and IgG4 subclasses and mask the Fc portion to prevent opsonization & phagocytosis. b) It can also bind with 'Von Willebrand factor', a protein found in the endothelium. Thus 'protein-A' helps in attachment of the bacteria to cause endovascular diseases. c) It helps in biofilm formation of MRSA strains (*ica* independent pathway)
'SecA' secreation system	Precursor proteins of the bacteria are transported into their destinations through this secreation system which also changes the protein structure to make it active.

'Microbial surface components recognizing adhesive matrix molecules' (MSCRAMMs)

They are cell wall anchored proteins produced by 'Sec A' secreation system. There are total 21 proteins identified till date.

Important ones are discussed below

Virulence factors	Function
a) Fibronectin binding protein (FnbpA and FnbpB). It is encoded by *fnbA,B* gene.	It helps in attachment of bacterial cells to an extra-cellular matrix component, fibronectin. Its binding with fibronectin interacts with the host cell integrin. Integrins initiate a signaling pathway causing rearrangement of the host cell actin filaments and helps in bacterial uptake (Staphylococci can survive within certain kind of cells like fibroblasts, osteoblasts, keratinocytes and endothelial cells). Binding of *S. aureus* FnBPA to human fibronectin is a primary step in pathogenesis of prosthetic device infections.
b) Collagen binding protein (Cna). It is encoded by *cna* gene.	It is necessary for adherence of *S. aureus* to collagenous tissues and cartilages.
c) Clumping factor A and B (ClfA and ClfB), encoded by *clfA,B* gene.	They can mediate clumping and adherence of bacterial cells to fibrinogen in the presence of fibronectin. ClfB is also found to help in adherence with nasal epithelium (it specifically binds cytokeratin-10 ligand).
d) Plasma-sensitive surface protein (Pls)	It participates in binding of the bacteria to both the fibrinogen and fibronectin
e) Polysaccharide intercellular adhesin (PIA / ica)	It helps in 'biofilm' production after attachment of Staphylococci with the surface of biomaterials. 'Biofilm' is a shelter for pathogenic bacteria making them inaccessible to host defence and antibiotics. Biofilms are commonly seen in intramammary devices, milking machine, catheters for urinary bladder etc. Biofilms are made of complex bacterial populations within a polysaccharide matrix, composed of poly-*N*-acetylglucosamine (PNAG). This PNAG production is induced by *ica* locus composed of *icaR* (regulatory) and *icaADBC* (biosynthetic) genes.
f) staphylococcal respiratory response regulator (SrrAB)	The *ica* locus is upregulated during anaerobic condition, suitable for biofilm production. SrrAB helps in PIA induction under anaerobic conditions through binding with a DNA sequence present at the upstream of icaADBC operon.

Virulence factors	Function
Rbf, Spx (global regulator of stress response), *arlRS* two-component system, staphylococcal accessory regulator (sarA), sigB operon	Regulator of biofilm formation
Biofilm-associated protein (Bap)	Formation of biofilm (*ica* independent pathway)
cidA protein	Cell lysis and DNA release which helps in biofilm formation
Accessory gene regulator (agr) quorum sensing system (RNA II, RNA III and AIP)	RNA II helps in Agr-sensing mechanism transcribed by genes *agrA*, *agrC*, *agrD* and *agrB*. RNA III acts as intracellular effector molecule which upregulates transcription of extracellular protein genes and downregulates surface protein Genes. AIP (autoinducer protein) regulates exotoxin production and biofilm dispersal.
Ribosomal protein L2 (RAP)	alternative 'agr' activator during early growth phase
Autolysin (Atl)	It helps in cell wall turnover, cell division, cell separation, lysis of bacteria required during biofilm formation
SERAMs (Secreatable Expanded Repertoire Adhesive Molecules)	After secreation from the bacterial cell they can bind fibrinogen, fibronectin, prothrombin, vitronectin. Then they rebind to *S. aureus* and mediate adhesion by acting as a bridge between bacteria and the host cells.

Pathogenesis

Transmission

S. aureus is mostly transmitted in human and animals by direct contact with contaminated living or non-living objects and indirectly through ingestion. The bacteria are common resident of bovine udder and external nares, nasal passage, skin, perineum, external genitalia, respiratory and intestinal tract of human and animals. Loss of skin barrier, presence of immunocompromising diseases such as diabetes and HIV, defects in neutrophil function are predisposing factors. Most of the animal infection is endogenous in nature.

The contaminated food items including infant milk are considered as potent source of food-borne *S. aureus* in human. In hospitals droplets, stools and skin cells of infected patients, medical instruments, beddings, clothing, furniture, toiletries and the atmosphere can spread MRSA. Occupational exposure to contaminated animals and raw meats was detected as a source of livestock-associated MRSA (LA MRSA).Airborne MRSA transmission through dust particles originated from animal farms was detected among the farm workers.

Pathogenesis (bovine mastitis)

The bovine mastitis caused by *S. aureus* is mostly subclinical in nature. The colonization of *S. aureus* at the tip of the damaged bovine teat initiates the infection. In the intact teat the bacteria exist as distinct micro colonies (biofilm) in skin layers specially in stratum corneum. Formation of biofilm is associated with staphylococcal proteins such as intercellular adhesion (*ica*), biofilm-associated protein (*bap*), accessory gene regulator (*agr*), staphylococcal accessory regulator (*sar*). The biofilm is impermeable to antibiotics or natural defense and hence the bacteria can persist for prolonged period.

The mechanism of penetration via the teat duct is not fully understood. Once the organisms pass the barriers of the teat duct, adhesion to the alveolar epithelial cells takes place. Adhesion of the bacteria is mediated by a group of bacterial surface proteins known as 'microbial surface components recognizing adhesive matrix molecule (MSCRAMM)'. The infection progresses through the teat and udder cisterns to reach the milk ducts. The organisms may be swept away during outflow of the milk from the udder without adhesion.

The spread of staphylococci is mediated by the production of different toxins and enzymes. The beta-haemolysin helps in bacterial multiplication in the udder. The toxins and cell wall components stimulate leukocytes and epithelial cells in the mammary gland to secreate pro-inflammatory cytokines and chemoattractants. The leukocyte activation by cell wall components of Gram-positive bacteria seems to be toll like receptor 2 (TLR2) dependent. The released cytokines like tumor necrosis factor (TNFα) and interleukin (IL1) are central mediators of inflammatory events during intra mammary infection. The chemoattractants trigger the migration of leukocytes, mainly polymorphonuclear neutrophils (PMN) from the blood and it increase their presence from a basal level of 5-25% to approximately 90% of total cells in the milk. It is the reason for increased somatic cell count of mastitic milk. The main functions of PMN are to engulf pathogens and destroy them via oxygen-dependent and oxygen independent mechanisms. At the same time, PMN can potentially harm the mammary gland although the exact mechanism is still not fully understood. Possible way of damage is degranulation and granular enzyme release. Bovine PMN can secreate different enzymes such as elastase and cathepsin G present in the PMN granules. The elastase is found more in milk PMN than blood PMN probably due to increased level of pro inflammatory cytokines. The proteases released by PMN are likely to be involved in udder tissue damage during mastitis.

Disease produced

Bacteria	Host	Disease produced
Staphylococcus aureus	Cattle	a) Bovine mastitis (subclinical or chronic) b) udder impetigo c) pustules at the base of the udder d) wound infections and abscess formation e) skin infection
	Sheep	a) Mastitis (acute and per acute) b) Tick pyemia: A pyemic condition of lambs which are infested with ticks (Ixodes vicinus), specially found in summer and spring seasons. The ticks are not the vector of the bacteria. The wound produced by ticks helps in dissemination of the infection. Abscesses are found at various sites specially in joints. Death may occur due to toxaemia. c)wound infections d) Eczema / dermatitis
	Goat	Mastitis
	Pig	a)Mastitis b)Endometritis c) Udder impetigo due to abrasions by the teeth of piglets during suckling
	Horse	a)Botryomycosis: Chronic granulomatous condition in the spermatic chord that occurs after castration b) Arthritis c) Mastitis
	Dog	a) Pyoderma b) Urinary tract infection
	Poultry	a) Bumblefoot: Suppurative granulomatous lesion in feet b) Arthritis and septicaemia c) Omphalitis (rare)
S. intermedius	Dog, cat	Otitis externa (associated with other pathogens)
S. pseudintermedius	Dog, cat	Primary cause of pyoderma. Pyoderma is characterized by superficial bacterial folliculitis, pruritis, alopecia, erythema and swelling of the skin. It occurs as secondary complication after atopic dermatitis (AD), flea allergy dermatitis, demodicosis and hypothyroidism. Canine AD is characterized by a type I hypersensitivity reaction (IgE mediated) to environmental allergens such as house dust mites, plant pollens and moulds

Bacteria	Host	Disease produced
S. hyicus	Pig	a) Exudative epidermitis ('greasy pig disease'): It occurs in young pigs (less than 7 weeks old). Skin lesions with brownish exudates are found in face and ear. b) polyarthritis
S. epidermidis	Cattle	mastitis
S. haemolyticus	Cattle	mastitis
Staphylococcus schleiferi subsp. *coagulans*	dog	Otitis externa
S. delphini	Dolphin	Skin lesions

Immunity

Humoral immunity plays a major role in clearance of the infection. Although cured animals are not fully resistant to the re-infection.

Diagnosis

Animal clinical samples are mastitic milk, pus and exudate from lesion, skin scrapings, urine and affected tissues. Clinical samples from human include swabs from nose and skin lesions. Cold chain should be maintained during transport without direct contact to the ice or coolants to prevent freezing of the collected samples.

Laboratory Examinations

Somatic cell count (SCC)

Enumeration of somatic cells in milk is the dependable and easy technique for diagnosis of subclinical mastitis. It can also give an indication about the microbiological quality of milk which is important from food safety perspective. The number of somatic cells less than 1,00,000 cells / ml indicates normal milk collected from healthy cattle. The SCC greater than 2,00,000-2,50,000 cells / ml specifies significant infection in udder. The SCC also increases although after calving during colostrum production or end of lactation. The SCC can be measured by California mastitis test (CMT) available commercially as a kit (MAST INDEX).

Direct Examination

A smear can be prepared from clinical samples or tissues and stained by Gram's Method. Staphylococci appear as gram positive cocci arranged in classical grape like bunch (Figure 1). Although the smear from the colony reveals gram positive cocci randomly distributed over the field.

Isolation of Staphylococcus

The media and conditions for isolation of *Staphylococcus* are described earlier.

Serological tests

a) Latex agglutination test

b) An agar diffusion method using micro titer plates is used to detect antibodies to the DNases produced by *S. aureus.*

c) Enzyme-linked immunossorbent assay (ELISA)

Tests for pathogenicity

a) Coagulase test: Detection of coagulase enzyme produced by *S. aureus* either in bound or free form is used as pathogenicity test although now a day coagulase is not considered as exclusive virulence marker of *S. aureus*. The bound coagulase is detected by the slide test and the free coagulase is detected by the tube test.

   i) In slide coagulase test, a loop full staphylococcal culture is placed over a drop of normal saline in a slide. Equal amount of rabbit plasma is added and mixed gently. In positive case clumping will be visible under naked eye. Fibrinogen of the plasma is converted into fibrin by coagulase and clumping is produced.

   ii) In tube coagulase test, 1:5 diluted rabbit plasma is placed into two sugar tubes. Now five drops of overnight grown culture is poured into one tube. Another will act as control. Both the tubes are incubated at 37°C. In positive cases clot will be produced within 1-3 hours or longer. In the control tube no clot will be detected.

b) PCR can be used to detect the genes for major virulence factors

Typing of S. aureus isolates

a) Capsular serotyping of the isolates is performed by the use of direct cell agglutination and immuno-precipitation of cell extracts with antisera specific for 12 capsular types.

b) Phage typing: It is carried out with the help of different bacteriophages capable of lysing *Staphylococcus*.

c) Molecular techniques such as pulsed-field gel electrophoresis (PFGE), multilocus sequence typing (MLST) and DNA sequencing of the X region present in the protein A gene (spa typing) are used for *S. aureus* typing.

The same *S. aureus* isolate can be designated by different nomenclature systems depending on the test used for typing. *S. aureus* isolates are named as CMRSA1, ST followed by a number and 't' followed by a number in PFGE, MLST and spa typing, respectively. PubMLST (https://pubmlst.org/) and SpaServer (https://spaserver.ridom.de/) maintains the MLST and spa-type details of *S. aureus* strains isolated from diverse sources throughout the world.

Molecular Biology

PCR assay is developed with the oligonucleotide primers for the detection of *Staphylococcus* specific 16S ribosomal RNA and the *nuc* gene (*S. aureus*–specific).

Prevention and control

For prevention of bovine mastitis and other clinical infections in animal farms associated with *S. aureus* following measures can be implemented.

a) The farm premises, mangers, stalls, beddings should be cleaned or disinfected in a regular interval because a clean stress-free environment decreases pathogen load

b) The animals should be provided with a balanced diet because appropriate amount of energy and protein are needed to develop a strong immune system. Feeding should be monitored carefully specially during dry period as underfeeding (negative energy balance) will generate different metabolic disorders (e.g. ketosis).

c) Feeding lactic acid bacteria (LAB) in cattle during dry period acts as immunomoduator to boost the immunity. Use of LAB increases IgG in blood and milk and stimulates lymphocyte proliferation. In experimental studies it is observed that IgG can recognize *S. aureus* epitopes and neutralize the bacteria after inoculation of LAB.

d) Internal teat sealants (bismuth subnitrate) are used in dairy cows during dry or periparturient period to prevent the occurrence of mastitis. The meta-analysis showed that use of internal teat sealant can reduce the occurrence of new intramammary infection and clinical mastitis

e) The udder should be examined properly before milking for the presence of cracked and bleeding teats. The bleeding teats should not be used for milking.

f) Teat of the cows should be cleaned and dried with a sterile cloth before milking. The environmental bacteria present in dirt can enter the teats during milking and initiate an infection. Germicidal teat dips available commercially can be used before and after milking. The teats should be dipped for at least 20 seconds. The dips cover the teat surface in a more effective way than sprays. The dip cups should be cleaned between each milking. The dips remaining in the cups after each milking should be discarded to prevent the spread of pathogen between the animals. In few commercial dairies double dip before milking is preferred. Mostly the commercial teat dips consist of iodine, chlorhexidine, sodium hypochlorite etc. The chemical disinfectants may pass through the milk as residue which is considered as a health hazard for the consumers. Currently the herbal ingredients such as turmeric (*Curcuma longai*), Indian Barberry (*Berberis lyceum*), Blue gum-tree (*Eucalyptus globulus*) are focused for development of teat dips with zero health hazard.

g) Vaccine: Bovine mastitis is multi-etiological complex infection which is difficult to control with vaccine. The experimental and commercially available vaccines against *S. aureus* contain either the whole organism (cellular lysates, inactive, attenuated vaccines) or subunits (toxins, surface proteins, polysaccharides).The experimental trials with commercially available vaccine consist of *S. aureus* SP 140 and *E. coli* J5 and recombinant *Staphylococcal* enterotoxin Type C mutant vaccine produce inconsistent results in improving udder health, milk production and prevention of bovine mastitis.

9

Streptococcus

Rivolta (1873) first described the chain forming cocci in pus collected from the equine infection. Rosenbach (1884) established the genus *Streptococcus*'. Nocard and Mollereau (1887) first observed the relationship between the bovine mastitis and *Streptococcus agalactiae*. Lancefield (1933) classified beta-haemolytic streptococci on the basis of group specific-carbohydrate antigens.

Properties of genus

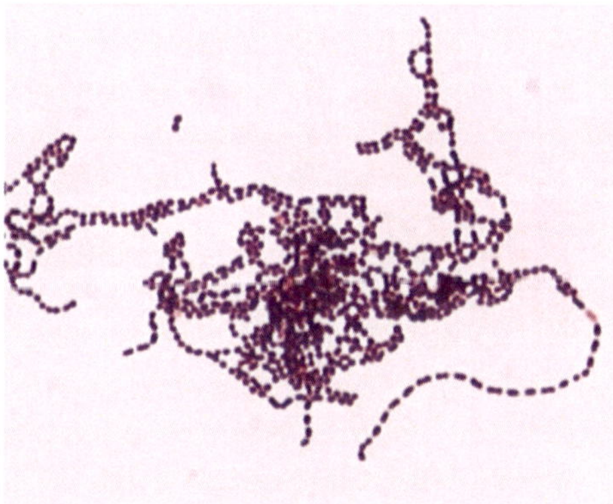

Fig. 1: Gram stained smear of *Streptococcus pyogenes*, 100X
(*Courtesy*: Neal Chamberlain, A. T. Still University of Health Sciences, USA)

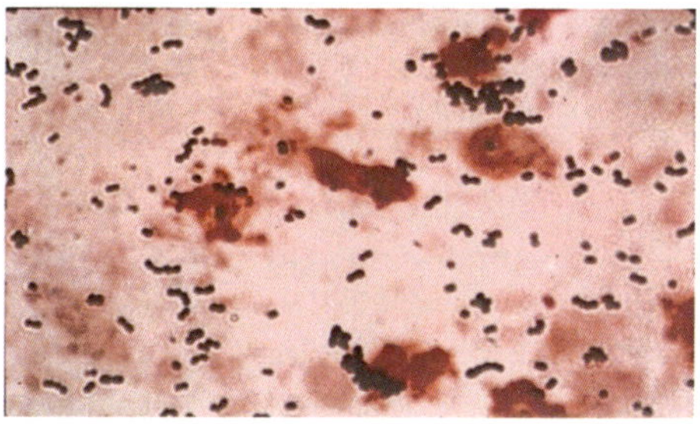

Fig. 2: *Streptococcus agalactiae* in stained smear of sputum
(*Courtesy*: Rebecca Buxton, American Society for Microbiology)

1. *Morphology*: Streptococci are gram positive cocci, capsulated, non-sporing and non-motile. Each coccus cell is 1µm in diameter. They are arranged in a pair or chain of cells as the cell division occurs in one plane (Figure 1& 2). The chain formation and the chain length are variable. *Streptococcus equi* ssp. *equi* is a constant chain producer. Young cultures are gram positive whereas bacteria present in the pus and older cultures in the laboratory are often stained as gram negative.

   Streptococcal capsule is polysaccharide in nature. The capsules of *S. equi, S. pyogenes* are made of non-antigenic hyaluronic acids containing repeating units of glucuronic acid and *N*-acetyl-glucosamine. Synthesis of the polymer is associated with three genes (*hasA*, *hasB*, and *hasC*) present in same operon.

In group A Streptococci, underneath the capsule, the cell wall is present. The cell wall has three layers. Outer most layer contains three major surface proteins i.e. M, T and R. Among them M-protein is antiphagocytic and the major virulence factor. It is encoded by *emm* gene. The M-protein structure consists of A, B, C, and D repeat regions followed by the protein anchor and pepsin cleavage site. The anchor region contains the LPXTGX motif required to anchor gram-positive proteins in the host cell membrane. Middle layer of the cell wall consists of group specific carbohydrate antigen (C-substances). Inner layer of the cell wall contains peptidoglycan. Peptidoglycan can stimulate the production of endogenous pyrogen and act as chemoattractant for leukocytes. Teichoic acids are found in the cell wall of streptococci like other gram positive bacteria.

2. Streptococci are aerobe or facultative anaerobe and require enriched specific media for growth.

3. *Classification*: *Streptococcus* belongs to *Micrococcaceae* family and the genus *Streptococcus* consists of 104 recognized species, both commensal and pathogenic. Major pathogenic species for human and animals are *S. pneumoniae*, *S. pyogenes*, *S. dysagalactiae* ssp. *dysagalactiae*, *S. equi* ssp. *equi, S. equi* ssp. *zooepidermicus*, *S. gordonii*, *S. parasanguinis*, *S. sanguinis*, *S. mutans*. The species such as *S. dysgalactiae* ssp. *dysgalactiae*, *S. iniae, S. agalactiae* and *S. parauberis* are considered as fish pathogens. 16S rRNA based phylogenetic typing identified five clusters namely *S. mitis*, *S. mutans*, *S. salivarius* (viridians streptococci), *S. agalactiae* and *S. pyogenes* (pyogenic group) which correlated with earlier clustering based on ecological niche and pathogenicity.

4. *Resistance:* Streptococci are heat sensitive (56°C for 30 minutes). The bacteria can withstand drying for several weeks specially with pus. Streptococci are lysed by 6.5% salt, 40% bile (except *S. agalactiae*), 0.1% methylene blue and common disinfectants. They are resistant to 0.02% sodium azide which can be added into media to isolate streptococci (azide blood agar).

5. *Natural habitat:* Streptococci are ubiquitously present in the nature specially in the soil, water and air. All warm blooded animals and human can act as reservoir. Bacteria can reside in the mucous membranes of upper respiratory, lower genital and alimentary tract, skin, nose, mouth and throat of human and animals. *S. pneumoniae* is carried by young children (40-60%), older children (12%), adolescents (6-10%) and

adults (3-4%) in their nasopharynx. Colonization is also influenced by overcrowding, winter season, passive smoke, viral respiratory tract infection and maternal pneumococcal carriage. Oral streptococci (20% of total oral bacteria) can colonize and produce biofilm on the surface of teeth.

6. *Genome: S. agalactiae* genome is circular and 2 Mbp in size. It contains approximately 2100 protein coding sequences as well as structural and regulatory RNAs. The genome also contains certain regions that share few properties with pathogenicity islands (PAI). The islands contain genes for surface proteins and putative virulence factors. The islands also contain mobile genetic elements such as prophages, plasmids, and conjugative transposons, suggesting that they have been laterally transferred from other sources.

Isolation, growth and colony characteristics

Streptococci cannot be isolated in ordinary bacteriological media. They are fastidious and auxotrophic for a number of amino acids. Presence of salt (6.5%), bile (40%), bacitracin and high pH (9.6) can inhibit the streptococcal growth. Blood agar with sodium azide, Columbia blood agar, Edwards medium can be used for isolation. Group D Streptococci can be isolated in Bile-aesculin media, eosine methylene blue agar (EMB), citrate-azide-tween-carbonate-agar (CATC), kanamycin-aesculin-azide-agar (KAA). Fish associated strains of *Streptococcus dysgalactiae* ssp. *dysgalactiae* (GCSD) are isolated in Todd-Hewitt agar containing congo red and oxolinic acid. Majority of them do no grow in MacConkey agar. Incubation temperature is 37°C, however thermophilic strains prefer higher temperature like 42°C for growth.

After overnight incubation, translucent, convex 1-2 mm diameter colonies are produced. The varieties of haemolysis observed in blood agar are described below (Figure 3).

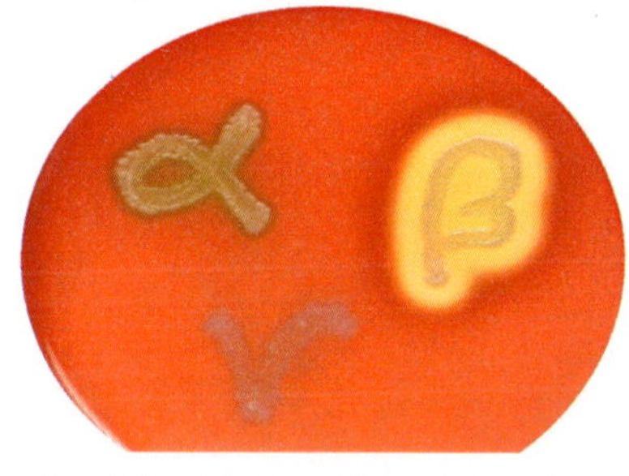

Fig. 3: Alpha (α), Beta (β) and Non-hemolytic Gamma (γ) streptococci (transmitted light) (*Courtesy*: Rebecca Buxton, American Society for Microbiology)

a) Beta haemolysis (β-haemolysis):
A zone of complete haemolysis surrounding the colony is found. It is produced by *S. pyogenes, S. agalactiae, S. equi* ssp. *equi*.

b) Alpha haemolysis (α-haemolysis): A narrow zone of greenish partial haemolysis is observed adjacent to the colony which is surrounded by a clear zone of complete haemolysis. It is produced by 'viridans' group of streptococci (*S. gordonii, S. mitis, S. mutans, S. oralis, S. parasanguis*), *S. equinus, S. uberis* and *S. suis*. Due to greenish colouration of blood agar plates the streptococcal group is known as 'viridans' (in Latin 'vĭrĭdis' means green).

c) *α'-haemolysis (alpha prime):* A hazy zone of partial haemolysis adjacent to the colony which is less well demarcated from the rest of the medium.

d) *Gamma haemolysis (γ-haemolysis):* Non-haemolytic and mostly non-pathogenic strains are described as γ-haemolytic.

In a liquid medium, growth after incubation is characterized by either evenly dispersed turbidity or as sediment with clear supernatant. GCSD is excellent congo red binder and produces orange colonies in Todd-Hewitt agar containing congo red and oxolinic acid. The oxolinic acid is inhibitory for contaminant staphylococci and Gram-negative bacteria.

Biochemical characteristics

Table 1: *S. agalactiae* produces following biochemical reactions that can be used for detection of the organism

Biochemical test	Expected result
Catalase	(-ve)
Oxidase	(-ve)
Indole	(-ve)
Nitrate reduction	(-ve)
CAMP	(+ve)
Carbohydrate fermentation:	
Lactose	(+ve)
Raffinose	(-ve)
Trehalose	(+ve)
Sorbitol	(-ve)
Innulin	(-ve)
Gelatin hydrolysis	(-ve)
Hippurate hydrolysis	(+ve)
Aesculin hydrolysis	(-ve)
Growth in 6.5% sodium chloride	(-ve)
Optochin susceptibility	(-ve)
Bile solubility	(-ve)

CAMP test: The test is named following the initials of the scientists Christie, Atkins, Munch-Peterson (1944) who discovered it. It helps to detect the mastitis causing streptococci (*S. agalactiae* and *S. uberis*).The strain of β-haemolysin producing *Staphylococcus aureus* is streaked across the center of sheep blood agar plate. A suspected group B *Streptococcus* is streaked at the right angle and within 1-1.5 mm of the *Staphylococcus* culture. The plate is incubated at 37°C for 18-24 hours. Positive test shows an arrow head of complete haemolysis. Streptococci produce a diffusible metabolite that completes the haemolysis which is partially lysed by β-haemolysin of *Staphylococcus* at 37°C (Figure 4).

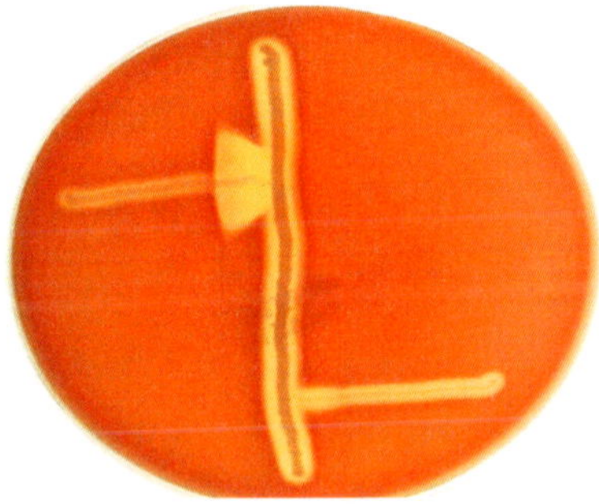

Fig. 4: CAMP test showing the arrow-shaped zone of enhanced hemolysis (positive result) of *Streptococcus agalactiae* and negative result of *Streptococcus pyogenes* when tested against *Staphylococcus aureus*
(*Courtesy*: Anne Hanson, American Society for Microbiology)

Antigenic Characteristics

On the basis of group specific carbohydrate antigen (C-substances) pathogenic streptococci can be sub divided into 21 serogroups. They are designated by letters of the alphabets (A to V, except 'I' and 'J'). This is known as 'Lancefield classification' as per the name of the discoverer, Rebecca Lancefield. The antigen can be extracted by hot hydrochloric acid, formamide or enzymes. The distribution of Lancefield group, streptococcal species and major virulence factors are described in Table 3. Some species such as *S. pneumoniae*, *S. uberis,* and *S. parauberis* are ungroupable.

Differentiation of streptococcal species into serotypes is based on 'type specific' antigen. Group-A streptococci (*S. pyogenes*) has more than 70 serotypes based on M-protein. Variability of the amino terminal region of M-protein is the basis of the typing. Currently *emm*-typing (M-protein encoding) is also used based on the variation of the hyper variable sequences of the *emm* gene. *Streptococcus suis* is classified into 35 serotypes based on capsular antigens. Among them, serotype 2 is most frequently associated with infections in pigs. The serotype 2 is also reported as zoonotic microbe causing human infections in Southeast Asia, Europe, North and South America, Australia and New Zealand.

Variations in capsular structure substantiated with molecular analysis differentiate pneumococci into 97 serotypes. The serotypes 1, 5, 6A/6B, and 14 are the predominant strains causing invasive pneumococcal disease (IPD) throughout the world. The most commonly detected serotypes are serotype 14 (India and Bangladesh), 1 (Nepal) and 19F (Sri Lanka and Pakistan). Introduction of pneumococcal vaccine in children recently changed the distribution of pneumococcal serotypes in the community ('serotype replacement'). For example, recent emergence of 19A replacing 19F is associated with 'capsular switching' (substitution of a particular capsule type gene with another). The newly emerged serotype can escape the vaccine because the vaccine does not contain the emerging serotypes.

Toxins and virulence factors

Toxins

a) Streptolysin-O (SLO): It is an oxygen labile haemolysin at room temperature. It is produced by Lancefield group A, C, and G of streptococci. It can lyse the red blood cells, leukocytes, platelets, and myocardial cells. It is lethal for mice, guinea pig and rabbit.

b) Streptolysin-S (SLS): It is an oxygen stable haemolysin at room temperature. It is produced by β-haemolytic streptococci.

c) Streptokinase: It is a type of fibrinolysin that helps in dissolving the fibrin clot. It is produced by Lancefield group A, C, and G of streptococci.

d) Erythrogenic toxin: It is produced by Group A streptococci, responsible for erythema production in scarlet fever of human. It is used as antigen in 'Dick test' for diagnosis of scarlet fever.

Virulence factors

Table 2: Virulence factors produced by Streptococcus spp.

Bacteria	Virulence Factors	Role of Virulence Factors
S. agalactiae	Capsule (capsular polysaccharide)	Human strains produce it to inhibit complement activation, C3 deposition and thus prevent opsonization and phagocytosis. However, bovine strains do not produce or produce fewer amounts.
	Pili	Pili help in adhesion with host cell surface and biofilm formation. Srt A (sortase transpeptidase) helps in assembly of the pili and Srt C helps in anchoring the pili with bacterial cell wall
	CAMP factor	Ceramide binding protein and lethal for mice. It potentiates the activity of haemolysin and it's cytotoxic to mammary tissues.
	R- protein [R28, member of alpha like protein (ALP) family]	Enhances colonization of the human strains to the epithelium, but its role in udder pathogenesis is not known
	Streptococcal C5a peptidase (scpA and scpB): surface-localized serine protease	a) It inactivates human C5a, a neutrophil chemoattractant produced during complement activation. This streptococcal enzyme contributes to virulence by interfering the neutrophil recruitment and results poor inflammatory response in the infected tissues. b) It can also bind fibronectin and promotes bacterial invasion of epithelial cells
	Neuraminidase Haemolysin Lipoteichoic acid	Exact role in pathogenesis in udder is un-established
S. dysgalactiae ssp. *dysgalactiae*	hyaluronidase	acts as 'spreading factor', enhances the tissue permeability of the bacteria by dissolving the hyaluronic acid
	streptokinase	As discussed above
	Fibronectin binding protein	It helps in attachment of bacterial cells to an extra-cellular matrix component, fibronectin.

Contd.

Bacteria	Virulence Factors	Role of Virulence Factors
S. equi ssp. *equi*	Capsule (non antigenic hyaluronic acid make)	Hyaluronic acid capsule enhances negative charge and hydrophilicity of the bacterial surface. So it can maintain the reducing environment adjacent to the bacteria to protect the oxygen labile toxins and enzymes released by it.
	M-protein (58 KDa): no antigenic variations is found in the M-protein of this Streptococcal species	Antiphagocytic because it can bind fibrinogen and complement control factor 'H'. These interactions mask C3b binding sites on the bacterial surface and inhibit the alternative C3 and classical C5 convertases. Thus it prevents the accumulation of complements on the surface and opsonization.
	Streptokinase	a) It helps in dissemination of the bacteria within the tissue b) It activates complement and produces low molecular weight nitrogenous substrates for bacterial growth
	Streptolysin-O	As discussed above
	IgG binding protein	It binds Fc region of Ig-G. Probably it masks the Fc portion to prevent opsonization & phagocytosis.
	Leukocidin	It can destroy leukocytes
	Bacterial peptidoglycan	a) It activates alternative complement pathway and produces C3a, C5a that acts as chemoattractant for neutrophils. It has major pathological consequences in the disease production. b) It acts as pyrogen by release of cytokines like IL-6, TNF from leukocytes and is responsible for fever in the course of the infection
S. equi ssp. *zooepidemicus*	M-protein, haemolysin, streptokinase	As discussed for S. equi ssp equi
S. equisimilis	M-protein	As discussed above
S. canis	M-protein, Streptolysin-O	As discussed above
S. suis	Capsule	As discussed above
	100 KDa and 136 KDa soluble proteins	Exact mechanism of action is not known, but they are required for full expression of virulence
S. porcinus	Capsule, streptokinase, M -protein	As discussed above
S. pneumoniae	Capsule	As discussed above

Bacteria	Virulence Factors	Role of Virulence Factors
	Pneumolysin	A toxin which is similar to the streptolysin- O, has cell membrane damaging effects and slows the ciliar beat to reduce bacterial clearance
	neuraminidase	It removes N-acetyl neuraminic acid from the oligosaccharides present in the mucosal cells, alters its structure and thus exposes receptors for bacterial attachment.
	Ig-A protease	It can destroy Ig-A antibody present in the secreation
S. uberis	Capsule, hyaluronidase	As discussed above
	65 kDa protein (R-like protein, trypsin resistant)	antiphagocytic
	uberis factor	Analogous to the CAMP factor
	Plasmin binding protein	It binds with plasmin and helps in invasion of the bacteria

Pathogenesis

Transmission

Streptococci are transmitted by ingestion, inhalation, congenital routes and coitus in animals and human. *S. agalactiae* are common in bovine gastrointestinal tract and in the environment of dairy cows. It can be transmitted into cattle mostly through faeco-oral route particularly through contaminated drinking water and sometimes through contaminated milking machines.

S. equi ssp. *equi* transmission takes place through contaminated discharges (nasal secreations) from infected horses via direct or indirect contact. The nasal shedding of *S. equi* ssp. *equi* begins 2-3 days after onset of fever and continues for 2-3 weeks. Recovered horses can shed the bacteria up to 6 weeks through nasal secreations. Few carrier horses can periodically shed the bacteria even after full recovery throughout the life because the bacteria can persist in guttural pouches. Direct contact with infected horses takes place when the horses are kept together with healthy horses. Indirect transmission occurs with the sharing of contaminated housing, beddings, drinking water, feed, utensils, clothing and equipments of attendants and veterinarians.

S. equi ssp. *zooepidemicus* resides on the tonsil, upper respiratory tract, skin and urogenital tract of horses. The infected horses may excreate the bacteria through nasal discharge or during the shedding of the abscess content. It can enter through the oral or nasal cavity of the healthy horses.

Pneumococci are transmitted from person-to-person by direct contact with respiratory secretions, saliva or mucus. Transmission of *S. pyogenes* occurs by inhalation, ingestion of contaminated and untreated foods (salads, milk, and eggs), direct contact with nasal discharges and skin lesions of infected persons, and direct contact with skin, vagina, anus and pharynx of carrier peoples.

Transmission of *S. equi* ssp. *zooepidemicus* to human occurs by inhalation, ingestion or through skin contact. Transmission of *S. suis* and *S. canis* from infected pigs and dogs, respectively to human can take place through direct contact. Fish associated streptococci (*S. iniae*) are transmitted through abraded skin during handling of live or freshly killed fishes.

Pathogenesis

S. agalactiae (bovine mastitis)

After transmission the bacteria can adhere to the gland sinus epithelium. Flushing of the milk during milking can remove the organisms from the epithelial layer. The bacteriostatic long chain fatty acids and keratin, present in the epithelium, prevents the bacterial penetration. Streptococci start to multiply over the epithelial layer. It causes slow progressing inflammation and fibrosis. Rarely the organisms can invade the epithelial barrier and through the lymphatics enter the supramammary lymph nodes. The invasion of epithelium is more common in aged cows. After invasion the organisms are rapidly cleared by neutrophils. The dead neutrophils can secreate lysosomal enzymes which cause tissue damage and inflammation. Fibrin plugs are produced in the smaller milk duct which can cause involution of the secretory tissue and cessation of the milk production. The condition is referred as 'agalactia' from which the bacteria derive its name *S. agalactiae*. The bacteria can persist as biofilm with the evasion of the host immune factors and antibiotics to causes chronic mastitis.

S. equi ssp. *equi (Strangles / Equine distemper)*

S. equi ssp. *equi* adheres with the crypt of the lingual and palatine tonsils and adjacent follicular-associated epithelium of the pharyngeal and tubal tonsils after entry through mouth or nose of the horses. The cell surface proteins (e.g. SzPSe) act as ligand for the bacterial adhesion. Within few hours, it is found below the mucosa initially into the local lymphatics or lymph nodes of pharyngeal and tonsillar region and later in mandibular and retropharyngeal lymph nodes. The nasal discharges collected as clinical samples during early stage of the infection may be found false-negative. The bacterial peptidoglycan activates alternative complement pathway and produces C3a, C5a that acts as chemoattractant for neutrophils. Large numbers of neutrophils come into the site of infection but low level of phagocytosis is observed due to antiphagocytic nature of bacterial capsule, M-protein (SeM), H factor binding Se18.9, Mac protein as well as due to secreation of leukocidin. The bacterial toxins like streptolysin-O and streptokinase may cause tissue damage by injuring cell membranes. With the progression of infection more neutrophils accumulate into the lymph node and causes swelling and abscess formation. The abscess may rupture due to lysis of the abscess capsule and evacuation of the content takes place. Majority of the abscesses are found in the upper respiratory tract and associated lymph nodes. Abscess in retropharyngeal lymph nodes hampers the respiration process. Sometimes metastasis of the abscesses is observed through blood or lymphatic channel into the thorax, abdomen and brain. Death in severe cases is associated with pneumonia, asphyxia due to obstruction of upper respiratory tract and impairment of lung function, and rarely due to infarctive purpura hemorrhagica. The purpura develops as squeal to strangles because of high antibody titers produced against SeM protein.

Disease produced

Table 3: Major pathogenic streptococci, host, Lancefield group and disease produced

Bacteria	Lancefield Group	Host	Disease produced
Streptococcus pyogenes	A	human	Pharyngitis, impetigo, scarlet fever, rheumatic fever, glomerulonephritis, septic sore throat
S. agalactiae	B	Cattle, sheep, goat, camel	Chronic mastitis
		dog	Endocarditis, vaginal and skin infection
		horse	Genital tract infection (rare)
		Human	Neonatal pneumonia
S. dysgalactiae ssp. *dysgalactiae*	C	Cattle	Acute mastitis (synergistic infection with Arcanobacterium pyogenes), abortion
		Sheep, goat	Arthritis, meningitis
		horse	Abortion
		piglets	Arthritis
S. dysgalactiae ssp. *equisimilis*	C, G	Horse	Endometritis, mastitis
S. equi ssp *equi*	C	Horse	a) Strangles (Equine distemper): It is an infection of upper respiratory tract and associated lymph nodes characterized by fever, purulent nasal discharge, swelling of mandibular and pharyngeal lymph nodes b) Mastitis in foals c) Suppurative omphalophlebitis in foals
S. equi ssp. *zooepidemicus*	C	Horse	Opportunistic genital and wound infection (joint ill)
		Cattle, goat	mastitis
		lamb	Pneumonia, septicaemia
		chicken	Septicaemia, endocarditis
		Pig	Septicaemia, arthritis
S. equinus	D	cattle	mastitis
		pigeons	arthritis
S. suis	D, R, S, T	pig	Encephalitis, arthritis, meningitis, abortion, endocarditis
S. porcinus	E, P, U, V	pig	Abscess formation
S. canis	G	dog	Mastitis, lymphadenitis, pyometra, pyoderma, 'Puppy Strangle'

S. pneumoniae	Ungroupable	human	Pneumonia with sepsis in adults; middle ear infections, meningitis and pneumonia in children
		Horse and calves	Lower respiratory tract infection
S. uberis	Ungroupable	cattle	mastitis
S. parauberis	Ungroupable	cattle	mastitis
S. gordonii	Ungroupable	Human	Infective endocarditis
S. sanguinis	Ungroupable	Human	Infective endocarditis
S. parasanguinis	Ungroupable	Human	Infective endocarditis
S. mutans	Ungroupable	Human	Dental caries

Immunity

The protective immunity of colostrum against *S. agalactiae* is mainly Ig-A mediated. The serum antibodies have little or no protective effect. The horses (75%) recovered from *S. equi* ssp. *equi* develop a solid long lasting immunity ('convalescent immunity') to strangles. Mostly it is mediated by mucosal IgG and IgA, locally produced in the nasopharynx together with serum IgG. Mucosal antibodies are produced during early phase of the infection and prevent the adherence of the bacteria with the host cells. In 25 % of recovered horses possibility of second occurrence exists as the mucosal and systemic antibodies fail to maintain the optimum concentration required for protection. The colostrum and milk also contain protective antibodies (IgGb and IgA) that are transferred into suckling foals. The colostrum fed during first 24 hours of life can protect the foals for one week.

Diagnosis

Clinical Samples

The clinical samples include mastitic milk, pus and exudate from lesion, guttural pouch washings (horses), skin scrapings, cerebrospinal fluid, urine and affected tissues. It should be carried into the laboratory in transport medium maintaining the cold chain as streptococci are highly susceptible to drying.

Laboratory Examinations

Direct Examination

A smear can be prepared from centrifuged deposit of collected milk, urine, pus or exudate samples or tissues and stained by Gram's Method. Streptococci appear as gram positive cocci arranged in a pair or chain of spherical cells. The chains are mostly observed either in clinical samples or in the smear prepared from broth culture (Figure 1, Figure 2). All species of streptococci are not always chain producers (except *S. equi* ssp. *equi*). *S. pneumoniae* is generally found as pair of cocci.

Isolation of streptococci

Media, incubation condition and colony characteristics are described earlier.
Immunological tests

Latex agglutination test and ELISA are used for detection of *S. agalactiae* in the whey samples. The numbers of bacteria should be sufficiently high in the samples to be detected by immunological tests. An antigen capture-ELISA for detection of pneumolysin in urine of children is developed.

Molecular Biology

16S rRNA gene specific PCR (Fl-IMOD primers) is developed for detection of *S. agalactiae* in mastitic milk samples. It can detect 100 cfu of the bacteria present in 1 ml of milk. Different nested or semi-nested PCR assays for detection of *S. agalactiae* have also been reported. PCR targeting *ply* (pneumolysin) or *lytA* gene can confirm pneumococcal infection in suspected patients.

Prevention and control

Following measures should be implemented for prevention of strangles in horses.

a) Fresh horses should be quarantined for 3 weeks before introduction to the herd. During the quarantine the guttural pouch washings should be screened for presence of *S. equi* ssp. *equi* by culture or PCR in every week (3 times during quarantine period).

b) Vaccination of adult horses with M-protein based bacterins is debatable because it may produce serum antibodies but is unable to provide protection during natural exposure. The pectoral muscle is preferred for vaccination as inoculation at cervical region produces intense pain at the site of injection. Occurrence of purpura hemorrhagica sometimes takes place as a major side effect of vaccination with bacterins in horses. The use of live-attenuated vaccine prepared from *S. equi* (uncapsulated strain 707-27) as a nasal spray produced promising results against natural exposure even in pregnant mares. However intramuscular injection of the live vaccine produces abscess. The modified live vaccine inoculated into the submucosal tissues of the upper lip produces immunity of shorter duration.

c) Feeding of colostrum from naturally exposed or vaccinated mares provide antibodies (IgGb) to the foals which can protect the foals up to 4 months of age.

Following measures should be implemented after an outbreak of strangles in a stable.

a) Until the outbreak is checked the movement of horses should be stopped to and from the infected stable

b) Infected and their contact horses should be kept separately from the healthy horses

c) Recovered horses should be checked for *S. equi* ssp. *equi* in guttural pouch washings for 3 weeks (once in a week). The consistently negative horses are taken back into the shed of the healthy horses.

d) The attendants should wear protective cloth during handling of the horses. Healthy horses should be handled first before the infected horses.

e) The equipments, beddings and utensils of the infected horses should be destroyed

f) After removal of organic matters the stables should be disinfected with phenols regularly. All the faeces and organic matters should be deposited in an isolated place preferably into a pit.

10

Corynebacterium, *Trueperella* and *Rhodococcus*

Corynebacterium diptheriae was first observed by Klebs in 1883 and was described in details by Loeffler in 1884. So it is also known as 'Klebs-Loeffler bacillus'. In 1888, Nocard isolated a similar type of bacteria from cases of bovine farcy. In 1894, Preisz described it completely and revealed its similarities with the diphtheria bacilli. Later it was named as *Corynebacterium pseudotuberculosis* (Preisz-Nocard bacillus). Bollinger (1890) first reported *C. renale* from the cases of pyelonephritis in cows.

The genus *Trueperella* was proposed by Yassin and others (2011) to describe *T. pyogenes* previously known as *Arcanobacterium pyogenes* or *Actinomyces pyogenes* or *Corynebacterium pyogenes*. The genus *Arcanobacterium* was first described (Collins and others, 1982) to include the bacteria originally isolated as *Corynebacterium haemolyticum* from the wounds of American soldiers. On the basis of 16S rRNA comparisons and menaquinone and phospholipid compositions it is proposed that the species *Arcanobacterium pyogenes* should be reclassified as members of the new genus *Trueperella*.

The genus *Rhodococcus* was first introduced by Zopf (1891) as a soil bacterium used in horticulture. Magnusson (1923) described *C. equi* (*Rhodococcus equi*) from suppurative pneumonia of a foal.

Properties of genus

1. *Morphology*: *Corynebacterium* is a gram positive, pleomorphic bacterium ranging from coccoid to filamentous rod. The size varies from 0.5-0.6 μm × 1.0- 3.0 μm. Some of the species appear as packets of parallel cells (palisade arrangement) or 'V' shaped (Chinese letter arrangement) in the microscopic field (Figure 1). The cell wall peptidoglycan contains *meso*-diaminopimelic acid (*meso*-DAP) like bacterial spores. The arabinose and galactose are major cell wall sugars. Short-chain mycolic acids (corynomycolic acids, 22-36 carbon) are present. This kind of cell wall structure is impermeable to the hydrophilic compounds. However, the 'porin' present in the cell wall sometimes helps in import

of the hydrophilic substances. *Corynebacterium* is acid fast, non-sporulating, non-capsulated and non-motile bacterium (except *C. aquaticum*). The fimbriae / pili are present. Being gram positive, it's an exception of possessing fimbriae / pili which is generally observed in gram negative bacteria. The bacteria often contain volutin granules as phosphate reserve. They are known as 'metachromatic granules' or 'Babes Ernst granules'. The granules can be stained by Neisser's or Albert's stain.

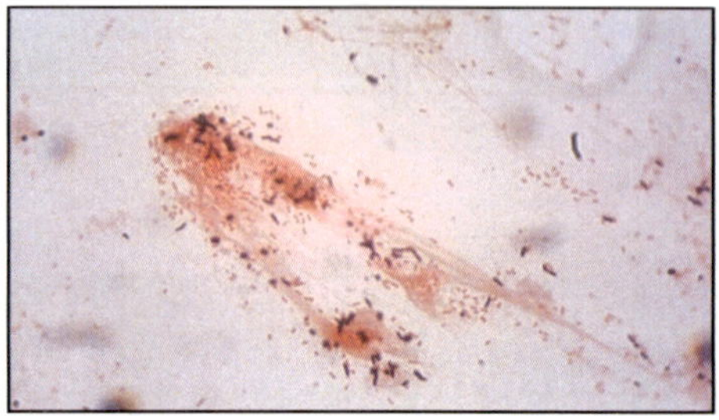

Fig. 1: *Corynebacterium diphtheriae* in skin swab smear (*Courtesy*: Rebecca Buxton, American Society for Microbiology)

Trueperella pyogenes is a Gram positive, non-motile, non-spore forming, short rod shaped bacterium. They are non-capsulated and do not contain metachromatic granules. Initially (during first 18 hour of growth) the bacterial cells may show characteristic 'Chinese letter arrangement'. Later the bacteria become granular and segmented and appear as small irregular cocci. The cell wall is devoid of mycolic acid and arabinogalactan. Cell wall peptidoglycan is composed of N-acetyl muramic acid and lysine. Being gram positive in nature, some strains exceptionally possess fimbriae.

Rhodococcus measures 1 µm × 5 µm. It has a life-cycle with two distinct forms i.e. coccus and rods. The coccal forms are found in pus samples and the solid media in the laboratory (Figure 2). In the liquid media the rods with mild branching are observed. They are encapsulated and weakly acid fast. Cell wall is like other coryneform members. They are non motile and some strains contain pili on their surface.

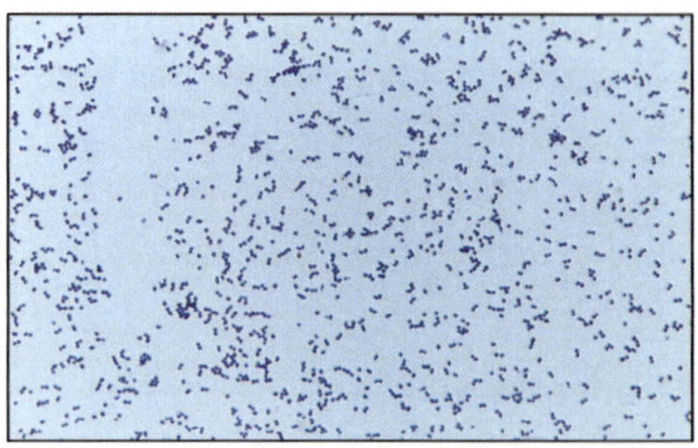

Fig. 2: Gram-stained image of *Rhodococcus equi* 100X (*Courtesy*: Rajesh Kumar Vaid, ICAR-National Research Center on Equines, Hisar, India)

2. *Corynebacterium* and *Trueperella* are facultative anaerobe. *Trueperella* shows fermentative metabolism and proteolytic activity.

3. *Classification: Corynebacterium* belongs to the family Actinomycetes. The family contains several other important genera like *Mycobacterium*, *Nocardia* and *Rhodococcus.* The group of bacteria is known as

'Diptheroidal / coryneform bacteria'/ 'CMNR group' / 'Mycolata'. They have common cell wall structure composed of peptidoglycan, arabinogalactan, mycolic acids and high (G+C) content in their genome.

The genus *Corynebacterium* contains 110 species of veterinary, medical and biotechnological relevance. Important species are *C. pseudotuberculosis, C. diptheriae, C. renale, C. cystitidis, C. pilosum, C. ulcerans,* and *C. bovis.*

The genus *Trueperella* consist *T. pyogenes*, *T. abortisuis*, *T. bernardiae*, *T. bialowiezense* and *T. bonasi.*

The only pathogenic species under the genus *Rhodococcus* is *R. equi* (previously *C. equi*).

4. *Resistance: Corynebacterium*, *Trueperella* and *Rhodococcus* are heat sensitive (60°C for 60 minutes) and common disinfectants (phenol, cresol etc). *Rhodococcus* are highly resistant to the environmental stress conditions like oxidative stress and low pH.
5. *Natural habitat: C. pseudotuberculosis* is commonly found in soil and intestine of healthy animals (sheep). *Trueperella pyogenes* is present as commensal in the skin and mucous membrane of the upper respiratory and urogenital tracts of cattle, sheep, goats and pigs. It is also isolated from the healthy udder and wall of rumen in cattle and stomach of pigs. *T. pyogenes* cannot replicate in the environment because it requires fermentable carbohydrates, inositol, proteins, hemin and temperature (20-40°C) for growth. *R. equi* is common in the soil, animal manure and intestine of mammals and birds. It prefers to grow with volatile organic acids present in the manure.
6. *Genome: Corynebacterium* consists of a single and circular chromosome. The size of the genome varies between 1.8 Mbp (*C. caspium*) and 15.8 Mbp (*C. striatum*). The GC content is 10.7 mol% (*C. striatum*) to 74.7 mol% (*C. sphenisci*). In total 2480 coding sequences (approximate) are present in *Corynebacterium* genome. The genus does not contain plasmids except few strains. Phylognetic studies reveal that most of the pathogenic species (*C. diptheriae, C. pseudotuberculosis, C. ulcerans*) are present in same group ('pathogenic clade'). The genome of pathogenic species contains pathogenicity island (PI) consists of the genes encoding toxins, siderophores, fimbrial proteins and adhesins. The PI of *C. diptheriae* also contains clustered regularly interspaced short palindromic repeats (CRISPR) regions.

Trueperella pyogenes genome contains a single circular chromosome (2.25-2.43 Mbp). The (G+C) mol% of the genome is high (59.4-59.8 mol %). The genome contains tRNA (most abundant), rRNA (3-9 in numbers), non-coding RNAs (1-3 in numbers), virulence associated genes, antibiotic resistance genes, housekeeping genes (*metG, tuf, gyrA,* and *fusA*), DNA gyrase subunit A (*gyrA*), methionine-tRNA ligase (*metG*) and high numbers of pseudogenes (27-191). The regulator genes (*luxS*, T4virus) for biofilm formation are also detected in the genome. Two plasmids (pAP1 and pAP2) are detected in *T. pyogenes.* The plasmid (pAP1) contains initiation of replication factor (*rep*) but does not possess any antibiotic resistance gene. Another plasmid (pAP2) contains *repA*, insertion sequence (IS6100) and antibiotic resistance genes [*erm(X)* and *tetA*].

The pathogenic strains of *R. equi* possess a plasmid (80-85 Kbp) encoding virulence associated proteins [VapA (15-17 KDa) and VapB (20 Kda)] which is absent in non-pathogenic strains. Highly pathogenic strains possess pVapA and intermediately virulent strains have pVapB. The pVapA possessing highly pathogenic *R. equi* strains are common in horses causing suppurative pneumonia ('horse-type'). The intermediately virulent *R. equi* strains with pVapB are frequently found in the lymph nodes of pigs and wild boars ('pig-type'). Recently, a novel linear virulence plasmid (pVapN) is characterized in cattle, goat, and human isolates ('bovine-type'). The non-pathogenic *R. equi* strains found in the soil do not have any type of pVap plasmid but the strains possess *traA* plasmid.

Isolation, growth and colony characteristics

Corynebacterium, *Trueperella* and *Rhodococcus* can be isolated in blood agar and nutrient agar. Nalidixic acid-novobiocin-actidione-potassium tellurite media (NANAT) can be used for isolation of *Rhodococcus equi.* The plates are incubated at 37°C for 24 - 48 hours. *Trueperella pyogenes* requires 5-10% CO_2 for growth. *Rhodococcus* can grow at wide temperature range (10 - 40°C). Optimum incubation temperature is 30°C.

The colonies of *C. pseudotuberculosis* are small, grey, granular and concentrically ringed. Colonies can be pushed across the agar without disintegration. Haemolysis on blood agar is variable, but large haemolytic zones develop in the presence of *Rhodococcus equi. C. pseudotuberculosis* is streaked in the center of the blood agar plate and *R. equi* culture is streaked at the periphery. Maximum haemolysis is observed where the diffusion zones of both the cultures overlaps. It is known as 'synergistic haemolysis'. In liquid medium granular deposits are found. The colonies of *C. diptheriae* are 1-3 mm in diameter, grey, convex and haemolytic. *C. bovis* produces circular granular colonies of 1-2 mm in diameter and cream coloured.

Trueperella pyogenes produces beta-haemolytic, circular, discoid, slightly raised, opaque and non-pigmented with butyrous consistency colonies on blood agar.

Rhodococcus produces irregularly round, smooth, semitransparent, glistening, coalescing, mucoid, teardrop colonies with entire edges after 48 hours of growth (Figure 3). The colonies vary in size from 2 to 4 mm. Sometimes two or more colonies adhere to produce large mucoid colonies (upto70 mm in diameter). The 'salmon pink' pigmentation is observed after prolonged incubation (4-7 days).

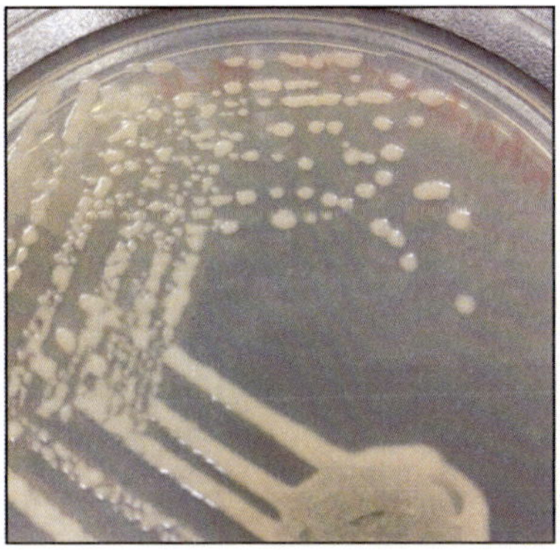

Fig. 3: Colonies of *Rhodococcus equi* in nutrient agar (*Courtesy*: Rajesh Kumar Vaid, ICAR-National Research Center on Equines, Hisar, India)

Biochemical characteristics

Table 1. *C. pseudotuberculosis*, *Trueperella pyogenes* and *R. equi* produce following biochemical reactions that can be used for detection of the organisms

Biochemical test	Expected result		
	C. pseudotuberculosis	*T. pyogenes*	*R. equi*
Catalase	(+ve)	(-ve)	(+ve)
Oxidase	(-ve)		(-ve)
Urease	(+ve)	(-ve)	(+ve)
Aesculin hydrolysis	(-ve)		(-ve)
Nitrate reduction	Variable [strains isolated from sheep, goat are negative]	(-ve)	(+ve)
Carbohydrate fermentation			
Glucose	(+ve)	(+ve)	No carbohydrate fermentation
Maltose	(+ve)	(+ve)	
Sucrose	(-ve)		
Casein digestion	(-ve)	(+ve)	(-ve)

Antigenic Characteristics

The exotoxin phospholipase D (*pld*) is considered as immunodominant antigen of *C. pseudotuberculosis.* The bacteria have two major serovars i.e. 'equi' and 'ovis'. They differ serologically, nitrate reduction pattern and in host specificity. The nitrate reducers are found in cattle and horses ('equi' serovar) and the non-reducers are found in sheep and goats ('ovis' serovar). The molecular tools like restriction enzyme analysis of chromosomal DNA, restriction fragment length polymorphism of 16S rRNA gene, pulsed field gel electrophoresis also supported the existence of two different serovars.

The 'pyolysin' produced by *T. pyogenes* can act as a protective antigen but due to toxicity it has limited value as a vaccine candidate without prior inactivation.

Rhodococcus has 27 serotypes (Prescott capsular serotype 1-27) based on the antigenic variation of the polysaccharide capsule. The serotype 1 is found worldwide and no correlation is found between the virulence and capsular serotypes.

Toxins and virulence factors

Toxins

Phospholipase D and C

It is the major exotoxin produced by *C. pseudotuberculosis.* It hydrolyses the sphingomyelin present in the eukaryotic cell membrane. It increases vascular permeability and it helps in spreading of the bacteria within the tissues. It is dermonecrotic and lethal for laboratory and domestic animals in higher doses. It causes lysis of equine macrophages (*in vitro*).

R. equi produces phospholipase C ('equi factor') as major toxin.

Toxic cell wall lipids

The extracted cell wall lipids of *C. pseudotuberculosis* is dermonecrotic in guinea pigs and cytotoxic for mice peritoneal macrophages. It is also antiphagocytic.

Pyolysin

It is 55 KDa oxygen-stable, heat-sensitive (56°C-100°C) haemolysin and protective antigen produced by *T. pyogenes.* The toxin is also sensitive to protease, trypsin, amylase, and extreme pH (3 and 11). Pyolysin is encoded by *plo* gene present in all wild type strains of the bacteria. It belongs to the toxin family cholesterol-dependent (cholesterol-binding) cytolysin (CDCs) and it has structural similarity (45%) with suilysin (*Streptococcus suis*), novyilysin (*Clostridium novyi*), botulinolysin B (*Clostridium botulinum*), and tetanolysin O (*Clostridium tetani*).The toxin lyses red blood cells (human, sheep, horse, rabbit, and guinea pig), polymorphonuclear neutrophils (PMNs), macrophages, epithelial cells, fibroblasts, and endometrial stromal cells. The toxin is dermonecrotic to guinea pigs and lethal to rabbits and mice if injected through intraperitoneal and intravenous routes, respectively.

The *plo* gene encoding pyolysin is situated in a genetic islet (*plo* islet, 2.7 kbp) in the bacterial chromosome. The islet consists of an open reading frame (orf121, 1605 bp), two promoter sequences (P1 and P2), three direct repeats (DR1-DR3) and a transcriptional terminator region. The islet is a conserved region and is found in both commensal and pathogenic strains of *T. pyogenes*. The expression of the *plo* gene is regulated at the transcription level by the promoters (P1 and P2) and direct repeats present in the islet.

The pyolysin is secreted into the extracellular environment by *T. pyogenes*. The toxin (PLO domain 4) can bind the cholesterol present in the cellular membrane and the binding stimulates oligomerization of the toxin monomers. The oligomers are inserted into the cellular membrane bilayer and helps in formation of a transmembrane pore (less than 50 nm in diameter). The leakage of cytoplasmic molecules takes place through the pore and the lysis of the cell occurs. Although exact role of pyolysin in *T. pyogenes* pathogenesis is still not established.

Virulence Factors

Virulence Factors	Function
Pili / fimbriae [composed of major pilin (SpaA and SpaD), minor pilin (SpaB and SpaE) and tip pilin (SpaC, SpaF) proteins in C. pseudotuberculosis] [composed of FimA, FimB, FimC, FimE, and FimG in T. pyogenes]	Helps in adhesion of bacteria with host cells
Lipoarabinomannan (CdiLAM), lipomanna (LM), invasion associated protein (DIP1281), Cp1002 (PhoP protein) [produced by C. pseudotuberculosis]	Helps in adhesion of C. pseudotuberculosis with host cells
Iron acquisition factors [encoded by Fe acquisition gene (fag) in C. pseudotuberculosis]	C. pseudotuberculosis is intracellular pathogen. It requires iron for the survival. 'Fag' factors help in this iron acquisition
Extracellular matrix-binding proteins [fibrinogen-binding protein, Collagen-binding protein A (CbpA) produced by T. pyogenes]	Adhesion and colonization of T. pyogenes to the host cells
Neuraminidases [Neuraminidase H (NanH) and neuraminidase P (NanP), encoded by nanH and nanP genes]. Frequency of nanP genes is more than nanH in T. pyogenes strains isolated from cattle and pigs	a) Adhesion and colonization of T. pyogenes to the host cells b) It makes IgA more susceptible to proteolytic attack. So evasion of immune system becomes easier for the bacteria
Two-component regulatory system PloS/PloR	PloR up-regulates expression of biofilm in T. pyogenes
Capsule	The capsule of R.equi is antiphagocytic
Virulence associated protein (VapA): It is 15-17 KDa protein and trypsin sensitive. Its expression is temperature regulated. The foal body temperature helps its expression.	R. equi possesses this immunodominant protein in their surface. It prevents phagosome-lysosome fusion within the macrophages and help in intracellular survival of the bacteria
Mycolic acid	R.equi isolates with longer chain length of mycolic acids are more lethal for mice

Pathogenesis

Transmission

Transmission of *C. pseudotuberculosis* in sheep and goats occurs through contamination of superficial wounds during shearing, castration, ear tagging and trauma. Ingestion of contaminated feed can also transmit the infection. In cattle and buffalo mechanical transmission through house flies is also observed.

T. pyogenes infections are endogenous in origin as the bacteria are present as commensal in the skin and mucous membrane of the animals. Mechanical injuries of skin and mucous membrane (e.g. udder or hoof injury), inflammations of organs (e.g. metritis), defective surgical procedures (e.g. castration) can break the skin or mucous membrane barrier and helps in penetration of *T. pyogenes* into the deeper tissues. Rarely skin injury caused by ticks also favours penetration of *T. pyogenes*. The adult male deer are highly susceptible to *T. pyogenes* infection as the bacteria are present as commensal in the forehead of the deer and the males are prone to forehead injury during rubbing on trees or fighting. The possibility of exogenous transmission through contaminated fomites, utensils, equipments, or directly from animal to animal also exists. The biting flies play a major role in transmission of *T. pyogenes* causing summer mastitis in animals.

R. equi is transmitted through ingestion, inhalation and congenital route from mare to its foals. The soil containing contaminated animal manures is major source of the infection.

Pathogenesis

C. pseudotuberculosis (*Caseous Lymphadenitis / CLA*)

The bacteria entering through the skin (wounds) are phagocytosed and the bacteria can multiply within the phagolysosome. Intracellular survival of the bacteria is mediated by phospholipase-D (*pld*) and toxic cell wall lipids. The phospholipase-D can inhibit chemotaxis, degranulation, complement mediated opsonization, and suppression of host immunity through inhibition of lymphocyte activation (suppression of ORAI receptors).The phospholipase-D increases the capillary permeability and helps in dissemination of the infection to the regional lymph nodes and different organs. The dissemination into different organs such as spleen, lungs, and liver is more in sheep than the goats where the infection is mostly restricted to the superficial lymph nodes. It is related to more production of interferon-gamma (IFNγ) in goats than the sheep in response to the *C. pseudotuberculosis* antigens. Abscess is produced in superficial lymph nodes and subcutaneous tissues. The abscess may discharge caseous pus containing large number of the bacteria.

The pathogenesis of *T. pyogenes* in different animals is not fully established.

R. equi (*Chronic suppurative bronchopneumonia*)

The bacteria enter the macrophages through Fc-receptors after getting opsonized with antibodies. The Fc receptors can induce phagosome-lysosome fusion and lysis of the engulfed bacteria. In susceptible foals (4-12 weeks old) the maternal antibodies are limited. So the bacteria can also use non-Fc receptors (complement receptors like CR1, CR3, and CR4) for their entry into the macrophages which helps in their intracellular survival. This kind of receptor mediated entry does not produce phagosome-lysosome fusion and 'oxidative burst' required for bacterial lysis. *R. equi* can produce catalase, superoxide dismutase, alkyl hydroperoxide reductase and thiol peroxidase to survive in presence of reactive oxygen and nitrogen species (RONS) during phagocytosis. The protein-repairing genes encoding mycothiol and mycoredoxins (Mrx) exclusively found in Actinobacteria also helps in intracellular survival. The virulence associated protein (Vap-A) of *R. equi* plays a major role in intracellular survival by reducing cellular lysosomal function and preventing the fusion of lysosome with the phagosome containing *R. equi.* Further it causes non-specific degranulation of lysosomes. It induces neutrophil influx and tissue destruction with advanced lung lesions.

Disease produced

Bacteria	Host	Disease produced
Corynebacterium pseudotuberculosis	Sheep, goat (ovis serovar)	Caseous lymphadenitis (CLA): It is characterized by chronic abscess in peripheral lymph nodes and subcutaneous tissues specially in the legs causing lameness. Nodules are formed. The nodules may rupture discharging thick greenish pus sometimes with blood. The abscesses are also developed internally in organs (lungs, kidneys, liver and spleen) and the condition is known as visceral CLA
	Horse (equi serovar)	Ulcerative lymphangitis ('Pigeon fever'): It is characterized by formation of nodules and ulcers in lower limbs of horses which causes lameness. It is common in summer and monsoon during presence of insects. Draining abscess is produced at ventral abdomen and pectoral region. If not treated it becomes chronic and relapsing. In Western United States, large abscesses looking like pigeon's breast are produced at chest and abdomen of affected horses. It is called 'pigeon fever'. Ulcerative lymphangitis is also reported from cattle, buffalo, camels, alpacas and llamas. In cattle ulcerative skin lesions are observed. Rarely mastitis and abortion are produced
	Human	Diptheria (rare)
C. renale	Cattle, sheep, horse, dog, pig, human	a)'Pizzle rot' / 'Sheath rot'/ 'Enzootic balanoposthitis': Preputial ulcerative dermatitis is observed in castrated sheep and goats. Mild ulcers develop at the preputial orifice. It occurs within 1-2 weeks of diet change (into protein diet). Untreated cases may spread into preputial mucosa with crusting swelling and painful micturition b) Cystitis, pyelonephritis
C. cystitidis	Cattle, sheep, goat	Renal infection
C. pilosum	Cattle	Renal infection
	Human	Cystitis
C. diphtheriae	Human	Diphtheria: Respiratory tract infection which produces a pseudomembrane over tonsils and pharynx. It is characterized by fever, dysphagia, headaches, sore throat, lymphadenitis and death
C. pseudodiphtheriticum	Human	Nosocomial Pneumonia, Bronchitis
C. ulcerans	Human, cattle	Pharyngitis and diptheria (human), mastitis (cattle)
C. bovis	Cattle	Mastitis (rare)

Contd.

Bacteria	Host	Disease produced
C. propinquum	Human	Urethritis
C. ulceribovis	Human	Ulceration
C. urealyticum	Human	Urinary tract infection
C. ureicelerivorans	Human	Septicemia
Trueperella pyogenes	Cattle	Summer mastitis (Holstein udder plague): It is a synergistic infection of T. pyogenes and Streptococcus dysgalactiae, Peptococcus indolicus, Fusobacterium necrophorum and Prevotella melaninogenica. It occurs in lactating and dry cows, heifers and young calves. It can be transmitted through contaminated milk, milking machines and biting flies. The term 'summer mastitis' is a misnomer as it can take place throughout the year specially during dry period in late autumn, winter and spring. Abscess is formed containing pus, which is discharged to the exterior through the fistula. Sometimes the exudate remains stagnant in the ducts. There is sloughing, fibrosis of the udder causing cessation of milk production
	Cattle	Liver abscess, bovine interdigital phlegmon, pneumonia, encephalitis, pyelonephritis, kidney abscesses, lymphadenitis, endocarditis
	Cattle and sheep	Abortion: T. pyogenes acts as primary pathogen. The abortion is generally sporadic but sometimes the whole herd is affected. Abortion may occur at any stage of gestation but is usually in the last trimester. Dams may be ill following abortion, and some die with suppurative endometritis, arthritis, or mastitis. The gross lesions are visible in the placenta, foetal trachea and lungs. The placenta is often retained
	Pigs	Pneumonia, pleuritis, endocarditis, osteoarthritis, polyarthritis, mastitis, reproductive tract infections, septicaemia
	Sheep and Goats	Abscess (primary pathogen), pneumonia, lymphadenitis, arthritis, osteomyelitis, reproductive tract infections, mastitis, septicaemia (associated with other microbes)
	Horses	Metritis, orchitis, mastitis, septicaemia, umbilical infection
	Dogs and Cats	Otitis externa, cystitis, lung abscess, feline pyothorax,
	Turkey	lameness and osteomyelitis
	Human	Endocarditis, endemic leg ulcers, pneumonia, arthritis, sepsis and abscesses in immunocompromised patients

Bacteria	Host	Disease produced
Rhodococcus equi	Foal	Chronic suppurative bronchopneumonia (Pyogranulomatous bronchopneumonia): It occurs in foals aged up to 6 months. Detection of clinical signs is difficult until it is severe. Subacute to chronic suppurative bronchopneumonia, pulmonary abscessation, and suppurative lymphadenitis are observed.
	Pig	Cervical, submandibular and mesenteric lymphadenitis
	Dogs	Skin lesions, tracheitis, vaginitis
	Human	Pyogranulomatous pneumonia in immunocompromised patients (e.g. AIDS patients)

Immunity

Due to facultative intracellular nature of *C. pseudotuberculosis* the protective immune response is Th1dependent. Experimental studies showed that the virulent strains can induce the production of Th1 associated cytokines (IFNγ) in murine splenocytes. Peak production of antibodies (IgG1 and IgG2a) was detected in mice 60 days after experimental inoculation of *C. pseudotuberculosis*. The phospholipase D (pld) is the immunodominant antigen of *C. pseudotuberculosis* and anti-pld antibodies are used as biomarkers in serodiagnosis of the infection in sheep and goats.

Immunity to *R. equi* pneumonia in foals depends on both the humoral and cell mediated immunity. However, the foals born to vaccinated mares are not protected against infection in spite of passive transfer of *R. equi* antibody.

Diagnosis

Clinical Samples: Pus, aspirates from the abscesses for diagnosis of *C. pseudotuberculosis* can be collected as ante-mortem samples. Mastitic milk, aborted foetus and aspirates from the abscesses can be collected aseptically for diagnosis of *T. pyogenes*. The transtracheal aspirates and bronchoalveolar lavage are collected for detection of *R. equi.*

Laboratory Examinations

Direct Examination: The smear is prepared on a clean glass slide from the collected samples and stained with Gram's stain. Characteristic appearances are observed under microscope (Figure 1).

Isolation of Corynebacterium, Trueperella and *Rhodococcus*: Media, incubation condition and colony characteristics are described earlier.

Serological tests: ELISA, Immunodiffusion test, complement fixation test, haemolysis inhibition test can be used for detection of both *Corynebacterium* and *Rhodococcus*. The ELISA can effectively detect the cases of visceral CLA or subclinical carriers where no specific clinical signs are found. The gamma interferon-ELISA appears to be more sensitive than the normal antibody ELISA in detecting prior infection in goats and it is not affected by vaccination in sheep. For detection of *R. equi* by ELISA, sonicated or Tween extracted bacterial antigen provides better result.

Immunological test: A lymphocyte stimulation assay with *R. equi* antigens and peripheral blood lymphocytes can detect the animals with *R. equi* pneumonia. The test is not useful in animals older than 2 months because the response of lymphocytes from healthy foals or adult horses sometimes exceeds that of sick foals.

Strauss reaction: The male guinea pigs (n=5) are inoculated intraperitoneally with the suspected material. A localised peritonitis and orchitis ('Strauss reaction') will be developed in positive cases. Isolation of bacteria from the infected testes is required to confirm the infection as several bacteria such as *C. pseudotuberculosis*, *Burkholderia mallei*, *Actinobacillus* produce positive Strauss reaction.

Molecular biology: A multiplex PCR is developed for detection of *C. pseudotuberculosis* from clinical cases of CLA targeting three genes i.e. 16SrRNA, *pld*, *rpoB*. The detection limit in clinical samples was estimated to be 10^3 c.f.u. and *C. pseudotuberculosis* can be detected directly in pus samples. PCR is developed for the rapid and reliable identification of *T. pyogenes* and *R. equi* based on the amplification of *plo* gene and fragment of the *choE* gene encoding cholesterol oxidase, respectively.

Prevention and control

Following measures can be taken to prevent caseous lymphadenitis in sheep and goats.

a) Quarantine of newly purchased animal before introduction into the herd or flock

b) Culling of infected animals

c) Disinfection of shearing, castration and ear tagging instruments to prevent the transmission of infection between the animals. The lambs should be sheared first and it is followed by shearing of ram and animal with palpable lesions

d) Personal hygiene of the animal handlers should be maintained

e) Housing should be free of sharp objects to prevent the injuroes

f) External parasites should be controlled

g) Vaccine: Formalin inactivated *C. pseudotuberculosis* culture supernatants containing phospholipase D is used as vaccine in many countries but the vaccine failed to give 100% protection against natural infection specially in goats

11

Listeria and *Erysipelothrix*

Murray (1926) and Pirie (1927) first described *Listeria* independently. In India, animal listeriosis in sheep was first reported by Mahajan (1936) in Andhra Pradesh.

Robert Koch first isolated *Erysipelothrix* in 1876 from a mouse he inoculated with putrefying blood. Koch initially named the bacterium "Bacillus of mouse septicemia". Pasteur and Dumas (1882) first isolated *Erysipelothrix* from the infected pigs. Friedrich Löffler (1886) first experimentally produced the infection in pigs. Rosenbach (1909) first described human erysipeloid. The nomenclature of the bacterium is changed several times and *Erysipelothrix rhusiopathiae* was finally accepted by the scientific community in 1966. The name is originated from Greek words such as 'erysipelas' (red skin), 'trix' (hair), 'rhusius' (reddening) and 'pathus' (disease).

Properties of Genus

1. *Morphology*: *Listeria* is gram-positive coccobacilli or small rod shaped intracellular bacterium (Figure 1). It shows typical 'palisade arrangement' under microscope. Rough form of the bacteria may become filamentous in nature. The bacteria are non-acid fast, non-sporing and non-capsulated.

   Erysipelothrix are gram positive, thin, rod shaped, non-motile, non-sporing, non-acid fast bacteria present in pair or in group or in a chain. Rough form is filamentous without branching. Capsule is present. Old cultures appear as gram negative, as it is easily decolourized.

2. *Listeria* are aerobic or microaerophilic in nature. *Erysipelothrix* are aerobic in nature and the growth is improved with 5-10% CO_2 tension.

3. *Listeria* is motile at 22°C (room temperature) with the help of peritrichous flagella. The motility is poor or absent at 37°C (mammalian body temperature). The motility is end to end tumbling type with intermittent period of rest.

4. *Classification*: *Listeria* belongs to Listeriaceae family. The genus *Listeria* has 17 species in total. The important species (8) are *Listeria monocytogenes*, *Listeria ivanovii* (previously known as *Listeria monocytogenes* serotype 5), *Listeria innocua*, *Listeria grayi*, *Listeria murrayi*, *Listeria welshimeri*, *Listeria denitrificans* and *Listeria seeligeri*. Among the eight species, first two are considered as pathogenic for man and animals.

   Erysipelothrix belong to the family Erysipelothrichaceae, order Erysipelotrichales and class Erysipelotrichia. It has eight species i.e. *E. rhusiopathiae*, *E. tonsillarum*, *E. inopinata*, *E. larvae*, *Erysipelothrix* species 1, *Erysipelothrix* species 2, *Erysipelothrix* species 3 and *E. piscisicarius* sp. nov. Among them *E. rhusiopathiae* is widespread among the mammals, birds and fishes.

5. *Resistance: L. monocytogenes* is sensitive to heat (55°C for 40 minutes) and common disinfectants. It can tolerate 0.04% potassium tellurite, 0.025% thallium acetate, 3.75% potassium thiocyanate, 10% sodium chloride and 40% bile.

   Erysipelothrix is resistant to drying, salting, pickling and during production of meat products. It can tolerate antibacterials such as 0.1% sodium azide, 0.05% potassium tellurite and 0.001% crystal violet.

6. *Natural habitat*: *Listeria* are commonly found in soil (soils closer to water bodies and pastures, soils with higher moisture, recently cultivated soils), silage, sewage and stream water. They are also isolated from the human (2-10% asymptomatic carriers) and animals like ruminants, pigs, horses and birds. The bacteria grow better in poor quality silage (pH more than 5.5) and sometimes in apparent good quality silage within the pockets of aerobic deterioration. The area of aerobic deterioration is common at the top few inches of the surface in plastic-covered clamps where the air has circulated under the plastic. Contamination of silages with soil (ash content of greater than 70 mg/kg dry matter) also increases the occurrence of *Listeria* in the silage. So, animal listeriosis is also known as 'silage disease'. *Listeria* is common contaminant bacterium of meat and milk products used for human consumption. It can survive low temperature pasteurization of milk. Most of the human listeriosis is food-borne in nature because many strains of *Listeria* are resistant to high salt or acidity in food and low humidity or low oxygen in food environments. The bacteria are transmitted from ready-to-eat foods (processed meats, soft cheeses, smoked fish, butter, milk, coleslaw) that are kept at refrigeration temperature (-0.5°C to 9.3°C) for prolonged period. The prolonged refrigeration favours the growth of *Listeria*. In

food producing plants, few strains of *Listeria* are persistent in cracks and crevices of surfaces and seals/gaskets due to biofilm formation capacity, increased tolerance to disinfectants and increased adhesion of the strains. Persister cells (dormant and non-dividing state) of *Listeria* are also detected in the environment which can resist the temperature and high pressure. The long-term survival in the environment is associated with transition of morphology from rod to cocci shape by an unknown mechanism. Few persister *Listeria* strains are also associated with clinical outbreaks producing prolonged incubation period.

Erysipelothrix is commonly found in sewage, abattoirs, surface slime of fresh and saltwater fish and soil. It is commonly isolated from the tonsil and lymphoid tissues of the pigs (most common reservoir) and intestine, liver and caeca of sheep, cattle and turkey. It is also detected in arthropods.

7. *Genome*: The size of *Listeria* genome is 2.8-3.2 Mbp. The GC content of the genome is 36-42 mol%. *Listeria* strains can be grouped into four evolutionary lineages (I, II, III and IV) based on genome characteristics. Lineage I is associated with human clinical infections and lineage II is sporadically isolated from humans and animals. Lineage III and IV are mostly identified in animals. The strains of lineage I show high sequence similarities and is descendants of a virulent clone. The plasmids are more common in lineage II strains. Whole genome sequencing (WGS) and subsequent genomic analyses can differentiate the evolutionary lineages.

The first complete genome sequence of *E. rhusiopathiae* strain Fujisawa was published from Japan and the strain was originally isolated from clinically infected pigs. The genome size was 1,787,941 bp and GC mol % was 36.6. The genome consists of 1704 coding sequences of which 1332 sequences encode the functional proteins. The genome contains the genes encoding peptidoglycan biosynthesis enzymes, two-component regulatory systems, virulence factors, capsule and adhesins. However, the genes encoding enzymes required for fatty acid, amino acid and vitamin synthesis are not detected. Further genomic studies confirmed that *E. rhusiopathiae* is generated by extensive homologous recombination.

Isolation, growth and colony characteristics

Initially the clinical samples with contaminating bacteria are incubated at 4°C. The low temperature prevents the growth of other bacteria and help *Listeria* to proliferate only. This method of enrichment for isolation of *Listeria* from clinical samples is known as 'cold enrichment'. The enrichment before isolation of pure culture from food items is done at 37°C for 48 hours as per the food and drug administration (FDA) bacteriological and analytical methods (BAM) and international organization of standard (ISO) 11290 methods. The common enrichment mediums for isolation of *Listeria* are electrical broth, Fraser media and University of Vermont broth (UVMII). The enrichment media contains bacteriostatic agents (nalidixic acid and acriflavine) along with antifungal (cycloheximide). After enrichment, *Listeria* can be isolated in commonly used bacteriological media like blood agar, trypticase soya agar, brain heart infusion agar by incubating at 37°C under aerobic condition. Some strains of the bacteria require increased carbon-di-oxide concentration for growth. The selective media for isolation of *Listeria* are McBride agar, polymyxin-acriflavine-lithium chloride-ceftazidime-aesculin-mannitol (PALCAM) agar, Oxford agar, *Listeria* agar with Ottaviani and Agosti (ALOA), BCM *Listeria* agar, CHROM agar-*Listeria*, potassium tellurite broth, lithium chloride phenylethanol moxalactum medium. *Listeria* are resistant to high salt concentration and can grow at pH 5-9. Required temperature for growth is 4°C-45°C.

In common bacteriological media, *Listeria* produces small translucent colonies within 24-48 hours of incubation. The colonies produce 'bluish green sheen' under artificial light. *Listeria monocytogenes* are haemolytic on blood agar with narrow zone of haemolysis surrounding the colony. It also produces positive CAMP reaction with *Staphylococcus aureus*.

Erysipelothrix can be isolated in commonly used bacteriological media like blood agar with streptomycin and vancomycin at 37°C (15-44°C) under aerobic condition. The selective media are *Erysipelothrix* selective broth, Packer's medium containing crystal violet and sodium azide, modified blood azide agar. Some strains of the bacteria require carbon-di-oxide (5-10% concentration) for growth. Required pH for growth is 7.2-7.6. The bacterial growth is enhanced with 5-10% serum, 0.1% Tween 80 (polyoxyethylene sorbitan) and 0.1-0.5% glucose. However, higher concentration of glucose and oleic acids are inhibitory for growth.

Erysipelothrix from acute and chronic infection produces smooth and rough colonies, respectively. The smooth colonies are convex with an entire edge and the rough colonies are slightly larger with an irregular edge. Initially after 24 hour of growth the smooth colonies are non-haemolytic. The partial haemolysis (α-haemolysis) is found after 48 hour of growth. The rough forms are non-haemolytic throughout the incubation period.

Biochemical characteristics

Table 1: *Listeria monocytogenes* and *Erysipelothrix rhusiopathiae* produce following biochemical reactions that can be used for detection of the organisms

Biochemical test	*Listeria monocytogenes*	*Erysipelothrix rhusiopathiae*
Catalase	(+ve)	(-ve)
Oxidase	(+ve)	(-ve)
Indole	(-ve)	(-ve)
Voges- Proskauer	(-ve)	-
Urease	(-ve)	(-ve)
H_2S production	(-ve)	(+ve)
Nitrate reduction	(-ve)	-
Carbohydrate fermentation		
Glucose	(+ve)	weak (+ve)
Maltose	(+ve)	-
Rhamnose	(+ve)	-
Trehalose	(+ve)	-
Lactose	(+ve) [late fermentation]	weak (+ve)
Sucrose	(+ve) [late fermentation]	-
Sorbitol	(+ve) [late fermentation]	-

Antigenic Characteristics

Listeria has two major types of antigens i.e. somatic (O-antigen) and flagellar (H-antigen). On the basis of antigenic variation *L. monocytogenes* and *L. ivanovii* have 16 and one serotype, respectively. Most of the human infection is caused by *L. monocytogenes* serotypes 4b, 1/2a, 1/2b and 1/2c. The serotypes 4b, 1/2a, 1/2b and 3 are associated with animal infections. The serotype 4b is more resistant to pasteurization because it can reside and replicate within macrophages or monocytes more efficiently. In India, serotype 1 and 4 of *L. monocytogenes* are most prevalent.

Erysipelothrix can be divided into 28 serovars based on somatic antigen (polysaccharide complexes). The serotyping is performed by double agar-gel precipitation test. The serovars are designated by numerical (1, 2, 3 etc. according to the serial of discovery) whereas the subtypes are designated by small alphabets (a, b, c etc.). Non-typeable serovar is called 'N' which is generated following mutation of other serovars. *E. rhusiopathiae* consists of the serovars 1a, 1b, 2, 4, 5, 6, 8, 9, 11, 12, 15, 16, 17, 19, 21, 23 and N whereas, the serovars 3, 7, 10, 14, 20, 22, 24, 25 and 26 are associated with *E. tonsillarum*. Most cases of swine erysipelas are associated with the serovars 1a, 1b and 2. The SpaA of *E. rhusiopathiae* was identified as major protective antigen. The protein is highly conserved in *E. rhusiopathiae* strains and it has three types i.e. SpaA, SpaB, and SpaC. The SpaA and SpaC are associated with farm animals and fishes, respectively. Other protective antigens of *E. rhusiopathiae* are RspA (rhusiopathiae surface protein A), CbpB (choline-binding protein), and GAPDH (glyceraldehyde-3-phosphate dehydrogenase). These proteins are exposed to the bacterial surface which is easily opsonized and phagocytosed by the macrophages.

Toxins and virulence factors

Toxins

Listeriolysin

Listeria produces a cholesterol dependent cytolysin (haemolysin), known as 'listeriolysin-O' (LLO, encoded by *hlyA*). It is reversible oxygen sensitive. It is structurally related to streptolysin-O, pneumolysin and perfringolysin. It can bind with the cholesterol of the cell membrane and produce a transmembrane pore. During infection LLO helps in escape of the bacteria from the phagocytic vesicle. It is an immunodominant protective antigen due to its rapid degradation and efficient procession.

No exotoxin is produced by *Erysipelothrix*.

Virulence Factors

The virulence factors produced by *Listeria* are internalins [internalin A (InlA) and internalin B (InlB)], surface actin assembly-inducing (ActA) protein, phospholipase (plcA and plcB), metalloprotease (mpl), Vip protein, bile exclusion system (BilE) and bile salt hydrolase (functions are described in pathogenesis).

The capsule, adhesins and neuraminidase enzyme act as virulence factors of *Erysipelothrix*. The neuraminidase enzyme can remove N-acetyl neuraminic acid (NANA) from mucin, fibrinogen and erythrocytes which causes reduced protection to the host offered by the molecules. It also adversely affects calcium exchange in heart. It helps in bacterial tissue penetration and increases haemolysis.

Pathogenesis

Transmission

Animal listeriosis is more common in temperate countries than tropical or sub-tropicals. In temperate countries the occurrence is seasonal and is associated with silage feeding. *Listeria* is transmitted through oral route, damaged mucosal surface (buccal mucosa) and dental plates. Oral route is the most common route of entry. Poor nutritional status, changes of weather, flooding, stress associated with overcrowding, transport, pregnancy and parturition act as predisposing factors for animal listeriosis.

Erysipelothrix can be transmitted by oral, cutaneous or respiratory route. Ingestion of contaminated feed and direct contact with contaminated fishes or fish meals are the common routes of transmission.

Pathogenesis

During transmission through oral route *Listeria* invades intestinal epithelial cells (M-cells) with the help of 'internalin' (80 Kda) protein present on the bacterial cell surface. The bacteria enter the host cells by phagocytosis after successful adhesion. Within the cell cytoplasm, *Listeria* escapes vacuole (phagosome) by secreation of listeriolysin-O, phospholipase-C [phosphatidyl choline specific phospholipase (PC-PLC) and phosphatidyl inositol specific phospholipase C (PI-PLC)]. The enzymes are secreated through extracellular vesicles (EVs) of the bacteria to lyse the vacuole (phagosome) membrane. Escaping phagosome is required for intracellular survival of the bacteria. After bacterial multiplication in the cell cytoplasm *Listeria* express surface protein (ActA, 90 KDa). The ActA protein motivates the host cell actin filaments to propagate the bacteria near the periphery of the cell. As at 37°C or normal body temperature the bacteria are non-motile or poorly motile in nature. The bacteria cannot move themselves near the cell periphery. After the bacterial propagation a projection is produced at the cell periphery that invaginates the adjacent non-infected cell along with the bacteria. The bacteria can enter the adjacent cell by lysing the membrane of the projection with the help of the lecithinase enzyme. Again the bacterial multiplication starts and the infection spread into different tissues. Other routes of entry provide the bacteria the direct access to the central nervous system through peripheral nerve ending (specially trigeminal ganglia).

After transmission, initially *Erysipelothrix* are found in the small intestine of the host. The bacteria adhere to the epithelium with the help of heat labile trypsin sensitive bacterial adhesin. *Erysipelothrix* can penetrate the intestinal wall and enter into the bloodstream and reach the site of predilection such as heart, joint, skin etc. Higher permeability of these tissues, passive supply of blood plasma favours the bacterial entry into the sites. The bacteria can multiply and produce endocarditis, arthritis etc. Antiphagocytic activity of virulent strains due to presence of capsule helps in survival and multiplication of bacteria. Deficiency of direct blood supply in the tissues helps in retention of bacterial antigen. Arthritis is produced due to prolonged retention of bacterial antigen into the joint tissues although the bacteria cannot be demonstrated.

Disease produced

Bacteria	Host	Disease produced
Listeria monocytogenes	Ruminants	It causes septicaemia, spinal myelitis, gastroenteritis, uveitis, mastitis in ruminants. The encephalitic form is known as 'Circling Disease' (Silage disease). The affected animal circles in one direction only. Other symptoms include unilateral facial paralysis, difficulty in swallowing, fever, blindness, head pressing against solid objects, death within 2-3 days. In cattle it can also localize in placentomes and multiply to cause abortion after seventh month of pregnancy. It is also responsible for sub-clinical mastitis, septicaemia.
	Human	It causes dermatitis, meningitis and endocarditis. It is transmitted to human by unpasteurized milk, dairy and meat products.
Erysipelothrix rhusiopathiae	Pigs (3-18 months old)	Swine Erysipelas: The term 'erysipelas' is derived from the ancient Greek word 'εrusíp+laς' which means 'rose' or 'red skin'. The disease has three clinical forms such as acute septicaemic form, sub-acute urticarial form, chronic endocarditis and/ polyarthritis. Acute septicaemic form shows acute death, fever, withdrawal from the herd, squealing, stiff stilted gait, depression. In sub-acute urticarial form, red diamond-shaped patches are formed on the skin which may become gangrenous. It is also known as 'diamond skin disease'. In chronic form, arthritis (stiffness, enlargement) as early as three weeks after initial infection, cardiac insufficiency with sudden death, reduced growth, abortions, increased pre- and postpartal vulval discharge, longer furrowing interval, reduction in litter size are observed in breeding sows.
	Sheep	Polyarthritis with post dipping lameness (2-6 months aged lambs), chronic ovine erysipelas (subchondral bone)
	Dogs	Septicaemia and endocarditis
	Turkey, chicken, ducks, geese, pheasants, quails, emu and wild birds	Reduced egg production, conjunctival edema, lack of coordinated movement, severe hemorrhages in breast and leg muscles in young birds, vegetative endocarditis followed by sudden death (turkey), septicaemia with swollen snood (turkey)
	Human	'Seal finger' / 'whale finger'/ 'blubber finger'/ 'fish hand'/ 'fish poisoning'/ 'fish handler's disease'/ 'pork finger': It is an occupational hazard for veterinarians, farmers and fishermen, homemakers having direct contact with animal or fish or their products. Localized allergic reaction ('erysipeloid') is developed. It chiefly occurs in the hand and fingers. It is manifested by local swelling, itching and burning pain. Rarely bacterimia causes infection to heart and joint.

Immunity

The immunity against *Listeria* is chiefly cell mediated due to intracellular nature of the bacteria. This kind of immunity persists for 2-4 weeks. Cell mediated immunity against *Listeria* is T_{H1} mediated that activates the phagocytes to destroy the ingested microbe. Antibodies against the bacteria are not always protective.

The humoral and cell mediated immunity play role in protection from *Erysipelothrix*. Anti-neuraminidase antibodies are experimentally found protective. In vaccinated pigs IgM and IgG can be detected between 7 and 21 days post vaccination. The experimental vaccine against *Erysipelothrix* can induce interferon-γ and TH1 activation in cetaceans (aquatic mammal).

Diagnosis

Clinical specimens: The clinical samples and post-mortem specimens include spinal fluid, blood, brain tissue, spleen, liver, and half of the brain in 10% formalin. In suspected 'erysipeloid' lesions the bacteria reside at the bottom of the tissue. The entire edge of the lesion should be collected aseptically.

Laboratory Examination

Direct Examination: A smear can be prepared from tissues of suspected animals to stain by Gram's Method (Figure 1). In encephalitic form of anima listeriosis very few numbers of bacteria can be observed. The negative finding is inconclusive. The clinical samples from acute *Erysipelothrix* infection reveals gram positive rods, whereas, the samples collected from chronic infections demonstrates the filamentous form of the bacteria.

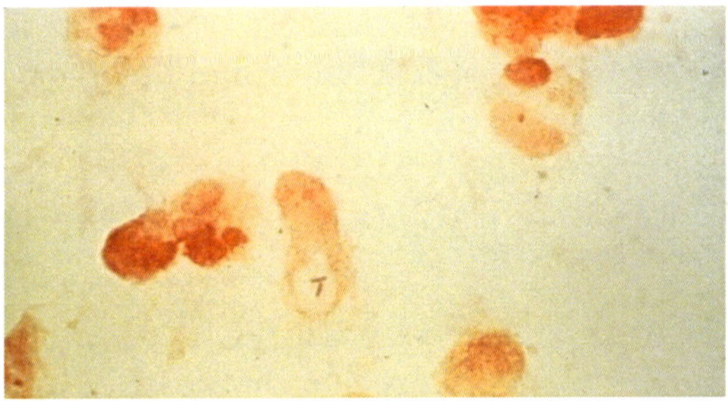

Fig. 1: *Listeria monocytogenes* within neutrophil in cerebrospinal fluid of meningitis patient (*Courtesy*: Rebecca Buxton, American Society for Microbiology)

Isolation of bacteria from clinical samples: Media and incubation condition are described earlier.

Serological tests: The serological tests for detection of *Listeria* are not so much useful as the bacteria are ubiquitous in nature and the positive titer may be present in clinically normal animals. As well as the cross reaction may occur with *Staphylococcus aureus, Arcanobactrium pyogenes, Enterococcus* sp. The seroprevalence rate cannot be correlated with the true infection without any clinical sign. However, slide agglutination test using heat killed cell suspension may be used for detection of anti-*Listeria* (somatic antigen) antibody. As well as, complement fixation test (CFT), ELISA can be used. Immunohistochemical detection of *L. monocytogenes* in formalin-fixed tissue is more sensitive than other serological tests.

Animal inoculation technique (Anton's eye test): Suspected clinical sample for animal listeriosis is instilled into the conjunctival sac of the experimental rabbits. In positive case, purulent conjunctivitis is produced within 24-48 hours followed by keratitis.

For diagnosis of *E. rhusiopathiae*, a group of mice is subcutaneously inoculated with 24 hour grown suspected broth culture and equine hyper immune serum against *E. rhusiopathiae*. Another group of mice is inoculated with same culture without serum. In positive case the second group of mice will die within 5-6 days, while the first group will remain alive due to lack of protection offered by the serum in second group.

Molecular biology: Polymerase chain reaction (PCR) can be performed to detect *Listeria* using listeriolysin gene (*hlyA*), invasion associated P60 protein (*iap*) as target. Subtyping of *Listeria* isolates is useful for outbreak investigation in man and animal. *Listeria monocytogenes* can be subtyped by different molecular methods including multilocus enzyme electrophoresis (MEE), DNA restriction enzyme analysis, pulse-field gel electrophoresis (PFGE), nucleic acid sequencing-based typing, microarray analysis, amplified intergenic locus polymorphism (AILP) and random amplification of polymorphic DNA (RAPD).

Polymerase chain reaction (PCR) can be performed to detect *Erysipelothrix* using primers on a region of 16S rRNA gene as target. PCR specific for *E. rhusiopathiae* using the primer for detection of their virulence factor has also developed. Both of these PCRs can rapidly confirm swine erysipelas from all kinds of clinical samples.

Prevention and Control

For prevention and control of *Listeria* and *Erysipelothrix* following measures may be adapted in animal farms.

a) Change of silage based diet should be introduced slowly

b) The silage should be monitored regularly to avoid the feeding of spoiled areas of silage and soil contaminated silage

c) The silage removed from the pit should be fed immediately to the animals

d) Live attenuated and killed vaccines against listeriosis in sheep are used in few countries which reduced the incidence rate.

e) The breeding herds of the major pork producing countries are regularly vaccinated against swine erysipelas. Generally pigs in grower stage are avoided for vaccination due to presence of maternal antibodies. Three types of swine erysipelas vaccines are commercially available i.e. attenuated (serotype 1a), killed/bacterin (serotype 2) and subunit vaccine (SpaA protein of serotype 1a /2). Breeding turkey flocks are vaccinated four weeks before onset of egg production with attenuated vaccine (serotype 1a) or bacterin (serotype 2).The ewes before lambing are vaccinated with bacterin (serotype 2) to prevent arthritis in lambs through maternal antibodies.

Differences of *Listeria* and *Erysipelothrix*

Characteristics	*Listeria*	*Erysipelothrix*
Motility	Motile at 4°C	Non-motile
Catalase production	+	–
Growth at 4°C	+	–
Methyl Red test	+	–
Voges Proskauer test	+	–
Type of haemolysis	Beta haemolytic	Alpha haemolytic
Growth on nutrient agar with 8.5% NaCl	+	–
Hydrolysis of tween 20, 80; aesculin and hippurate	+	–
H_2S production	+	–
Susceptible laboratory animals/ birds	Guinea pigs	Pigeons
Antibiotic susceptibility	sensitive to neomycin	resistant to neomycin

12

Bacillus

In 1850, *Bacillus anthracis* was first reported by three individuals in two different countries i.e. Delafond and Davaine in France, and Pollender in Germany. They could not establish the relationship of the bacterium with the infection. Absolute proof of the anthrax etiology as *B. anthracis* was established by Robert Koch during 1876-77. The name *Bacillus anthracis* was first coined by Cohn (1875) and the disease 'anthrax' was first named by Hippocrates (5th century B.C.). In Greek language meaning of 'anthrax' is 'coal' referring to the black coloured skin or blood in affected animals.

B. anthracis has following historical importance.

a) Anthrax is the first disease identified to be caused by a bacterium.

b) Robert Koch first isolated the bacteria and reproduced the disease in experimental animals. He proposed his postulates (Koch's postulates, 1876) based on his experiments related to this bacteria. The postulates later became a fundamental milestone of all microbiological works related to the infectious diseases.

c) Louis Pasteur first used heat attenuated culture of *B. anthracis* as vaccine in a group of sheep in 1881 at Pouilly-le-Fort (France). He cultured the bacteria at 42-43°C in presence of oxygen. The bacteria did not produce spores and became attenuated.

d) First concept of bacterial antagonism was provided by Louis Pasteur and Joubert based on their work on *B. anthracis*. Injection of unidentified bacteria along with *B. anthracis* can prevent anthrax in animals.

e) Metchnikoff (1905) worked on *B. anthracis* to determine the role of macrophages in cellular immunity

Properties of genus

Morphology: *Bacillus anthracis* is a gram positive, sporulating, non-motile, capsulated organism. They are typical rectangular shaped rods with square cut ends ('box-car shape', Figure 1). They measure about 1 μm × 3-5 μm. Within the tissues, they may produce long chain like arrangement.

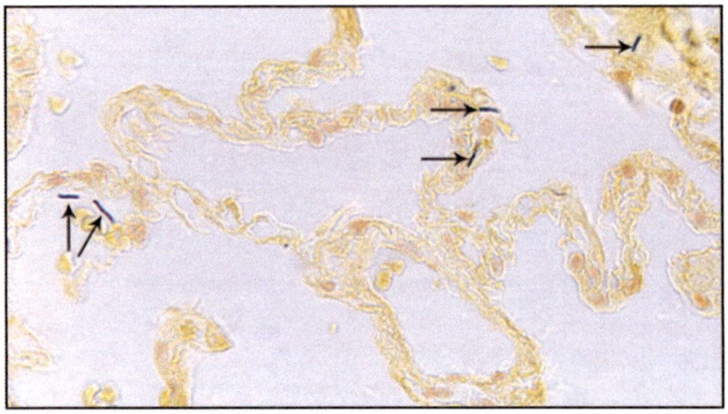

Fig. 1: *Bacillus anthracis* in infected human lungs (*Courtesy*: Public Health Image Library, American Society for Microbiology)

Bacterial endospore

No spores are produced within the host tissues. The spores are produced in the environment in presence of oxygen and low CO_2 tension. So, the sporulation is observed during opening of the anthrax infected carcass by scavengers or human. The spores are oval, 0.75×1 µm in size. The spores do not bulge the parent cells. The spores have no measurable metabolism, little or no water, no ATP, no macromolecular synthesis machinery and no active enzyme system. The spores are highly resistant to heat, cold, drying and disinfectants. It can survive in the environment for decades and in favourable conditions, it can regenerate into the vegetative bacteria.

Cell cover

The cell cover of *B. anthracis* consists of four layers from outside to inside i.e. a) capsule b) S-layer c) peptidoglycan and d) cytoplasmic membrane. Presence of both capsule and S-layer in same bacteria is an exceptional example.

a) *Capsule*: The capsules are produced within the host (under increased CO_2 tension) to protect the bacteria from phagocytosis. The capsule is protein in nature, not carbohydrate, exception of bacterial capsule structure. It is a polymer of D-glutamic acids and peptide bonds are formed between γ-carboxyl and α-amino groups. The capsule synthesis is regulated by plasmid encoded (pxO2) gene locus [*cap* or *pgs* (poly glutamate synthesis)] containing *capA, capB, capC, capD* and *capE* genes. Among these five gene products capD protein also helps in anchoring the capsule with underlying layer. The capsule is antiphagocytic and prevents the bacterial opsonization.

b) *S- layer* (*surface layer*): It is also a protein layer covering the cell and situated just beneath the capsule. It is composed of two major proteins: Sap (S-layer associated protein) and EA1 (extractable antigen), encoded by chromosomal genes, *sap* and *eag*, respectively. The Sap protein forms a network near the surface whereas EA1 forms patches in different directions. The S-layer also helps to prevent the phagocytosis.

c) *Peptidoglycan*: Like other gram positive bacteria, it is also 20-50 nm thick layer composed of glucosamine and muramic acid (β, 1-4 glycosidic linkage) along with cross linked amino acids. The cross linkage is found between meso-DAP (di amino pimelic acid) and D- alanine at 4th position. Unlike other gram positive bacteria, N-acetylation of glucosamine and muramic acids are not detected, responsible for lysozyme resistance of the bacteria. The neutral polysaccharide is immunogenic and helps in identification of the bacteria in Ascolis test. The teichoic acid is absent. Different proteins are covalently or non-covalently attached with the neutral polysaccharide of peptidoglycan.

d) *Cytoplasmic membrane:* The cytoplasmic membrane is composed of phospholipids and membrane proteins. The phospholipids provide resistance to cationic antimicrobial peptides (a component of host innate immunity). There are 25 membrane-associated proteins with 1-10 transmembrane fragments and 13 lipoproteins. At transcription level, the toxin and capsule synthesis is stimulated by presence of bicarbonate-CO_2. There is a bicarbonate transporter system (ABC transporter) present in the cytoplasmic membrane which helps in transport of bicarbonate within the cell. This system is composed of transmembrane proteins (e.g. permease). Without this system the bacteria cannot synthesize toxins and capsule and may become non-pathogenic.

2. *Bacillus* are facultative anaerobic in nature

3. *Classification*: The genus *Bacillus* belongs to Bacillaceae sensu stricto family. The members of *Bacillus* genus include *B. anthracis*, *B. cereus*, *B. thuringiensis*, *B. mycoides*, *B. pseudomycoides*, *B. weihenstephanensis*. *B. anthracis* is considered as the most potent animal and human pathogen. The different species of *Bacillus* genus other than *B. anthracis* is known as 'anthracoid' organisms. The anthracoids and *B. anthracis* can be differentiated (Table 1). *B. anthracis* is one of the most monomorphic species. Serological, biochemical, phage typing and recent molecular tools failed to identify the strain variation of the organism.

4. *Resistance*: The vegetative bacteria are killed by exposure to heat (60°C for 30 minutes). The bacterial spores are destroyed by moist heat like autoclaving (120°C for 15 minutes) and dry heat (150°C for 60 minutes). The heat fixation of smear during preparation of slide for staining cannot kill the spores. Aldehydes, beta-prpiolactone, ethylene oxide, chlorinating disinfectants are useful against the spores.

5. *Natural habitat*: The alkaline and calcium rich soil, flooded periodically, is the major reservoir of *B. anthracis* spores for decades. The spores may have positive buoyancy and float on the surface during the flooding of the soil. Other species of *Bacillus* are saprophyte and mainly found in air, soil and water.

6. *Genome*: *B. anthracis* genome contains single circular chromosome and two circular virulence plasmids (pXO1 and pXO2). The genomic DNA has a higher buoyant density and lower melting temperature due to presence of adenine and thymine in greater amount. The best characterized bacterial genome is possessed by 'Ames ancestor strain' of *B. anthracis*. The Ames genome is 5,503,926 nucleotides in size with 5,775 protein coding genes. In total, 33 ribosomal RNA genes (23S, 16S and 5S) and 95 tRNA genes are found on the chromosome.

Two types of plasmids are found in *B. anthracis*, pXO1 and pXO2, encoding genes for toxin and capsule, respectively. The strains of *B. anthracis* can be classified on the basis of plasmid possession. 'Sterne' type strains (first described by M. Sterne in 1939, examples are – Sterne, 34F2, STI, Weybridge) possess only pXO1 plasmid and uncapsulated in nature. Whereas 'Pasteur' type strains (6602 and 4229) possess pxO2 only. Sterne strains are used in preparation of live vaccine against *B. anthracis*. However another vaccine strain is known as 'Carbosap' (Italy) in which both plasmids are present. The toxin plasmid (pXO1) contains a 44.8 kb 'pathogenicity island', known as Tn*XO1*. It carries the genes for a transposase, a site-specific recombinase in addition to a germination operon (*gerX*) that is associated with spore germination within the macrophages. The pathogenicity island also includes the toxin units such as *pagA* (protective antigen), *lef* (lethal factor), and *cya* (calmodulin-sensitive adenylate cyclase, edema factor), and *atxA*, a major virulence gene regulator.

Isolation, growth and colony characteristics

B. anthracis can be isolated in routinely used bacteriological media like nutrient agar, 5% sheep blood agar, serum agar, and polymyxin-lysozyme-EDTA-thallous acetate agar (PLET). The carbohydrates and amino acids are used as carbon and nitrogen sources, respectively. Methionine and thiamine are also required for bacterial growth. PLET agar is used for isolation of *B. anthracis* from contaminated samples. The plates are incubated at 37°C for overnight in blood agar and 48 hours in PLET agar.

In solid media, small, grey coloured, non-haemolytic, 0.3-0.5 mm diameter colonies are produced. Prolonged incubation may produce α-haemolysis. Older colonies have rough irregular edges producing 'ground glass' or 'frosted glass' appearance. Microscopically, at the edge of the colony there are numerous chains of bacteria, protruding from the center producing classical 'Medusa head' or 'spiked' or 'judge's wig' appearance. If the bacteria are grown under *in vitro* capsule producing conditions (serum agar incubation with 0.7% sodium-bicarbonate and 20% CO_2), the mucoid colonies are produced.

In contrast, *B. cereus* produces β-haemolytic dry colonies with hairy edges. *B. licheniformis* produces opaque colonies with rough surfaces.

'String of pearls' reaction: The young culture of *B. anthracis* is streaked on tryptose agar containing 0.5 unit of penicillin per ml of the medium and incubated at 37°C for 3 to 6 hours. A cover slip was placed over the streaked area and examined under the oil immersion or high dry objective for the presence of enlarged, round, cellular forms characteristic of the positive reaction. As the round cells are present in chain it is known as 'string of pearls' (Figure 2).

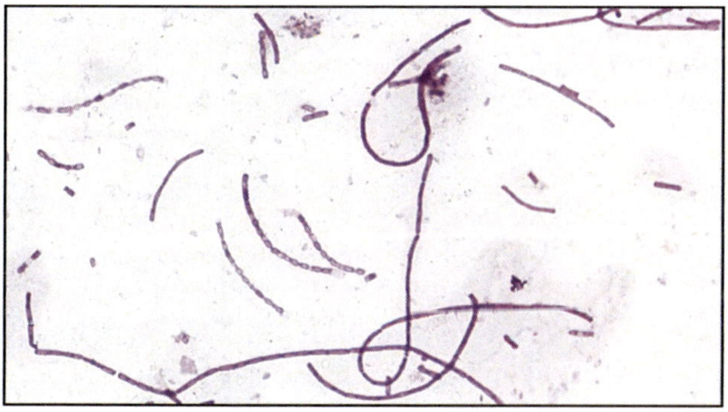

Fig. 2: *Bacillus anthracis* string of pearls
(*Courtesy*: Neal Chamberlain, American Society for Microbiology)

Biochemical characteristics

B. anthracis produces following biochemical reactions that can be used for detection of the organism.

Biochemical test	Expected result
Catalase	(+ve)
Oxidase	(+ve)
Indole	(-ve)
Methyl red	(+ve)
Voges- Proskauer	(+ve)
Citrate Utilization	(-ve)
Urease	(-ve)
H_2S production	(-ve)
Nitrate reduction	(+ve)
Casein hydrolysis	(+ve)

Biochemical test	Expected result
Starch hydrolysis	(+ve)
Carbohydrate fermentation:	
Glucose	acid without gas
sucrose	acid without gas
Maltose	acid without gas
Levulose	acid without gas
Trehalose	acid without gas
dextrin	acid without gas
Gelatin liquefaction	slow ('Inverted fir tree appearance' in gelatin stab culture)

Antigenic Characteristics

Three kinds of antigens are detected in *B. anthracis*. The antigens are capsular polypeptide, somatic protein and somatic polysaccharide (neutral polysaccharide). *B. anthracis* is antigenically correlated (except capsular antigen) with *B. cereus* and *B. thuringiensis* which creates hindrance in serodiagnosis.

Toxins and virulence factors produced

Toxins

This plasmid (pXO1) encodes a tripartite (3 subunits) A-B toxin that is an essential virulence factor for the development of anthrax. The toxin comprises two alternative A-subunits, edema factor (EF/Factor-I, 89 KDa), lethal factor (LF/ Factor III, 82 KDa) and a single B-subunit, designated as protective antigen (PA/Factor II, 83 KDa). EF is a calcium and calmodulin-dependent adenylate cyclase. LF is a proteinase that inactivates cellular signaling pathways through proteolysis of mitogen activated protein kinase (MAP kinase). The PA combines with LF to form lethal toxin (LeTx), and with EF to form edema toxin (EdTx). The lethal toxin causes death, if experimentally injected into laboratory animals. Fischer 344 rat is the most sensitive to the lethal toxin. The edema toxin is responsible for edema formation at the site of infection. Neither LF nor EF is active without PA.

Mechanism of action of anthrax toxin

The anthrax toxin acts in a sequential way. The PA binds with the host cellular receptors. Two kinds of receptors are identified i.e. ANTXR1 [also known as tumor endothelial marker-8 (TEM8)], and ANTXR2 [capillary morphogenesis protein 2 (CMG2)]. After binding with the receptors, PA is cleaved by the cellular protease or the cell surface furin (a protease which helps in converting the inactive protein into active one) to generate activated PA (63 KDa). The activated PA (PA_{63}) forms a heptamer ('prepore') and can bind with EF/LF in the cell surface. The complex enters the cell by endocytosis through the clathrin coated vesicles. The membrane proteins like LRP6 (lipoprotein-receptor-related protein) also become a part of the toxin receptor complex and helps in endocytosis. The clathrin coated vesicles shed off their coats and fuse with early endosome and toxin-receptor (PA+LF/EF + receptor) complex. The acidic pH of the endosome helps in insertion of PA heptamer into the membrane of intraluminal vesicles. Partial unfolding of LF/EF also occurs due to acidic pH. The unfolded EF/LF enters the lumen of the intraluminal vesicles through PA channels. Thus it is protected from direct contact with lysosomal proteases and it becomes safe from degradation. In this endocytic pathway late endosomes are developed, in which these intraluminal vesicles can undergo back fusion with the limiting membrane and release the EF/LF into the cell cytoplasm.

The EF produces intracellular cyclic adenosine mono phosphate (cAMP) in the presence of calcium or calmodulin (eukaryotic calcium binding protein). Accumulation of cAMP induces interleukin (IL-6) production and suppression of tumor necrosis factor (TNF-α) production by monocytes. Phagocytosis and respiratory burst is also inhibited resulting increased susceptibility to different infections.

The macrophages are only found susceptible to the LF. The LF induces the synthesis of reactive oxygen intermediates (ROI) or superoxide anions. It up regulates the cytokine production like IL-1 that is accumulated within macrophages. Increased concentration of the LF and ROI lyses the macrophages and sudden release of stored IL-1 causes shock and death of the infected host. So the toxin unit is called 'lethal factor'.

Minor toxins

a) *B. anthracis* can produce a thiol-activated cytolysin known as 'anthrolysin-O'. It can lyse the host cells.

b) Several chromosomally encoded proteins have been detected which may contribute to pathogenicity, including haemolysins, phospholipases and siderophores.

Pathogenesis (*B. anthracis*)

Transmission

a) The infected animals excreate bacterial endospores through the faeces, blood and other body fluids into the environment. Industrial effluents specially from tanneries are important source of infection in the environment. The spores remain viable in the pastures for decades. Ingestion of spores from contaminated pastures with thorny vegetations is a way of transmission. As *B. anthracis* is non-invasive in nature a break in the mucous membrane made with thorny vegetation is required.

b) Inhalation of spores causing pulmonary form of the disease.

c) Biting flies like *Tabanus* or *Stomoxys* are responsible for outbreaks in livestock in India, Africa and USA. Non-biting *Chrysoma* (blowfly) can transmit the infection in southeastern Africa. The infection occurs in the peak season of flies. The tabanid flies can acquire the infection during feeding on the infected carcasses. However, no multiplication of the organism is detected in the gut of the flies.

d) Animal to animal transmission can take place through the ingestion of infected carcasses (carnivores).

Pathogenesis

The dormant endospores of *B. anthracis* are infectious in nature. The infection occurs only when the endospores enter into the host from the external environment. There is no well-documented case of vegetative anthrax bacilli occurring in a natural system. Following ingestion or inhalation, how the spores cross the intestinal or pharyngeal epithelium is still unknown. Irrespective of the route of entry, the spores are engulfed by the macrophages. The spores may remain dormant for a long time. The germination occurs within the macrophages with the help of the 'germination operon' of the bacteria (*gerX*) and the presence of germinants. The most common and well documented germinant is L-alanine. Triggering of the L-alanine receptor by its ligand is believed to activate its endogenous proteolytic activity, which converts the proenzyme 'germination specific cortex-lytic enzyme (GSLE)' into its active form. The active GSLE allows the spore cortex hydrolysis, uptake of water, swelling of the cortex, loss of endospore refractility, loss of resistance to damaging chemical and physical challenges and ultimately release of spore components and initiation of metabolism. The vegetative bacilli are released within macrophages and they can escape the killing mechanism of macrophages with the help of *atxA* (anthrax toxin activator) gene products. The bacteria start to multiply within cell cytoplasm and release toxin. The temperature and bicarbonate of the host activates the transcription of toxin and capsule genes. The infection may be localized (cutaneous anthrax) or spread into local or regional lymph nodes (gastrointestinal anthrax) with the help of toxin and capsule. The bacterial multiplication occurs in the lymph nodes, resulting toxaemia and bacterimia. The syndrome and fate of the infection depends on sensitivity of macropahges to LF and adenylate cyclase activity of EF.

Disease produced

Bacteria	Host	Disease produced
Bacillus anthracis	Cattle, sheep, goat, horses (Goat and horses are less susceptible and Algerian sheep is resistant)	Anthrax: It is characterized by high fever, anorexia, edema in neck, brisket, abdomen, respiratory distress, abortion, reduced milk production, blood stained milk, diarrhoea and death within 48 hours. There is oozing of dark coloured unclotted blood from natural orifices and absence of rigor mortis. In horses, only acute form is detected. The subcutaneous edematous swelling is more pronounced in horses.
	Pigs are relatively resistant. The dwarf pigs are fully resistant (natural resistance)	Anthrax (rare): The cellulitis (edema) of the neck and throat, bloodstained froth in mouth, diarrhoea and death with 12-36 hours are observed in pigs. Pulmonary and cutaneous forms are found. Cutaneous form is also known as 'Bullnose'
	Dogs and cats (relatively resistant)	Anthrax (rare)
	Birds (Free birds are resistant to anthrax except Ostrich)	Anthrax is found in birds kept in captivity including poultry, pigeon, eagles etc. Louis Pasteur correlated high body temperature of the birds with anthrax resistance
	Fish and reptiles (resistant to anthrax)	The body temperature of fish and reptiles is outside the range required for multiplication of anthrax bacteria
	Human	a)Pulmonary Anthrax (Wool Sorter's disease) b)Malignant carbuncle / malignant pustule (ulcerative inflammatory lesion covered with black scab)
Bacillus cereus	Human	Food Poisoning
	Cattle	Mastitis (rare)
Bacillus licheniformis	Human	Food Poisoning
	Cattle, sheep	Abortion (rare)
Bacillus subtilis	Human	Food Poisoning

Immunity

The Protective antigen (PA) of *B. anthracis* plays an important role in protection of anthrax. The antibodies against polysaccharide in the cell wall are not protective.

Diagnosis (*B. anthracis*)

Clinical specimens

a) Fresh blood collected from ear vein either puncturing the vein through syringe or inserting a dry swab into an incision in the vein is the most common clinical sample. It should be collected within 24 hours of death. After collection from incision a cotton ball soaked in alcohol is placed over the incision and ignited. It will seal the wound to prevent further environmental contamination. In all species of animals (except pig and carnivores) at the terminal stage blood comes out the natural orifices, if not treated. The peripheral blood contains huge number of organisms due to bacterimia. Minimum 5×10^4 numbers of bacteria per ml is required for its detection in blood. However, after 24 hour of death due to the presence of contaminants, the anthrax bacilli visualization becomes difficult.

b) Other body fluids collected through the fine needle aspirates of affected areas, such as submandibular swellings, regional lymph nodes and mesenteric fluid. This would be appropriate in pigs, carnivores or antibiotic treated animals in which terminal bacterimia is absent.

c) Milk can be collected for detection of anthrax

d) *Post-mortem samples*: In many countries post-mortem of anthrax suspected carcass is banned to avoid the environmental contamination through the infected body fluids. The sporulation of the bacilli may also occur due to exposure to oxygen. However, the materials may be collected with scalpel incision from a lymph node near the surface progressing to more internal organs such as mesenteric lymph nodes or spleen.

If the carcass is opened unknowingly about the anthrax and the disease is suspected later by observing the typical post mortem lesions like dark unclotted blood, markedly enlarged haemorrhagic spleen, thickened mesentery with excessive peritoneal fluid, petechial haemorrhages on many of the organs; the samples may be collected from spleen or lymph nodes. Special precaution should be taken to decontaminate the place of post mortem with all accessories. Proper disposal of anthrax carcass should be done immediately after post mortem. If the carcass is decomposed, recovery of the anthrax bacilli in laboratory needs special treatment of the samples like mixing with deionized water and keeping in water bath having 62.5 ± 0.5°C temperature (for 30–60 minutes) followed by dilution of the sample to avoid the saprophytic contaminants.

All the samples should be sent to the laboratory with proper labeling as 'anthrax suspect'.

Laboratory Examinations

As *B. anthracis* is world organization for animal health (OIE) risk group 3 organisms (it can cause severe human or animal infection and may spread into the community and/or animal population but for which usually effective prophylaxis and treatment is available), the laboratory should have suitable facilities to handle such containment group 3 organisms.

Direct Examination

a) A smear can be prepared from collected blood sample or tissue and stained by Gram's or Giemsa stain. *B. anthracis* appears as gram positive non-sporing rods with square cut ends arranged in singly or in pair or in long chain (Figure 1).

b) Capsule demonstration

i) *McFadyean's reaction*: The smear is prepared, heat fixed and stained with polychrome methylene blue for 1 minute. The capsule will appear pink and the bacilli are dark blue under microscope. Freshly collected blood or the bacteria grown in media containing bicarbonate and CO_2 in the environment will show the bacteria with capsule. Positive (Pasteur type strain) and negative control (Sterne stain) should be included with each test.

Polychrome methylene blue is a complex mixture of methylene blue and other homologous substances like azure A and azure B which are produced by oxidation (ripening) of methylene blue solution upon standing. Natural ripening takes a year or more to complete but can be hastened by addition of 1% K_2CO_3 to Loeffler's alkaline methylene blue solution. However, the polychrome methylene blue loses its affinity for capsule with the putrefaction of the carcass. For the samples collected from partially decomposed carcass Giemsa staining is better in demonstrating the bacteria than McFadyean's reaction.

ii) India Ink: The capsule can be observed as a halo surrounding the bacteria in an India ink stained smear.

Isolation of bacteria from clinical samples: Media and incubation conditions are described earlier. It is time consuming, laborious and detection is only successful in a high dose infection, where huge number of bacilli are present in the clinical samples.

Immunological tests: The antigen detection of *B. anthracis* lacks sensitivity and specificity, whereas, the antibody detection occurs efficiently only in the later stage of the infection.

a) *Ascoli's thermoprecipitation test*: This test was developed by Ascoli in 1911. It detects thermostable *B. anthracis* antigen in animal tissues or hides. Approximately 2 grams of tissue sample is added in 5 ml of sterile saline containing 1/100 final concentration of acetic acid and the mixture is boiled for 5 minutes. The resultant solution is cooled and filtered through the filter paper. A few drops of rabbit antiserum are placed in a small test tube. The filtrate from the previous step is gently layered over the top of the antiserum. A positive test is the formation of a visible ring at the junction of two liquid layers within 15 minutes.

b) *Immunofluorescence test*

c) *ELISA*: It is used to detect *B. anthracis* toxin proteins (EF, LF, PA) or polypeptide capsule. PA or LF can be detected in the later stage of the infection.

d) *Europium Nanoparticle based Immunoassay (ENIA)*: It is a recently developed highly sensitive assay for detection of *B. anthracis* PA.

Molecular Biology: Polymerase chain reaction (PCR) can be used to detect the virulence factors of *B. anthracis* like protective antigen (*pag*) and lethal factor (*lef*). Detection of these two genes is a reliable method, as they produce less nonspecific bands. Other potential targets include AC-390, 16 SrRNA and 16 S-23 S internal transcribed spacers. The PCR works well for cultured organisms and for body fluids but is less successful in the environmental samples due to inhibition by KCl, NaCl and other salts, ionic detergents such as SDS, phenol, bile salts, urea etc.

Real time PCR is also successfully used to detect *rpoB* (175 bp) sequence specific to *B. anthracis*. In a real time PCR, no preparation of amplicon like conventional PCR is required and there is less chance of cross-contamination as the amplification and detection takes place in the same chamber.

Prevention and control

During anthrax outbreak quarantine of the animal farm, destruction of the equipments and utensils and vaccination of the healthy animals is required. Infected carcasses should not be opened but the carcasses should be burned or buried together with equipments and utensils. The burial should be done at least 2 meter under the soil with quicklime at the top layer.

In most of the countries including India 'Stern spore vaccine' is used to prevent anthrax in cattle and sheep. It is a live vaccine and it offers protection for one year in cattle and 26 months in sheep. In endemic zone it is routinely used as a vaccine every year. The post-vaccination reactions include fever, decreased milk yield and abortion in sows. The milk of the vaccinated animals is discarded for 72 hours and the animal is withheld from slaughter for 45 days.

Differences of *B. anthracis* and anthracoid organisms

Characters	*B. anthracis*	Anthracoids
Pathogenicity	Pathogenic	Non- Pathogenic (with some exception)
Motility	Non-motile	Motile
Haemolysis	Non-haemolytic in sheep blood agar	Haemolytic in sheep blood agar
Lysis by gamma phage	Susceptible	Resistant
Polypeptide Capsule production in the media containing serum with increased CO_2 tension	(+ ve)	(-ve)
Growth in broth	No turbidity and pellicle	Often turbidity and pellicle
Growth in Gelatin stab	'Inverted fir tree' appearance	absent
Liquefaction of gelatin	slow	rapid
Growth in penicillin agar (10 μg/ml)	(-ve)	(+ve)
Reduction of methylene blue	weak	strong
Lecithinase production	Weak	Strong

13

Mycobacterium

In 1882, Robert Koch first isolated the bacterium, stained with alkaline methylene blue and vesuvin as counter stain and showed its etiologic relationship with tuberculosis. Ehrlich first developed acid-fast stain in 1882 and used for better staining of the bacteria which was adopted by Robert Koch. The acid-fast staining technique was modified later by Franz Ziehl and Friedrich Neelsen, accordingly, it is known as Ziehl-Neelsen (Z-N) staining. In 1890, Koch prepared a glycerine broth extract of the tubercle bacillus, known as 'tuberculin'. He tried to prepare it as a curative agent; but it was used later in diagnosis. In 1895, Johne and Frothingham described the first case of paratuberculosis in cattle which became known as 'Johne's disease'. The causative bacterium was later isolated by Twort and Ingram in 1910.

In India, bovine tuberculosis is reported from several states since 1959 (Dhanda and Lall, 1959). The bovine paratuberculosis in India was first reported by Nanda and Singh (1940) from Haryana.

Properties of genus

1. *Morphology: Mycobacterium* is gram positive, straight or slightly curved rod with occasional coccobacillary, club and branched form (Fig. 1). In the tissues, it measures 1-4 μm in length and 0.2-0.3 μm in width. It occurs singly, in pair or in bundle. The bacteria are non-motile, uncapsulated and non-sporing in nature.

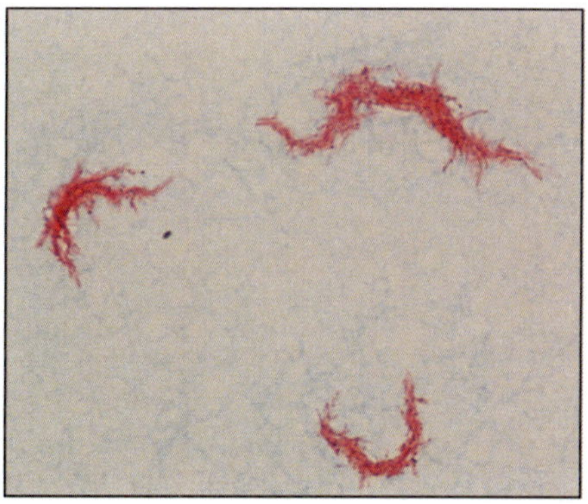

Fig. 1. *Mycobacterium tuberculosis* showing the growth in 'cords' or ropes (*Courtesy*: Sarah Zimmerman, American Society for Microbiology)

It is difficult to demonstrate their gram positive nature due to high lipid content of the cell wall. The stains are relatively impermeable to the bacterial cell. In acid fast / ZN method of staining, primary stains (strong carbol fuchsin) enter the cell with the help of the heat (mordant).

The bacteria are called acid fast (acid fast bacilli, AFB) because it can resist the decolourization by acid-alcohol mixture due to high lipid content of the cell wall.

The bacterial cell contains cytoplasmic membrane, periplasmic space, peptidoglycan and lipids. The outer most layer is a ribbon like structure, called 'mycoside', composed of glycolipids and peptidoglycolipids. Mycoside determines the colony characteristics, serological properties, helps in intracellular survival and it is antiphagocytic. There is a layer of long chain mycolic acid and esters below the mycoside. The mycolic acids are β-hydroxy acids substituted at α-position with alipathic chain and are responsible for acid fastness. It is attached with the underlying peptidoglycan layer by arabinogalactans (arabinose and galactan). The peptidoglycan is composed of N-glycosylmuramic acid and N-glycosylglucosamine. Mycobacterial peptidoglycan has adjuvant property.

2. *Mycobacterium* are aerobic or microaerophilic

3. *Classification*: The genus *Mycobacterium* (Actinomycetes family) currently contains 200 species and sub-species. Some species are pathogenic for man and animals which grow slowly in artificial media in the laboratory (slow growers) than the others (fast growers, *M. smegmatis*). Previously, slow growing *Mycobacterium* can be sub divided into three types based on their host specificity, i.e. human type, bovine type and avian type. Runyon classified non tuberculous *Mycobacterium* [NTM / atypical mycobacteria / mycobacteria other than TB (MOTT)] into four major groups (photochromogens, scotochromogens, nonphotochromogens and rapid growers). The photochromogens produce yellow or orange coloured pigment during exposure to light (*M. phlei, M. kansasii*), scotochromogens produce yellow pigment constitutively (under light or dark) and non-photochromogens do not produce any pigment (*M. avium*, *M. intracellularae*).

Recent taxonomic classification shows that slow growing mycobacteria (pathogenic) are composed of several species. The most important group of species is *M. tuberculosis* complex (MTBC). The complex consists of *M. tuberculosis*, *M. bovis*, *M. bovis* bacille Calmette-Guérin (BCG), *M. caprae*, *M. africanum*, *M. pinnipedii*, *M. microti*, *M. orygis*, *M. mungi*, dassie bacillus, chimpanzee bacillus, and smooth colony morphology tubercle bacillus named *M. canettii*.

'Environmental *Mycobacterium*' contains both slow and fast growers, as well as pigmented or non-pigmented colony producers. *M. avium-intracellulare* complex (MAC) is a major group of environmental *Mycobacterium*. MAC is composed of two major species- *M. avium* and *M. intracellulare*. *M.*

avium is subdivided into four subspecies (ssp.) i.e. ssp. *avium* (Maa), ssp. *paratuberculosis* (Map), ssp. *silvaticum* and ssp. *hominissuis*. *M. avium* ssp. *paratuberculosis* (Map) is the etiological agent of paratuberculosis or Johne's disease in ruminants and Crohn's disease in humans.

4. *Resistance*: *M. tuberculosis* can be killed by exposure to heat (60°C for 15 minutes). *M. tuberculosis* is also susceptible to ionic detergents, sunlight, pasteurization and phenolic disinfectants. *M. avium* ssp. *paratuberculosis* (Map) can survive the low temperature holding method (63°C for 30 minutes) and to some extent high temperature short time method (72°C for 15 seconds) of milk pasteurization. The Map remains viable for long time in soil, putrefying materials, faeces and sputum. *M. bovis* is found more resistant to sunlight than *M. tuberculosis*.

5. *Natural habitat*: Infected animals and humans are the major sources of *Mycobacterium*. Different discharges from infected hosts make the environment infective. Survival of the bacteria in the environment like soil and water for long time occurs due to impermeable cell wall and slow growth. Cattle, buffaloes and goats can act as reservoir of *M. bovis*, while, the pigs, cats, dogs, horses and sheep are considered as 'spillover hosts' (to whom infection occurs sporadically and persistence of infection takes place only when there is an existence of reservoir host in nearby environment). In addition to the domestic animals, wildlife like African buffalo, bison and deer can act as reservoir and baboon, black bear, cheetah, lion can act as spillover hosts.

Environmental mycobacteria like MAC can be isolated from soil, wastewater, water tank, municipal water, aerosols, protozoa, deep litter, fresh tropical vegetation in addition to the animals and humans. MAC can utilize variable nutrients for their growth. However *M. avium* ssp. *paratuberculosis* is a host dependent bacterium. It can survive in the environment but requires host cells (macrophage) for its replication. Natural reservoir of MAC includes domestic birds, chickens, cattle, swine, farmed deer, sheep, goats, horses, dogs and cats. Wildlife like white tailed deer, bison, boar, wild rabbit act as reservoir of *M. avium* ssp. *paratuberculosis*. Whereas, wild boar, deer, kangaroo are the reservoir of *M. avium* ssp. *avium*.

6. *Genome*: The evidence suggests that *M. tuberculosis* complex (MTBC) is originated from a common ancestor *Mycobacterium canettii* thousands of years ago. The mycobacterial species under MTBC have almost similar genome (> 99 % similarity) with absence of horizontal gene transfer and recombination events. The evolution of individual species of the complex took place through single nucleotide polymorphism (SNP), small insertions and deletions ('indels'), insertion sequences (IS), duplication of paralogous

gene families and large size deletions (up to 25 Kbp). The large size deletions generate 'regions of difference' (RD) in the genome which can differentiate the mycobacterial species. It is a useful diagnostic tool for identification of the mycobacterial species. The average size of *M. bovis* genome is 4.3 Mbp which contains approximately 4200 genes, including each of the ribosomal RNA genes (5S, 16S, 23S) and 45 tRNAs. The genome has high GC content (65 mol%) and great numbers of repetitive elements such as mobile genetic elements (insertion sequences), proline-glutamate (PE) or proline-proline-glutamate (PPE) family genes (10% of genome), integrase, phage sequences, clustered regularly interspaced short palindromic repeats (CRISPR), and 13E12 repeat family genes. The PE-PPE gene gamily is associated with pathogenesis and the repetitive elements are useful for molecular typing of the isolates.

Isolation, growth and colony characteristics

M. bovis and M. tuberculosis

The tissue samples are homogenized with the solution of hypochlorite (1:1000) for 4-16 hours. It is decontaminated by the addition of acid (5% oxalic acid), alkali (2-4% sodium hydroxide) or detergent (0.375–0.75% hexadecyl-pyridinium-chloride, HPC). The acid or alkali mixture is neutralized, centrifuged and the sediment is used for culture. A slope (agar slant) of the solid medium is prepared into a tightly screw capped glass tube for inoculation. Minimum 8-12 week incubation at 37°C is required. Carbon-di-oxide (5-10%) can be added for enhancing the growth of *M. tuberculosis*. The slopes are visualized from outside for appearance of colonies at intervals. The media used are Lowenstein-Jensen (LJ), Herrold's and Middlebrook's (7H10, 7H11) agar. The LJ is an egg based agar medium. Middlebrook's agar is an example of non-egg based medium. Glycerol can stimulate the growth of *M. tuberculosis* (eugonic), not *M. bovis* (dysgonic). Stonebrink's medium, containing inspissated egg with malachite green to prevent the contaminant growth, can be used for isolation of *M. bovis*. The LJ and Stonebrink media contain pyruvate as growth enhancer.

M. bovis produces smooth, non-pigmented buffy or off-white coloured colony. In liquid medium it forms fungus like pellicle at top layer unless tween-80 (detergent) is added reducing the surface tension and submerges the growth.

M. avium ssp. *avium*

It can be isolated in Dorset egg medium, Lowenstein-Jensen (LJ), Herrold's and Middlebrook's (7H10, 7H11) medium containing pyruvate. Glycerol and 'mycobactin' are also added as growth enhancer. Mycobactin extracted from the environmental mycobacteria, acts as siderophore helping in acquisition of iron. Mycobactin is produced by all cultivable mycobacteria except *M. avium* ssp. *avium* and *M. avium* ssp. *paratuberculosis*. So, both of these mycobacteria require mycobactin from external sources. Incubation period is 8 week at 40°C. Even it can grow at 42-43°C. It produces smooth or rough types of colonies. In liquid culture a radiometric method using ^{14}C labeled substrate can be used for rapid detection (BACTEC system).

M. avium ssp. *paratuberculosis*

Commonly used media for isolation are Lowenstein-Jensen (LJ) medium with mycobactin, Herrold's egg yolk medium with mycobactin, modified Dubos's medium, modified Middlebrook 7H10. The oxalic acid, sodium hydroxide may be used for decontamination of samples before inoculation into LJ medium. The slopes in screw capped tubes are incubated for at least 4 months at 37°C. The sheep-associated strains may require 12 months incubation for visible colony formation. Occasionally the colonies are observed after 6 weeks of incubation. Initially the tubes are placed horizontally with loose screw caps for one week to evaporate the moisture. After 1 week, the slopes are kept in vertical position with tightened cap.

Young colonies are smooth, glistening and convex. Later they become raised, cream coloured and rough. The colony diameter may be changed from 0.25-1mm (primary) to 2 mm (older).

Non-cultivable *Mycobacterium* is *M. leprae*, causative agent of human leprosy. *M. leprae* cannot be grown by routine bacteriologic media, automated detection systems and cell culture. It can only be grown in nine banded armadillo or mice footpad.

Biochemical characteristics

Different biochemical tests like niacin production, nitrate reduction, urease production test, deamination of pyrazinamide can be conducted for detection and differentiation of mycobacterial species.

Toxins and virulence factors produced

Toxins

No true exotoxins are produced by *Mycobacterium*.

Virulence factors

Mycobacterial virulence factors/ antigens

Virulence factors (antigen)	Location in cell	Function
Mycoside	Outer most layer of cell wall	antiphagocytic
Dimycolyl trehalose or Trehalose-6-6'-dimycolate (cord factor)	cell wall	It stimulates the granuloma formation, used as an adjuvant. It can also inhibit chemotaxis by neutrophils and disrupts mitochondria causing inhibition of oxidative phosphorylation.
Sulfolipid and phospholipid (phosphatidylinositol mannoside)	cell wall	It prevents respiratory burst, phagolysosome fusion, disrupts reactive oxygen intermediate function; thus helps in intracellular survival of the bacteria
Phenolic glycolipid (PGL)	cell wall	It induces chemokine (CCL) and recruits macrophages in which mycobacterial multiplication can occur
Phthiocerol dimycocerosates (PDIMs)	cell wall	It masks pathogen associated molecular pattern (PAMP) of M. tuberculosis surface and helps in immune-evasion
Heparin binding haemagglutinin (HBHA)	Surface of cell wall	It helps in bacterial adhesion with host cells
Glycopeptidolipid (Glycopeptidolipids typically consist of a lipopeptide core that is N-linked to a mono-or di-unsaturated long chain fatty acid)	Found in MAC group of bacteria	It can activate antigen presenting cells as adjuvant that mediate CD1 expression through Toll-like receptor 2 (TLR 2)
Heat shock protein (α-crystalline, HSP 65)	Cell bound antigen	It protects bacteria from the reactive oxygen intermediates, myeloperoxidase based killing mechanism during respiratory burst of the macrophages. It helps in intracellular survival of the bacteria and its latency maintenance.
Catalase (KATG)	Cell bound antigen	It lyses reactive oxygen intermediates (ROI) and prevents killing by phagocytosis.
Fibronectin binding protein		It binds fibronectin making it unavailable for binding and activation of T cells and macrophages.

Virulence factors (antigen)	Location in cell	Function
ESAT-6 CFP 10	Secreated protein	They are highly immunogenic T- cell antigen and help in evasion from phagosome within the macrophages. It is encoded by RD-1 region of the genome. ESAT-6 also causes apoptosis of macrophages and re-phagocytosis by new macrophages
Ag85A, Ag85B	Secreated protein	They are Mycolyl transferase enzymes, involved in the coupling of mycolic acids with arabinogalactan. They are Highly immunogenic and abundant proteins
noxR1, noxR3 and ahpC		Antioxidant enzymes prevent the oxidative stress within macrophages. It helps in intracellular survival and latency maintenance
dosRS (devRS) regulon		Helps in survivality of the bacteria under hypoxic condition

The major variations found in antigen production between *M. bovis* and *M. tuberculosis* are

a) *M. bovis* produces more MPB 70 and MPB 83. MPB83 is a glycosylated cell wall-associated protein, while MPB70 is a secreated protein. Exact functions are unknown, but the proteins play role in host preference.

b) ESAT 6 proteins are altered in *M. bovis*

Pathogenesis

M. bovis

Transmission

a. *M. bovis* is excreated through the urine, faeces, milk and semen of infected animals and thus contaminates the pastures. The ticks of the infected cattle skin can also carry the bacteria. *M. bovis* is transmitted between cattle and other animals through inhalation, ingestion and vertical way. The inhalation is the most common route of transmission through droplets, eructation during rumination, and dust particles. The healthy cattle can acquire the infection from pastures, where the infected cattle grazed even several weeks earlier. The survival of bacteria in pastures is increased during hot and humid weather. Vertical way is less commonly found between the domestic animals. Pseudo-vertical transmission is another rare possible route that occurs through the ingestion of tuberculous milk from the sub-clinically infected cows, typically excreating tuberculous bacteria (10^3 cfu/ml) in the milk.

b. From wildlife, *M. bovis* can be transmitted into domestic animals through direct contact, inhalation and predation, whereas, the *vice-versa* takes place through direct contact and inhalation only.

c. *M. bovis* infection of human from domestic animals may occur by the inhalation of aerosols or through the consumption of contaminated milk or unpasteurized dairy products. Human to human spread is rare and it is possible only in the immunocompromised hosts.

Pathogenesis

The primary lesion varies according to the route of transmission into the host. The lesions in the respiratory tract and mesenteric lymph nodes are observed in infection through inhalation and ingestion route, respectively.

The mucus and cilia present in the upper respiratory passage attempts to clear *M. bovis* during entry through the inhalation route. The bacteria, attached with dust or droplets may avoid the collision with mucociliary layer and pass through the terminal bronchioles to enter the alveolar space. The bacteria are phagocytosed by alveolar macrophages. There are two types of macrophages available in the airway i.e. microbicidal macrophages ('primed') and microbial-growth permissive macrophages. The microbicidal / primed macrophages are recruited through toll-like receptors (TLRs) mediated signaling and the signaling pathway is activated by mycobacterial molecular patterns (PAMPs) present on the bacterial surface. However, the mycobacterial surface lipid, phthiocerol dimycoceroserate (PDIM) can mask the PAMPs to avoid the contact of primed macrophages. Instead, another surface lipid, known as phenolic glycolipid (PGL) can enhance the release of chemokine (CCL2) to attract growth-permissive macrophages. The strategy to avoid primed macrophages is not so effective in upper airways where other commensal bacteria may trigger the TLR signaling. The alveolar space of the lower lung is preferred by mycobacteria due to presence of very few commensals.

M. bovis and other pathogenic mycobacteria can survive and replicate within the growth-permissive macrophages which is a distinguishing feature of pathogenic mycobacteria from the environmental non-pathogenic groups. The pathogenic mycobacteria can bypass the phago-lysosome fusion or can multiply within the phago-lysosome (acid resistant strains). Few strains can burst the phagosome and survive in the cytosol. The mycobacterial strategies for intracellular survival include the use of different virulence factors like sulfolipid, phenolic glycolipid, heat shock protein (Table 1). *Mycobacterium* spp. can synthesize own tryptophan which helps to survive under intracellular tryptophan starvation. Recent study identified the role of efflux pumps in intracellular survival of mycobacteria by providing protection from antimicrobial peptides of the macrophages. This is considered as probable reason for mycobacterial preference of macrophages, not neutrophils. The efflux pumps are also associated with antibiotic resistance of mycobacteria.

After 10-14 days of the infection, cell mediated immunity (CMI) develops. This CMI is primarily mediated by lymphocytes. The lymphocytes secreate lymphokines and the lymphokines attract more mononuclear cells at the site. It causes cell death and caseous necrosis. Sometimes activated macrophages along with mycobacteria enter the regional lymph nodes like bronchial and mediastinal lymph nodes through the lymph vessels. The lymph nodes are commonly infected than other tissues because all the fluids in the body pass through the nodes where the meshwork of trabeculae entraps the bacteria.

The enlarged activated macrophages provide a suitable environment for mycobacterial growth and granuloma formation. Microscopically, a granuloma (tubercle) contains caseous necrosis in its central area surrounded by zones of epithelioid cells, granulocytes, and lymphocytes. The epithelioid cells are aggregate of macrophages whose membranes become tightly adhered like epithelial cells. Minerals are present at the necrotic center. Multinucleated giant cells are found near the necrotic foci. Outer boundary of the granuloma is formed by a fibrous connective tissue. The apoptosis (programmed cell death) of macrophages occurs when the numbers of mycobacteria within it reaches the maximum limit. The dead macrophages with live mycobacteria are re-phagocytosed by new macrophages to initiate the granuloma formation. The apoptosis and re-phagocytosis of macrophages is controlled by mycobacterial secreation system (ESX-1/ESAT-6) which induces host matrix metalloproteinase 9 (MMP9) for recruitment of new macrophages. The secreation system (ESX-1/ESAT-6) is still not detected in *M. avium* which may use different mechanism for granuloma formation. Granulomas are produced in response to several causes both infectious and non-infectious, other than mycobacterial infection. It is a beneficial trial of the host to restrict the infection from spreading and to activate the defense mechanism for destruction of the bacteria. In many cases, the infection is restricted within this granuloma and symptoms are only produced during reactivation of the infection, when the body defense is weakened. The persistence of infection is characterized by positive skin test or culture without any visible lesion (NVL).

Reactivation of infection may occur during viral immunosuppression (bovine viral diarrhoea, bovine leucosis), metabolic imbalance, postpartum period, use of corticosteroids. The 'necroptosis' of the macrophages present in granuloma occurs due to excess of TNF in the body of the host. It is also a programmed cell death which causes lysis of the macrophages. The excess host TNF causes the activation of the reactive oxygen species in the macrophage through RIP1 and RIP3 kinases. The reactive oxygen species can kill both the macrophages and the residing mycobacteria. The few surviving mycobacteria are released extracellularly which can multiply rapidly because the necrosed debris ('caseum') acts as an ideal bacterial growth medium. The 'serpentine cords' are also observed during this phase. In some cases, dissemination of infection continues through blood causing 'miliary tuberculosis'. It causes granuloma formation in different vital organs and it is common in deer.

Through ingestion route of entry, the lymph nodes, associated with gastrointestinal tract are commonly infected. Bovine tonsil is rarely infected because it locates sub-epithelially and it is devoid of afferent lymph vessels. The retropharyngeal lymph node is the most common site of infection in the head. In intestine, mesenteric lymph nodes are commonly infected. Localized granuloma in the mucous membrane of intestine is not observed suggesting that the organisms can diffuse into the lymphatics of lamina propria and are transported by phagocytes into the mesenteric lymph nodes.

MAC

Transmission

MAC members are transmitted between animal and avian hosts by both vertical and horizontal way (ingestion and inhalation route).

M. avium ssp. *avium* is excreated through the faeces of infected birds and survive in soil and water for a long period. Ingestion is the major route of transmission. From wildlife, the birds can acquire the infection by ingestion of infected feed, water or inhalation of contaminated dusts.

M. avium ssp. *paratuberculosis* occurs in young animals which are below 30 days old. It is transmitted mainly through ingestion route. Faeces excreted from infected animals are major source of infection in the environment. Vertical and pseudo-vertical (through infected milk or colostrum) transmissions are also observed. Calves can also acquire infection during suckling of teats contaminated with infected faeces. Rarely semen of infected bull, embryo transfer and wildlife can transmit the infection.

Potable water and aerosols are considered as the primary source of MAC infection in immunocompromised human patients.

Pathogenesis

M. avium ssp. *avium (Maa)*

Maa is responsible for causing avian tuberculosis in birds. The primary lesions of tuberculosis in birds are common in intestinal tract. Such lesions can take the form of deep ulcers filled with caseous material and numerous bacteria. Typical lesions are also found in the liver and spleen, and these organs become enlarged due to the formation of new tuberculous tissue. The lungs are generally free from the lesions.

M. avium ssp. *paratuberculosis (MAP)*

MAP after entry within the body interacts with the mucosa associated lymphoid tissue (MALT) and penetrates the intestinal epithelial layer through M-cells. It is phagocytosed by sub epithelial and intra epithelial macrophages. Within the macrophages, the bacteria can replicate and survive through the mechanisms described earlier. The cell mediated immunity (CMI) causes granuloma formation in the lymph nodes associated with the intestine. The granulomas are diffused with little or no necrosis in the cattle. Initially, there is accumulation of lymphocytes and epithelioid cells in lamina propria followed by the accumulation in the submucosa, like a band with the advancement of the disease. In sheep and goats, caseous necrosis is observed within granuloma.

The battle between the bacteria and the host defense system continues, causing intestinal damage with thickening and corrugation of the tissues. There is continuous excreation of epithelioid cells filled with bacteria through the faeces. The clinical stage lasts for 3-6 months or more.

Disease produced

Bacteria	Host	Disease produced
Mycobacterium bovis	Cattle, deer, elk, buffalo, sheep, goat, horse, dog, cat and poultry	Tuberculosis: It is a chronic, contagious disease characterized by granuloma formation in lungs or other organs, continuous weight loss, respiratory distress, diarrhoea, bloody faeces, irregular estrus cycle, abortion, tuberculous mastitis etc. It can be transmitted to primates and human from the infected animals.
	Human	Tuberculosis
Mycobacterium tuberculosis	Human	Tuberculosis: It is a chronic infection characterized by cough with sputum and blood at times, chest pains, weakness, weight loss, fever and night sweats. According to world health organization (WHO), 10 million cases of TB and 1.3 million deaths occurred during 2017.
	Cattle, goat, pig, dog and poultry	Tuberculosis
Mycobacterium caprae	Goats	Caprine Tuberculosis
Mycobacterium avium complex (MAC)	Human	The most common presentations of MAC lung infections in immunocompetent hosts are TB-like apical fibrocavitary disease or interstitial nodular infiltrates and bronchiectasis. MAC can also be associated with hypersensitivity pneumonitis, known as 'hot tub lung'. The syndrome is a combination of inflammatory reactions and infectious mechanisms and is the result of exposure to contaminated indoor spa or showers. In children, cervical lymphadenitis is the most common presentation

Bacteria	Host	Disease produced
Mycobacterium avium ssp. *avium (serovar 1,2,3)*	Chicken (backyard), turkey, wild birds kept in captivity, parrots, cockatoos, budgcrigars, finchcs, flycatchers, canaries, sparrows, crows, barn owls, cowbirds, blackbirds, eastern sparrow hawks	Avian tuberculosis (avian mycobacteriosis): It is a chronic contagious infection characterized by progressive loss of weight; atrophy of breast muscles with prominent keel; disappearance of body fat; dull and ruffled feathers; pale comb, wattle, and earlobes; unilateral lameness; jerky, hopping gait; nodular lesions in intestine; decreased egg production
	Pig	Swine mycobacteriosis: Granulomas are confined within cervical and mesenteric lymph nodes only and miliary form is not found. Pig to human transmission is rare
Mycobacterium avium ssp. *paratuberculosis*	Cattle, sheep, goat, horse, pig	Paratuberculosis /Johne's disease: There are four stages of the disease. In the first stage, no visible signs are found. In the second stage, antibodies are detected. No signs are found. In the third stage clinical signs like weight loss and dirrhoea appear. The final stage is characterized by emaciation, dehydration and faecal shedding of the bacteria. The infceted animals should be discarded.
	Human	Crohn's disease (inflammatory bowel disease)
M. avium subsp. *hominissuis*	Human	Disseminated disease in humans (AIDS patients with low CD4 counts), chronic lung diseases in patients with cystic fibrosis (CF) or bronchiectasis, cervical lymphadenitis in children
Mycobacterium intracellularae	Poultry, cattle, sheep, goat, pig, dog, cat	Tuberculosis
	Human	Respiratory distress
Mycobacterium leprae	Human	Leprosy: It is a chronic granulomatous disease that affects the skin, peripheral nervous system, mucous membrane. Paucibacillary (low numbers of organisms) form of leprosy is the milder form and is characterized by one or more skin macules. Multibacillary (large numbers of organisms) leprosy is associated with symmetric skin lesions, nodules, plaques, thickened dermis, and frequent involvement of the nasal mucosa.

Bacteria	Host	Disease produced
Mycobacterium farcinogenes	Cattle	Bovine Farcy: Chronic suppurative infection which begins at the lower limb. Nodules are formed along the lymphatics of the extremities or in the lymph glands of the head region. Nodules may rupture and produce ulcers. The disease is commonly found in the tropical countries. Previously Nocardia asteroides (N. farcinica) was considered as etiological agent.
Mycobacterium ulcerans	Human	'Buruli ulcer'/'Bairnsdale ulcer': Localized nodule or ulcer to widespread ulcerative or non-ulcerative infection including osteomyelitis is detected. In Africa, the disease is known as 'Buruli ulcer', while in Australia, it is called 'Bairnsdale ulcer'. The infection due to M. ulcerans is the third most common mycobacterial disease in the world
Mycobacterium marinum	Human	'Swimming pool' / 'fish tank' granuloma: It occurs due to trauma at finger, hand, arm, elbow, knee, toe soft tissue in freshwater or saltwater due to punctures from fins of fish or shrimp

Immunity

An excessive cell mediated immune response or the virulence of mycobacterial strain decides the fate of the infection. In susceptible hosts, the interaction of mycobacteria with immune cells results in the granuloma formation. The neutrophils are the first inflammatory cells to arrive at the bacillus multiplication site, followed by natural killer (NK) cells and macrophages. The NK cells can destroy the pathogens directly or cause lysis of infected monocytes. T-cells are among the first cells involved in granuloma formation. All of the major T-cell subsets (γδ T-cells, CD4+ and CD8+ αβ T-cells) have been shown to be involved in the immune response in cattle. There is a balance between mycobacterial killing and survival in granuloma that results in eradication, persistence or progression of the infection. It depends on cytokine production by the host (Th1 and Th2 mediated). More production of Th2 cytokines is associated with the disease progression.

Anti-mycobacterial antibodies are not correlated with resistance of natural infection. Generally, antibodies are produced at later stage of the infection when CMI response wanes.

Diagnosis

M. bovis and *M. avium* ssp. *avium*

Clinical specimens

Ante-mortem clinical specimens include saliva, aspirates from cavities, lymph nodes, biopsies and milk. Whereas, lymph node, lung in 10% formalin are collected as post mortem samples for detection of *M. bovis* and *M. avium* ssp. *avium*. All the specimens should be immediately sent to the laboratory following the regulations for sending biohazardous substances. If there is delay in sending, refrigeration of the samples should be done to prevent the growth of contaminants. Addition of 0.5% boric acid may preserve the specimens for at least one week, if refrigerator is unavailable.

Laboratory examination

As *M. bovis* is OIE risk group 3 bacteria (organisms that can cause severe human or animal disease and may spread in the community and/or animal population but for which effective prophylaxis and treatment is available), the laboratory should have suitable facilities to handle such containment group 3 bacteria. The laboratory should be created following the guidelines of international organization for standardization (ISO) 15189 standard.

Direct Examination: A smear can be prepared from collected sample or tissue and stained by Ziehl-Neelsen method. *Mycobacterium* appears as red coloured slender rods singly or in bundle (Figure 1). Fluorescent acid fast stain may also be used for better detection.

Isolation of bacteria from clinical samples: Processing of clinical samples and media / incubation conditions are described earlier.

Immunological tests

a) *Tuberculin test:* Tuberculin is mycobacterial extract, protein in nature, originally prepared by Robert Koch for treatment of tuberculosis. 'Old tuberculin' was prepared by evaporating a broth culture 1/10th of its volume. Along with active principle it also contains non-specific substances. Currently, the bacteria are grown in synthetic glycerinated medium and the active principle is extracted by trichloro-acetic acid. It is known as 'purified protein derivative (PPD)'. Throughout the world, the PPD is generally prepared from *M. bovis* AN5 strain, originally isolated in United Kingdom in 1948. The strain (AN5) is selected for high yield of cell mass on glycerinated media. In genomic analysis, it is observed that the strain does not have any substantial difference with others isolated from different parts of the globe.

Tuberculin test is found 68-95% sensitive and 96-99% specific. Tuberculin is inoculated into the suspected cattle by intradermal route at mid neck or caudal fold of tail. Middle neck is more sensitive area. The site should be clipped and disinfected before inoculation. The clipped area is measured with calipers prior to injection. Dose is 0.2 ml containing 2000 IU of bovine tuberculin. The skin fold swelling is measured after 72 hours to read the test result. In poultry, 0.05-0.1 ml (2000 IU tuberculin) is inoculated into the wattles or combs of the suspected birds. Bare skin area is chosen as inoculation site in ducks. In turkey and other birds, wing web is the preferred site for inoculation. However, the sites other than wattle produce unsatisfactory results. The reading is taken after 48 hours.

In positive cases in cattle, the skin fold is increased by 4 mm or more and there are clinical signs like extensive edema, exudation, necrosis, pain or inflammation of the lymphatic ducts in inoculated region or of the lymph nodes. It occurs due to delayed-type hypersensitivity reaction associated with an influx of sensitized T-lymphocytes and monocytic cells into the site of inoculation. Test result in cattle is inconclusive with the skin fold increase between 2-4 mm without any clinical signs. The result in cattle is negative with the skin fold increase less than 2 mm without any clinical signs. In poultry, swelling is developed at the site ranging from small nodule to large edema extending into other wattle or neck. The positive result should be supported by other tests. Inconclusive and negative results should be re-tested after 40-60 days (double intradermal test).

False Positive reaction may occur due to

i) Infection with other *Mycobacterium* like paratuberculosis, skin mycobacteria etc.

ii) Infection with non-mycobacterial species having similarity in cell wall structure

iii) Local inflammation

False negative reaction may occur due to

i) Very early *M. bovis* infection

ii) Generalized *M. bovis* infection contributing to ‘anergy’ (immunological tolerance)

iii) Stress associated with poor nutrition, transportation, parturition

iv) Concurrent viral infection

v) Use of immunosuppressive drugs

vi) Incorrect test procedure

b) *Interferon-gamma assay*: The principle of the test is based on the fact that when sensitized T-lymphocytes from blood of an *M. bovis*-infected animal are re-exposed to antigens from *M. bovis*

(PPD) for 16-24 hours, the cells will release the cytokine interferon gamma (IFN-γ). The freshly collected blood sample is required for the test. The IFN-γ is detected by ELISA. In addition to PPD, now a day ESAT-6, CFP-10 is also successfully used as antigen.

Advantages

i) As it is a laboratory based test the animal is handled only once during the collection of blood. There is no need to maintain the animals. It is less hazardous in comparison to tuberculin test.

ii) Highly sensitive

iii) Detects *M. bovis* infection earlier than the tuberculin skin test

Dis-advantages

i) Non-specific responses in animals (specially those are <15 weeks old)

ii) The blood is perishable and it should be transported at 10-26°C temperature.

iii) Human error

c) *Lymphocyte proliferation assay*: Like Interferon gamma test it is also performed using freshly collected whole blood. It is suitable for diagnosis of *Mycobacterium* in wildlife and zoo animals.

d) *Rapid whole blood agglutination test*: Avian tuberculosis can be detected by rapid whole blood agglutination test using coloured antigen. Smooth strains of *M. avium* ssp. *avium* are used as antigen containing 1% malachite green. A drop of antigen in white tile is mixed with equal volume of whole blood collected from the suspected birds. In positive cases, the agglutination develops showing the accumulation of malachite green stained antigen surrounding the droplet with a red coloured center. The test is commonly used for screening of the flocks.

5. *Serological test:* For detection of *Mycobacterium*, the serological tests are not so useful specially in early stage of the infection. However, in anergic stage of the infection it can be used. Recently an animal-side serological test is developed having application for *on-farm* diagnosis (diagnosis without laboratory). The test involves the use of a small plastic cassette to which a few drops of serum are added and the result is obtained within 20 minutes.

6. *Molecular Biology*: Rapid identification of *M. tuberculosis* complex (MTBC) can be made by polymerase chain reaction (PCR) targeting the genes for 16S-23S rRNA, insertion sequences (IS6110, IS1081) and *M. tuberculosis*-complex-specific proteins (MPB70).Specific identification of an isolate as *M. bovis* can be made using PCR targeting a mutation at nucleotide position 285 of *oxy*R and at position 169 of *pncA* gene. The sequencing of heat shock protein (hsp65) to distinguish between subspecies of *M. avium* has been found useful. Molecular typing of mycobacterial strains can be done with restriction endonuclease analysis (BstEII, PvuII, and BclI enzymes),pulsed-field gel electrophoresis (PFGE), IS*6110*-restriction fragment length polymorphism (IS*6110*-RFLP), polymorphic GC-rich repetitive sequence-restriction fragment length polymorphism (PGRS-RFLP), spoligotyping (based on variable presence of spacers in the direct repeat region of genome, also known as 'spacer oligotyping'), variable number tandem repeat (VNTR), mycobacterial interspersed repetitive units-variable number tandem repeat (MIRU-VNTR), and whole-genome based multi-locus sequencing typing (core genome / cgMLST and pan-genome/ pgMLST schemes). The PFGE is not very useful in typing MTBC due to little discriminatory power associated with low number of polymorphic positions present in the strains and prevention of entry of lytic enzymes used in PFGE due to lipid rich cell wall. The spoligotyping is also less discriminatory for those MTBC strains which have lost the spacer sequences.

M. avium ssp *paratuberculosis* (MAP)

Clinical specimens: Faeces, blood as ante-mortem samples and tissue samples like intestine, lymph nodes are collected after post mortem. All the specimens should be immediately sent to the laboratory after collection. In the laboratory, tissue and faecal samples are preserved at -20°C and -70°C, respectively. No chemical preservatives are used.

Post Mortem findings: Post mortem is an important way of paratuberculosis diagnosis. Thickening and corrugation of mucosa specially in ileum region is pathognomonic. Mesenteric lymph nodes are enlarged. Smears prepared from affected mucosa and cut surfaces of lymph node can be stained by ZN method.

Laboratory Examination

1. *Direct examination*: In ZN stained slides; MAP appears as bundle of small red coloured acid fast rods. Presence of single rod is inconclusive.
2. *Isolation of bacteria from clinical samples*: To isolate the bacteria the tissue or faecal samples must be processed in proper way. Tissue samples are placed in sterile blender containing trypsin (2.5%). Sodium hydroxide (4%) is added for the pH adjustment and stirred for 30 min

at room temperature in magnetic stirrer. It is filtered through gauze and filtrate is centrifuged at 4000-5000 RPM for 30 minutes. The supernatant is discarded and the sediment is used as inoculum. Media and incubation condition are described earlier.

3. *Serological tests*

   a) ELISA: It is OIE prescribed test for detection of paratuberculosis. It can detect chronic carriers also.

   b) Complement Fixation test (CFT)

   c) Immuno- diffusion test: The antigen used is a protoplasmic extract of *M. avium* ssp. *avium* strain 18, prepared by disruption of cells in hydraulic press cell fractionators.

4. *Immunological tests*:

   a) *Delayed type hypersensitivity test (Johnin test)*: It is the same test like tuberculin. In this test, 0.1 ml of avian tuberculin or Johnin is inoculated intradermally into the middle neck region of suspected cattle. Test is read after 72 hours and 2mm increase in skin thickness is considered as positive reactor.

   b) *Interferon-gamma test*: The assay is based on the release of interferon gamma from sensitized lymphocytes during 18-36 hours incubation with specific antigen (avian PPD, bovine PPD or Johnin).

5. *Molecular Biology*: PCR is used successfully for detection of MAP using insertion sequence (IS*900*) as target gene. There are some unique sequences like ISMav2, f57 and ISMap02 detected by PCR as marker of MAP. Restriction enzyme analysis of insertion sequence (IS*1311*) which is common to *M. avium* and *M. paratuberculosis* can be used for species differentiation.

Prevention and control

Prevention of tuberculosis in cattle herd depends on removal of positive tuberculin reactors, testing of the newly purchased animals before introduction into the herd, and inhibition of transmission with hygienic measures. The animals detected as 'doubtful' in tuberculin test should be re-tested with confirmatory serological tests or tuberculin in every 3 months until the animal showed 'negative' results. The final testing should be conducted after 6 months and if the animals are found still 'negative', the herd is declared as 'tuberculosis free'.

The eradication of bovine tuberculosis is possible by ‘test and slaughter’ policy. The complete eradication is difficult to achieve due to presence of reactor animals with no visible lesions (NVL), false negative results in tuberculin test, difficulty in testing of all the cattle in a herd maintained by extensive system, and presence of wildlife reservoirs. If the test and slaughter policy is not feasible, annual vaccination of the herd with BCG vaccine can be conducted. The calves should also be vaccinated after birth. In endemic zone, the immunity is not solid against the infection and the vaccinated animals give false positive reaction in tuberculin test.

14

Clostridium

The genus *Clostridium* belongs to the family Clostridiaceae. The genus name was originated from the Greek word 'klo ster', which means 'spindle' referring to their individual rod shape. Clostridia are gram positive, large, sporulating anaerobic rods (except *C. piliforme* which is gram negative). At present, there are more than 200 numbers of species under the genus *Clostridium.* Among them, 15 species can produce potent toxins and are considered as pathogenic for animals and human. The animal pathogenic clostridia can be classified as neurotoxic, histotoxic and enteric.

A. Neurotoxic *Clostridium:*

   a. *Clostridium botulinum* (type A-F)

   b. *Clostridium tetani*

   c. *Clostridium baratii* (type F)

   d. Clostridium *argentinense* (previously *C. botulinum* type G)

B. Histotoxic *Clostridium:*

   a. *Clostridium perfringens* (previously *C. welchii*)

   b. *Clostridium septicum*

   c. *Clostridium chauvoei*

   d. *Clostridium novyi* (previously *C. oedematiens*)

   e. *Clostridium haemolyticum*

   f. *Clostridium sordellii*

   g. *Clostridium histolyticum*

   h. *Clostridium fallax* (clostridial myositis in horses)

C. Enteric *Clostridium*:

   a. *Clostridium difficile*

   b. *Clostridium colinum*

c. *Clostridium spiroforme*

d. *Clostridium piliforme* (Tyzzer's disease in laboratory mice, foals)

e. *Clostridium perfringens*

Clostridium perfringens **(*C. welchii*)**

The organism was first isolated and described by Welch and Nuttall in 1892 after its isolation from a human cadaver. It was named as *Bacillus perfringens* in 1898.

Properties of the genus

1. *Morphology: C. perfringens* are gram positive, straight rods measuring 2-6 μm in length and 0.8-1.5 μm in width. It occurs in single, pair or short chain. The bacteria are capsulated, non-motile and sporulating. The endospores are oval, central or sub-terminal in position and usually bulge the side of the bacillus. However, it is an inefficient sporulator. The spores are rarely found in the exudates.

2. *C. perfringens* is not a strict anaerobe (aerotolerant) unlike other clostridia.

3. *Resistance:* The spores are killed by boiling for 5 minutes. Type A and C of the bacteria produce little heat-resistant spores that can survive 100°C for 1 hour.

4. *Natural habitat*: It is one of the most ubiquitous anaerobic bacterium found in the environment. It is frequently isolated from soil, gastrointestinal tract of healthy man (10^3-10^4 c.f.u. per gram of faeces) and animals (carnivores and omnivores). During infection, more number of bacteria (10^9c.f.u./gm of faeces) is produced due to multiplication under favourable condition.

5. *Genome*: *C. perfringens* was the first gram-positive bacterium for which a genetic map was elucidated. It has a single circular 3.6 Mbp sized chromosome. The chromosome contains origin of replication (*oriC*) and 10 rRNA operons on either side. Several genes encoding extracellular toxins are clustered within a 250-kb region near *oriC*. Five toxin types of *C. perfringens* have similar genome organization. Acquisition or loss of toxin gene is responsible for difference in toxin production pattern by different types of *C. perfringens*.

Isolation, growth and colony characteristics

C. perfringens requires enriched medium for the growth. Blood agar, Robertson cooked meat broth (RCM) can be used for the isolation of the organism. The broth should be boiled at 100°C to reduce free oxygen and then cooled at 37°C prior to the inoculation. The clinical samples are inoculated into the blood agar or RCM and incubated anaerobically at 37°C. Sometimes 2-10% CO_2 can enhance the growth. An anaerobic jar with catalyst, indicator for anaerobic condition and an attachment delivering H_2 and CO_2 are satisfactory for the isolation.

The colonies are round, smooth, convex, 2-3 mm in diameter. The colonies are surrounded by a narrow zone of complete haemolysis and a wide zone of partial haemolysis (double haemolysis) in blood agar. Alpha and theta toxins of the bacteria can produce this type of haemolysis specially with sheep and ox red blood cells. Specifically, alpha and theta toxins are responsible for the outer and inner zone of haemolysis, respectively.

Biochemical characteristics

C. perfringens produces following biochemical reactions that can be used for detection of the organism.

Biochemical test	Expected result
Catalase	(-ve)
Oxidase	(-ve)
Indole	(-ve)
Casein digestion	(+ve)
Gelatin hydrolysis	(+ve)
Carbohydrate fermentation	
Glucose	(+ve)
Lactose	(+ve)
Sucrose	(+ve)
Maltose	(+ve)
Lecithinase production (in Egg Yolk Agar)	(+ve) Nagler reaction: The egg yolk agar plate is equally halved. In one half, 1% lecithinase antitoxin is added, other half remains free. Now the culture is streaked in both the halves. In antitoxin free part, 'zone of opalescence' is produced surrounding the colony due to lecithinase production by the bacteria. Whereas, in antitoxin added part, no such reaction is observed.
Lipase production (in Egg Yolk Agar)	(-ve)
Litmus milk	'Stormy clot' formation or 'stormy fermentation': Litmus milk medium contains lactose and casein. This sugar is fermented by C. perfringens to produce acid. This acid can coagulate casein and changes the pH (colour change is indicated by litmus as blue to pink). The acid clot is then broken by gas formation producing the 'stormy' appearance.

Antigenic characteristics: *C. perfringens* possesses somatic and polysachharide capsular antigens.

Toxins and virulence factors

Toxins

C. perfringens produces four major (α, β, ε, ι) and eight minor toxins (γ, δ, η, θ, κ, λ, μ, ν). On the basis of the major toxin production it can be classified into five toxinotypes i.e. A, B, C, D and E. It is noted that the bacteria can also produce enterotoxin (*C. perfringens* enterotoxin), *C. perfringens* β-2 toxin, *C. perfringens* necrotic enteritis toxin B-like (Net-B).

Alpha-toxin (α-toxin): It is a major toxin produced by all types (A, B, C, D, E) of *C. perfringens.* It is the first toxin identified as enzyme (lecithinase or phospholipase-C). It is a 43 KDa protein comprising 370 amino acids. It is encoded by *plc* gene. The protein comprises two domains. N-terminal domain (1-246th amino acid) is the active site of the enzyme and C-terminal domain (256-370th amino acid) helps in anchoring the toxin with the cell membrane (Ca^{++} dependent phospholipid binding). The N-terminal domain is responsible for the lysis of phosphatidyl choline (lecithin) and sphingomyelin, thus it acts as 'lecithinase'. It is also responsible for the 'Nagler's reaction'. The C-terminal domain makes the toxin lethal and haemolytic on red blood cells (except horse and goat). It is a 'hot-cold haemolysin' like *Staphylococcus* β-haemolysin. Incomplete haemolysis at 37°C is completed at below 10°C temperature. Alpha toxin is the major *C. perfringens* toxin responsible for gangrene. This toxin also helps *C. perfringens* to escape macrophage mediated phagocytosis and survive in the host tissues.

Beta toxin (β-toxin): The toxin is the major virulence factor of *C. perfringens* type B and C. It is heat labile and protease (trypsin) sensitive. The toxicity is restricted among the newborns in which the protease activity of the intestinal tract is comparatively low. It is a 34.8 Kda protein containing 336 amino acids. The gene encoding the toxin (*cpb*) is located in a plasmid containing the insertion sequence (IS*1151*).The toxin is dermonecrotic and lethal, not haemolytic. Edema and dermonecrosis is associated with the stimulation of sensory nerve ending releasing tumour necrosis factor (TNF-α). It is a pore forming toxin (PFT). It can produce cation selective pores in the phospholipid bilayer of the cell membrane.

Epsilon toxin (ε-toxin): It is a major toxin produced by *C. perfringens* type B and D. It is a 32.9 KDa protein, encoded by *etx* gene. It is secreated as inactive 'prototoxin'. It is activated by the protease enzyme (trypsin). So it has opposite characteristics of β-toxin. During its activation, the enzyme removes

40-42 amino acids from the protein. The size of the protein is reduced along with the conformational change. Specific glycoprotein receptor (34KDa) for the toxin is present on the cell membrane. A lipid environment is required for binding of the toxin with the receptor. After binding, the toxin produces anion selective pores on the cell membrane that changes the cellular permeability. The cell death occurs due to the necrosis, with reduction in nucleus size and without DNA fragmentation. The toxin induced cell signalling required for the necrosis is not fully understood. The epsilon toxin can alter the blood vascular endothelial cells and blood brain barrier. It can directly interact with the hippocampus neurons leading to the release of glutamate. The glutamate is responsible for the toxin induced nervous syndrome (excitation).

Iota toxin (ι-toxin): It is a binary toxin produced by *C. perfringens* type E. The toxin has two independent fragments (100 KDa and 45 kDa), not linked covalently. The larger fragment helps in binding of the toxin with the cell membrane, whereas, the smaller fragment has enzymatic activity. The binding and enzymatic components of the toxin are encoded by two closely linked genes (*ibp* and *iap*, respectively). The iota toxin is secreated as inactive protein. It is activated by proteolytic cleavage and removal of 20 KDa N-terminal peptide from the larger toxin fragment (100 Kda) and 9-11 N-terminal residues from the smaller toxin fragment (45 Kda). The active ‘binding component’ (80KDa) recognizes the specific receptor present in the cell membrane. Receptor mediated endocytosis of the enzymatic component takes place. The enzymatic component modifies cellular and muscular ‘actin’ molecules (ADP-ribosylation) and prevents polymerization of actin molecules. Due to actin depolymerisation, there is rounding of cells (*in vitro*), inhibition of leukocyte migration and activation, inhibition of smooth muscle contraction and cellular endocytosis. The iota- toxin producing *C. perfringens* type E causes enterotoxaemia in calves and other young animals.

Gamma –toxin (γ-toxin): It is a minor lethal toxin produced by *C. perfringens* type B and C. It is not histotoxic.

Delta toxin (δ-toxin): It is a 32 KDa protein, produced by type B and C of *C. perfringens.* It is a haemolysin, active against red blood cells of the even-toed ungulates (cattle, sheep, goat, pig). It is cytotoxic for macrophages and platelets. The cell surface receptor for the toxin is ganglioside (G_{M2}). It is also pore forming, but in contrast to β-toxin, it produces anion selective pores on the host cellular membrane. The delta toxin can potentiate the action of other toxins (β and ε).

Eta toxin (η-toxin): It is a minor lethal toxin produced by *C. perfringens* type A.

Theta toxin (θ-toxin / Perfringolysin): It is a 53 KDa protein, containing 472 amino acids. It is produced by most of the strains of *C. perfringens.* The gene encoding the toxin is '*pfoA*', found in the bacterial chromosome. It is a cholesterol dependent cytolysin like streptolysin-O, listeriolysin-O and other clostridial toxins. The toxin is elongated rod shaped, rich in β-sheets and hydrophilic. It contains four domains (1-4). The domain 4 binds with the cholesterol present in the cellular membrane. After the binding, there is a conformational change in other domains leading to assembly of 40-50 toxin monomers perpendicularly in the membrane. Later, it forms the membrane pore complex (300-450 Å diameter). The perfringolysin can potentiate the α-toxin in tissue necrosis during gangrene production. It contributes to the leukostasis in the blood vessels adjacent to the gangrenous lesions. It is toxic for leukocytes at high dose. It can also disrupt endothelial integrity causing local edema, systemic shock and multi organ failure.

Kappa toxin (κ-toxin): It is a type of collagenase (ColA) produced by some strains of *C. perfringens.* It is encoded by *colA* gene. It can also potentiate the alpha toxin in tissue destruction. Probably it is responsible for the 'pulpy muscle' observed in gas gangrene.

Lambda toxin (λ-toxin): It is a 36-kDa thermolysin-like zinc metalloprotease. It can lyse casein, gelatin, haemoglobin but not collagen. It is lethal and necrotizing. It is encoded by *lam* gene, found in plasmid. Exact role in disease production is not clear, but it can activate the major toxin (ε-toxin).

Mu toxin (μ-toxin): It is a hyaluronidase enzyme (endo-β-N-acetyl glucosaminidase) produced by *C. perfringens.* It is 114KDa protein and encoded by *nagH* gene, located in the bacterial chromosome.

Nu toxin (ν-toxin): It is a lethal deoxyribonuclease (DNAse).

C. perfringens β-2 toxin: It was first demonstrated in the *C. perfringens* isolated from a piglet that died of necrotic enteritis. The toxin is produced by all the toxinotypes of *C. perfringens.* It is a 27.6 KDa protein. The gene encoding the toxin is located in the same plasmid having the gene for beta toxin. Although, genetically both the toxins are unrelated and produce no immunological cross-reaction. *C. perfringens* can produce beta (β) and β-2 toxin separately or in combination. However, some common properties between both the toxins are sensitivity to trypsin, cytotoxicity for few cell types and production of necrotic enteritis.

C. perfringens necrotic enteritis toxin B-like (Net-B): It is produced by *C. perfringens* strains associated with avian necrotic enteritis. It is a 33 KDa protein, encoded by *netB* gene, located on an approximately 85 kbp plasmid.

Since the protein has similarity to *C. perfringens* β-toxin (38% similarity) it is designated as necrotic enteritis toxin, B-like (NetB). NetB is also a pore-forming toxin which produces plasma membrane pores with a pore diameter of 1.6-1.8 nm. The NetB pore diameter is slightly larger than the pore size produced by β-toxin (1.36-1.6 nm). The development of necrotic enteritis in chickens is dependent on the ability to produce functional NetB toxin.

Enterotoxin (C. perfringens enterotoxin): It is a 35.5 KDa protein, containing 319 amino acids. All *C. perfringens* strains, causing food poisoning in human, produce this toxin. During ingestion of the contaminated food, the bacteria may enter the stomach. Gastric acidity can kill most of them. The presence of 10^5 or more number of bacteria per gram of food can cause the infection. Multiplication and sporulation of the bacteria are prerequisite factors for this toxin production. The toxin is secreted during sporulation as inactive 'prototoxin'. It is activated by the trypsin enzyme. The toxin is encoded by '*cpe*' gene, located in either the bacterial chromosome or plasmid. The chromosomal *cpe* carrying strains are more resistant to heat, osmotic stress and associated with food poisoning.

The toxin can bind with its receptor (claudin) present at the cell to cell adhesion region ('tight junction'). The toxin and the receptor form an intermediate complex (135 KDa) which is followed by a large complex formation (200KDa). During the large complex formation, the toxin is inserted deep into the cell membrane. The large complex generates pore on the membrane. In addition, the large complex removes 'occludin' protein in the tight junction between two adjacent cells and increases the paracellular permeability. It is responsible for the intestinal fluid accumulation, epithelial cell desquamation, alteration of the intestinal motility and thus it causes diarrhoea. The enterotoxigenic *C. perfringens* can also cause antibiotic induced diarrhoea, chronic non-food borne diarrhoea in human and diarrhoea in pigs and foals.

Toxino types of *C. perfringens* and their major toxin production

Toxin / C. perfringens type	Type A	Type B	Type C	Type D	Type E
A	+	+	+	+	+
B	-	+	+	-	-
E	-	+	-	+	-
I	-	-	-	-	+

Virulence factors of *C. perfringens*

Virulence factors	Function
Neuraminidase	Neuraminidases are two types- small and large and they are encoded by nanH and nanI gene, respectively. Both can hydrolyze the sialic acid residues located on mammalian cell membranes.
'Bursting factor'	It causes typical muscle lesion in gas gangrene.
'Circulating factor'	It increases adrenaline sensitivity of the capillary membrane and prevents phagocytosis

Pathogenesis

C. perfringens type A

Necrotic Enteritis (Poultry): In poultry, *C. perfringens* type A is mainly transmitted from the environment, contaminated feed, water or any part of the broiler production unit in a farm. It is detected in eggshell fragments, chicken fluff and paper pads used to transport the chicks in the hatchery. Wild birds can also excreate the bacteria through the droppings to contaminate the environment.

The presence of the bacteria in the intestinal tract of the poultry is not the ultimate reason for the disease development. Predisposing factors like intestinal damage by *Coccidia* and diet are also important. The intestinal damage can release the plasma proteins into the lumen of the intestinal tract. The plasma proteins enhance the bacterial multiplication. The diet with high levels of water-soluble non-starch polysaccharides (rich in rye, wheat and barley) is known to increase the viscosity of the intestinal contents which can predispose to the disease.

Gas Gangrene: In human and animals, wound contamination (direct contact with contaminated soil and faeces) with *C. perfringens* type A and other clostridia causes 'gas gangrene' (clostridial myonecrosis). The injection wound in horses makes them susceptible for wound infection (malignant edema). Tissue damage in the muscle takes place by the bacterial toxins. Alpha toxin of *C. perfringens* plays primary role in pathogenesis in the following way:

- Lytic action of alpha toxin on phospholipid produces diacyl glycerol and ceramide that stimulates arachidonic cascade causing local edema and vasoconstriction. Vasoconstriction reduces the blood flow in the affected tissue causing rapid destruction.
- The toxin also enhances expression of adhesin molecules (ICAM-1) in the vascular endothelium causing hyper adhesion of leukocytes in the endothelium. It also helps in blockade of the blood vessel.
- The toxin produces superoxide anion via stimulation of a protein kinase.

The above mentioned conditions create anoxia (reduced O_2 tension) in the tissue promoting the clostridial growth and tissue necrosis. Other toxins such as kappa (collagenase) and mu (hyaluronidase) also helps in spreading the toxin and tissue necrosis. The leukocytes are not found in the gas gangrene lesion probably due to the leukocidin nature of alpha, theta and nu toxin of *C. perfringens*. The tissue necrosis is aided by gas formation due to bacterial fermentation. The pockets of gas produce sufficient pressure to interfere with the venous return from the muscle.

Haemorrhagic abomasitis: The calves can get the infection through ingestion of *C. perfringens* contaminated colostrum. Feeding large amount of frozen colostrum often results the condition (haemorrhagic abomasitis) in an organized dairy farm.

Necrotic Enteritis (Pig): The sows are the major source of the infection to the piglets during the first week after birth. Contaminated feed acts as the additional source. Pathogenesis is poorly understood. Attachment and invasion of the bacteria is uncommon. *C. perfringens* β-2 toxin plays important role in pathogenesis. The enterotoxin also causes villous necrosis and fluid secreation in the intestinal lumen.

Food Poisoning: In human, consumption of contaminated food (cooked poultry meat or beef, if stored for a long time after cooking without refrigeration) results 'food poisoning'. Failure to refrigerate after cooking may cause germination of spores and multiplication of vegetative cells. The vegetative cells sporulate in the gut and release enterotoxin after consumption.

C. perfringens type B

In the lambs, the infection can take place from the dam or the contaminated feed, drinking water and other environmental sources. The predisposing factors favour the rapid bacterial multiplication in the gut with production and absorption of large amount of the toxins (β-toxin). Excess milk consumption, migration of sheep to highland pasture during summer (hilly area) is associated with the disease.

C. perfringens type C

The faeco-oral route is the major transmission way in piglets (12 hours-3 days old). Small number of clostridia may eliminate other bacteria form the piglet intestine or there is absence of the established intestinal flora. Sudden change of diet also alters the existing intestinal flora. So, the clostridia can readily colonize the gut after entry. Piglet to piglet transmission can take place. Spores remain viable in the environment for the prolonged period.

After entry within the host, *C. perfringens* type C adheres with the jejunum at villous apices. It causes desquamation of the area. The bacterial proliferation occurs along the basement membrane. Proliferating bacteria liberate toxins (β and β-2 toxin). The beta toxin is lethal, necrotizing and causes tissue damage. The piglets are deficient in pancreatic secretion (containing protease) and the colostrums are rich in protease inhibitor. So, the beta toxin which is protease sensitive remains active in colostrums fed piglets. The toxin causes necrosis of the villous lamina propria. It is followed by necrosis of crypts, submucosa and muscular layer. The bacteria are shed into the intestinal lumen. The death of the lamb occurs due to intestinal damage and toxaemia. Beta toxin increases the capillary permeability which helps in the passage of the toxin into the blood circulation.

C. perfringens type D

In sheep, it is associated with the disproportionate growth and toxin production of *C. perfringens* type D that is normally present in the healthy gut as commensal. Due to change in diet from poor quality to palatable or continuous concentrate feeding, the rumen cellulose degrading bacteria are destroyed. Undigested feed, containing the starch passes into the intestine, which favours the growth of *C. perfringens* type D. So, the nfection is also known as 'overeating disease'. Continuous concentrate feeding reduces the acidity of the stomach and also favours the bacterial growth. After multiplication, the bacteria release epsilon (ε) toxin in the intestinal lumen as inactive prototoxin. Presence of digestive enzymes (trypsin and chymotrypsin) activates the toxin. The epsilon toxin has no direct effect on the intestinal mucosa. However, it is absorbed from the lumen into the blood circulation due to increased permeability of the mucosa. It can cross blood brain barrier and can interact with the hippocampus neurons leading to the release of glutamate. It is responsible for the toxin induced nervous syndrome (excitation) and sudden death. Other organs like lungs and kidneys are also affected. The kidney shows pulpy appearance during post mortem due to autolysis of the already damaged tissue by the toxin. So, the disease is also known as 'pulpy kidney disease'.

C. perfringens type E

It releases iota (ι) toxin that plays major role in the pathogenesis.

Disease produced

Bacteria	Host	Disease produced
C. perfringens type A	Poultry	Necrotic Enteritis: Sudden death (50% mortality rate) is the major feature. Clinical signs include depression, dehydration, ruffled feather, diarrhoea. Liver, kidney, caeca become thin walled, friable, filled with gas, covered with pseudo membrane. Cholangiohepatitis: It is the subclinical form of the infection, characterized by the focal necrosis of the intestinal mucosa, enlarged liver with a pale reticular pattern or sometimes with pale and stellate foci. Decreased feed consumption, weight gain is found.
	Human and animals	Gas Gangrene (Clostridial Myonecrosis): Wound contamination results gas gangrene. Incubation period varies from 24 hours-several days. Pain develops which is associated with edema, formation of gas bubble in the tissue, haemorrhagic exudates. The area becomes black. Toxaemia and shock may occur.
	Calves	Haemorrhagic abomasitis: Affected calves die rapidly showing bloating. Abomasum is dilated with thickened walls and folds. Severe necrosis with micro colonies of the bacteria is found. Mucosa and sub-mucosa are filled with gas bubble.
	Pigs	Necrotic Enteritis: It is characterized by the non-haemorrhagic mucoid diarrhoea in suckling and feeder pigs. Lesions are usually severe in small intestine, particularly jejunum and ileum. Mucosal necrosis may involve epithelium and lamina propria, but in contrast to type-C infection, it rarely affects other layers of the intestine. Pseudomembranous enteritis is also noted in piglets
	Neonatal foal	Haemorrhagic Diarrhoea
	Dogs	Haemorrhagic Canine Gastroenteritis
	Human	Food Poisoning: It is characterized by diarrhoea, vomition and general malaise. It is self limiting. Symptoms typically resolve within 24 hours
C. perfringens type B	Lambs (1-2 week old)	Lamb Dysentery: Haemorrhagic and fatal enterotoxaemia of lambs that is characterized by abdominal pain, bloody diarrhoea, recumbancy, coma or sudden death.
	Goats, calves, foals	Haemorrhagic Enteritis

Bacteria	Host	Disease produced
C. perfringens type C	Piglets (12 hours-3 days old)	Haemorrhagic or Necrotic Enterotoxaemia: Acute form is characterized by intense abdominal pain, depression and bloody diarrhoea, which begins 8 to 22 hours after exposure. It lasts for 1-2 days. Chronic form continues for 1-2 weeks with persistent diarrhoea without blood and dehydration. Fibrinonecrotic (pseudomembranous) enteritis with emphysema is found in jejunum.
	Lambs (1-10 days old), calves, foals, chicken	Haemorrhagic or Necrotic Enterotoxaemia (enteritis): In addition to other signs like piglets, tetany and opisthotonos are found (nervous syndrome).
	Sheep	'Struck': It is restricted to UK only. Sudden death of sheep occurs (like struck by lightning) due to toxaemia. Mucosal necrosis occurs without diarrhoea. Damaged ruminal or abomasal mucosa by rough feed encourages bacterial invasion.
	Children	Enteritis necroticans (Pigbel): It is found in Asia, Africa and characterized by segmental necrosis of the jejunum along with a high mortality rate if not diagnosed early.
C. perfringens type D	Sheep	Classical Enterotoxaemia (Sudden death, Pulpy kidney disease; Overeating Disease): It is found throughout the world in almost all age group of sheep (3-10 weeks old). It is characterized by mild diarrhea, convulsion, blindness, head pressing and sudden death.
	Goat	Enterotoxaemia: It is characterized by haemorrhagic enterocolitis without pulpy kidney.
C. perfringens type E	Lamb, calf, rabbit	Enterotoxaemia: Haemorrhagic necrotic enteritis occurs.
	Dog, Pig	Enteritis
Untyped *C. perfringens*	Cattle, Camel, rabbit, elk, cats and human	Enteritis in cattle, enterotoxemia in camels, enteritis in rabbits, enteritis in wild elk, cats and milk-borne disease in humans.

Immunity: The immunity to the infection is anti toxin antibody mediated.

Diagnosis

Clinical samples: The clinical samples include diarrhoeic faeces, intestinal contents of the affected animals and birds, liver, kidney, and caeca of poultry.

Laboratory Examinations

Direct Examination: Examination of smears of intestinal mucosa and intestinal contents reveals many large, gram-positive bacilli. A few of them may produce spores.

Isolation of bacteria from clinical samples: Media, incubation condition and colony characteristics are described earlier. The colonies can also be confirmed by tube biochemical tests or commercial system (API system).

Double haemolysis produced by the *C. perfringens* (98% isolates) is unique characteristics for its identification. The bacterial count should be 10^8-10^9 cfu / gm of the collected specimen to correlate with the etiology of the symptoms.

Immunological test: Commercial ELISA kits are available for the detection of *C. perfringens* enterotoxin and beta (β) toxin as antigen. The beta toxin is protease sensitive and highly labile. So, the negative finding is inconclusive.

Detection of toxins: *In vivo* assay for the toxin demonstration is currently not a common practice.

a) *Mice protection test*: For lethal activity, the supernatant of suspected culture or intestinal content (treated with trypsin and specific antitoxin) is injected intravenously into the laboratory mice (0.5 ml / mice). If there is no death of the mice within stipulated time, it is assumed that specific antitoxin neutralizes the toxin. Accordingly the toxin type is identified.

b) For necrotizing activity, suspected culture supernatant or intestinal content is injected intradermally into the guinea pigs for dermonecrosis.

c) *C. perfringens* enterotoxin can be detected by Vero cell assay.

Detection of the toxin does not confirm the existence of the infection. Often false negative results can take place as these toxins are highly labile (*C. perfringens* β toxin).

Molecular biology:

a) Colony DNA-DNA hybridization is an efficient technique to detect different toxins of *C. perfringens* including enterotoxin, sialidase.

b) Multiplex PCR is developed for the detection of the *C. perfringens* toxins including the enterotoxin. Generally all the toxin genes are expressed to produce the toxin [except enterotoxin gene (*cpe*) in *C. perfringens* type E]. The PCR can detect up to 5×10^2 cfu clostridia per gram of faeces.

Prevention and Control

Hygienic measures should be maintained during parturition, shearing of wool, castration and docking of the animals. Anti-*C. perfringens* antiserum can be used in sheep during clostridial outbreak as control measure. Type-B *C. perfringens* antiserum can produce cross-protection against type-C as both of them produce β-toxin. Anaphylaxis may occur during administration of equine origin antiserum. The animals should be monitored at least for 24 hours after administration of antiserum. The pregnant ewes should be vaccinated during the outbreak to transfer the passive immunity into the lambs. The ewes require at least two weeks to generate protective antibodies in the colostrum.

Vaccination of healthy ewes and sows is preferred in endemic zones for clostridial enterotoxaemia. The vaccination should be done with one / two month gap and the last dose should be given 2-3 weeks before parturition. Subsequently the ewes are vaccinated once just before lambing.

Pulpy kidney disease can be controlled by vaccination, administration of antitoxin and reduction of the food intake. Activated alum-precipitated toxoid or multivalent bacterin-toxoid is commonly used as vaccine in healthy sheep and calves in endemic zones. Presence of 0.15 Wellcome unit of epsilon antitoxin per milliliter of serum is protective to the sheep. Vaccination should be done at the base of the ear of sheep to avoid skin damage. Vaccination with toxoid against clostridial epsilon-toxin is not preferred in goats due to variable results. During outbreak, the antitoxin and toxoid are administered together. The toxoid is repeated after one month of the outbreak to the surviving animals, as the antitoxin is protective for one month only.

Clostridium tetani

In the old literatures of Hippocrates ('Corpus Hyppocraticum'), 'tetanus', caused by *Clostridium tetani* was mentioned. The 'tetanus' was originated from the Greek word 'tetanos' means 'contracture'. In 1884, Nicolaier first described the organism *Clostridium tetani* as long slender rods, isolated from the experimental rabbits inoculated with the garden soil. In 1889, Kitasato first isolated the organisms in pure culture. In 1890, Emil Von Behring and Kitasato demonstrated the toxic properties of the organisms. They also demonstrated that the animals can be immunized with tetanus toxin attenuated by iodine tri-chloride. The sera contained neutralizing antibodies against the tetanus toxin.

Properties of genus

1. *Morphology*: *C. tetani* are long, slender, gram positive rods measuring 2-4 µm in length and 0.5 µm in width with rounded ends. Filamentous forms are also found. The older cultures may appear as gram negative. They are non-capsulated, sluggish motile by peritrichous flagella and readily sporulating. The matured endospore is spherical, terminal and the presence of spore bulges the bacterium. The terminal spore containing

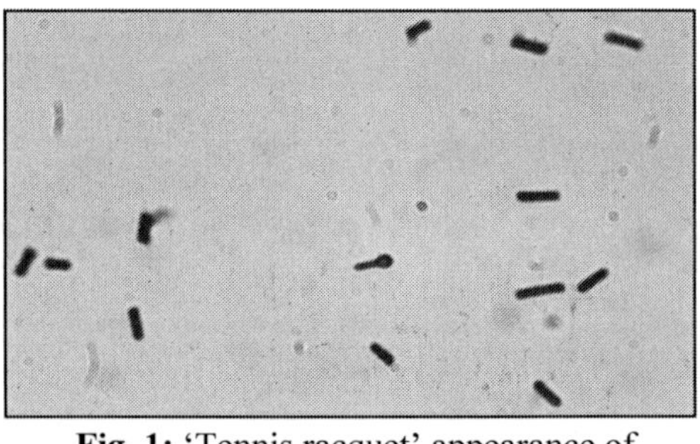

Fig. 1: 'Tennis racquet' appearance of *Clostridium tetani*
(*Courtesy*: Thomas Walton and Erica Suchman, American Society for Microbiology)

bacteria looks like 'drumstick' or 'tennis racket'. Sometimes the spores are sub-terminal producing 'dumb-bell appearance' (Figure 1).

2. *C. tetani* is a strict anaerobe

3. *Resistance*: The spores can tolerate the boiling for 15 minutes to two hours. Some strains are susceptible to moist heat (autoclave) and dry heat (hot air oven). Some strains can resist 5% phenol (for 10 days), lysol and formalin. The bacteria are susceptible to halogen compounds like 3% iodine and 10% hydrogen peroxide. In low oxygen tension (oxidation reduction potential below +0.01, e.g. wound in the body), the spores can germinate and the resultant vegetative bacteria multiply and can liberate the toxin.

4. *Natural habitat: C. tetani* resides in the soil and the intestine of man and animals like horses, cattle and sheep. Spores are commonly found in the alkaline soil that is rich in manure (human and animal faeces) and calcium. Uncultivated land and acidic volcanic soil rich in granite is more or less free of the spores. Spores are also present in the house dust, clothing etc. The house dust helps in rapid dissemination of the spores.

5. *Genome:* The genome of *C. tetani* consists of a 2,799,250 bp chromosome encoding approximately 2,372 genes. The tetanus toxin and the collagenase are encoded by a 74,082 bp plasmid. Some genes (collagenase, tetanolysin) are observed to be common between *C. tetani* and *C. perfringens*. The genome (G+C) content is 25-26 mol %.

Isolation, growth and colony characteristics

Blood agar and RCM are used for isolation of *C. tetani.* The optimum incubation temperature is 37°C, with the range of 14-44°C. RCM is also used for preservation of the culture. Pure anaerobic condition like 85% nitrogen, 10% hydrogen and 5% carbon dioxide is required for the isolation. In blood agar, round, translucent, grey, 2-4 mm diameter colonies are produced. Sometimes the edges of the colonies are filamentous producing 'fuzzy appearance'. The edges may further spread and produce a thin film over the surface (swarming). Individual colonies are found in the media with higher agar concentration (3%). Haemolysis is found beneath the colonies in the blood agar. In RCM, blackening of the meat particles is observed (proteolytic strains).

Biochemical characteristics

C. tetani produces following biochemical reactions that can be used for detection of the bacteria

Biochemical test	Expected result
Catalase	(-ve)
Oxidase	(-ve)
Indole	(+ve)
Casein digestion	(-ve)
Gelatin hydrolysis	(+ve) [slow]
Hydrogen sulphide	(+ve)
Carbohydrate fermentation	(-ve)
Litmus milk	(-ve) or delayed fermentation

Antigenic characteristics

C. tetani possesses somatic (heat stable) and flagellar (heat labile) antigens. On the basis of flagellar antigen, 10 serotypes are detected. The serotypes are designated by the Roman numerals (I, II, III, IV etc.). The serotype VI is non-flagellated. All the serotypes produce same type of toxin. Two types of somatic antigens are found, one is shared by all the serotypes, and the other is present in few serotypes (II, IV, V, IX) only.

Toxins and virulence factors produced

Toxins

C. tetani produces two kinds of toxins known as 'tetanus neurotoxin' (TeNT, tetanospasmin) and 'tetanolysin'.

Tetanus neurotoxin' (TeNT): It has structural similarity with the botulinum toxin. Both are secreated as an inactive precursor from the bacterial cell. The precursor toxins are activated by proteolytic cleavage either by clostridial protease or the protease present in the intestinal tract of the host animals. The active neurotoxin consists a light chain (50 KDa) and a heavy chain (100 KDa) joined by a disulfide bridge. It is encoded by *tox* gene present in a 75 Kbp plasmid.

C. tetani liberates the toxin in the wound after multiplication. The toxin diffuses into the extracellular fluid or passes through the lymph. It can target the nerve endings like sensory, adrenergic and motor neurons (motoneuron). Specific receptors at the nerve endings accept the TeNT. The receptors should contain ganglioside associated with a GPI anchored protein (15 KDa). Heavy chain domain of the toxin contains ganglioside binding ligands. After binding, the toxin enters through the receptor mediated endocytosis. The endocytic vesicles (non-acidified) can carry the toxin into the neurons of the spinal cord. The TeNT causes transynaptic migration and reaches the axon terminal. The terminal synapse into the motor neuron via acidified endocytic vesicles.

Acidified vesicles help in the release of light chain of the toxin into the cytosol of the neuron.

The light chain (Zinc mettaloprotease) of the toxin can cleave the 'synaptobrevin' (vesicular associated membrane protein, VAMP). Synaptobrevin is present in the synaptic vesicle membrane and helps in the neurotransmitter release. The cleavage prevents the release of inhibitory neurotransmitters like glycine and gamma amino butyric acid (GABA). Lack of inhibitory neurotransmitters causes the constant muscle contraction. It leads to 'tetanic spasm' causing tearing of tissues or breakdown of bones. Even only 0.09×10^{-3} μgm of toxin is lethal for a mouse (mouse lethal dose). Each milligram of toxin contains about 3×10^7 mouse lethal doses. The tetanus toxin affects both the somatic and autonomic nervous systems, but autonomic features (labile hypertension and tachycardia) are more common.

Tetanolysin: It is a cholesterol dependent cytolysin (48Kda) like streptolysin-O, listeriolysin-O and other clostridial toxins (perfringolysin). It is heat and oxygen labile. It can lyse a variety of cells such as erythrocytes, polymorphonuclear leukocytes, macrophages, fibroblasts, ascites tumour cells, HeLa cells and platelets. The toxin is lethal and cardiotoxic. It has no role in tetanus pathogenesis.

Pathogenesis

Transmission

Major route of transmission is wound or umbilicus contamination with the soil. Penetrating wounds produced by rusty nails, thorn or a dirty tissue abrasion is most preferred by the bacteria. Wounds produced during castration of goats and lambs are preferred site for the bacterial multiplication and toxin liberation. In underdeveloped rural areas, the castration is done by sharp bamboo made instruments. Ash or mud is later topically applied over the wound. This inhuman method is always at risk of getting the infection. *C. tetani* can also enter the uterus during dystocia in cattle and sheep.

Pathogenesis

Incubation period for tetanus in animals varies from 24 hours to 2 weeks. In the wounds or abraded tissues, anaerobic condition is produced with the help of facultative anaerobes. *C. tetani* spores can germinate in the favourable conditions. It produces vegetative bacteria. The vegetative form multiplies and liberates toxin (TeNT). The toxin spreads from the infected site (i) by diffusing into the adjacent muscle tissues, (ii) through the lymphatic system, or (iii) through the nerves. The toxin enters the blood circulation from the lymphatic system. Then it is distributed to all muscles and nerve endings. It attaches to a receptor (ganglioside and GPI anchored protein) on the nerve ending. A light chain fragment of the bound toxin is taken into the nerve cell. It enters the central nervous system by retrograde movement through the nerve axons. It prevents the release of inhibitory neurotransmitters like glycine and GABA (as described earlier). After the toxin-receptor binding, the antitoxin cannot neutralize the complex.

Two forms of tetanus are noted i.e. ascending and descending. In ascending form the toxin travels through the regional motor nerve of a limb. Signs are observed in the muscles of that limb. It spreads to the opposite limb and move upwards (ascending). This form is found in less susceptible animals (dog, cats). In descending form, the toxin circulates through the blood stream and enters into the nerve endings supplying head and neck. Consequently, the clinical signs are observed in the head and neck, followed by the limbs (descending). This form is found in more susceptible animals (horse, human) (Figure 2).

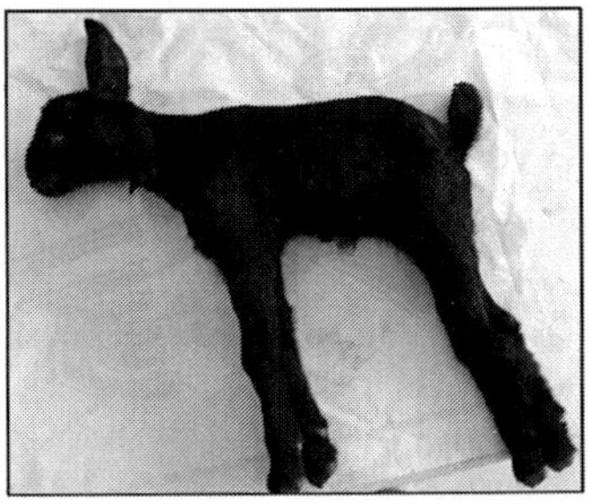

Fig. 2: A kid died due to tetanus (*Courtesy*: Shantanu Saha, Animal Resources Development Department, Government of West Bengal, India)

Disease produced

Bacteria	Host	Disease Produced
Clostridium tetani	Horses, lambs and human are most susceptible followed by adult sheep, goats and pigs. Dogs and cats suffer from the disease rarely. Poultry are relatively resistant. Variation in susceptibility occurs probably due to variation in toxin susceptibility among the species, difference in diet and management practices which favours the wound contamination.	**Tetanus (locked jaw):** It is initially characterized by mild stiffness, unwillingness to move. After 24 hours, general stiffness of the limbs, head and neck is found. In later stage of the disease, muscle rigidity extends from the limb to the trunk, dilation of nostril, erection of ear, protrusion of nictitating membrane followed by respiratory failure. At the terminal stage hypotension, pulmonary edema develops. Pneumonia is the most common cause of the death. The infected animals cannot open their mouth, so it's also known as 'locked jaw'.

Immunity: Blood brain barrier, uterine and intestinal barriers of the body offers major resistance against the tetanus neurotoxin (TeNT). The macrophages are the first line of defence against *C. tetani*. The toxin interfere the lysozyme release from the macrophages. In surviving patient, natural immunity against *C. tetani* is poor. As the immunogenic part of the toxin produced is very low in quantity and the toxin after production readily binds with its receptors and become unavailable to the host system for generation of the immunity. In the endemic zone, high level of tetanus antitoxin in sera of unvaccinated population is found. It occurs due to prolonged ingestion of *C. tetani* spores.

Diagnosis

Clinical samples: Necrotic tissues from the wound, exudate can be collected as clinical specimens. However tetanus is diagnosed on the basis of history, clinical signs. Laboratory examination aids confirmation.

Laboratory examination

Direct examination: The smear is prepared from the exudate, tissues and is stained by Gram's Method. Predominance presence of gram positive rods with 'drumstick appearance' in the microscopic field is observed. It is not confirmatory, as drumstick appearance is also shown by *Clostridium tetanomorphum* and *Clostridium tetanoides.*

Isolation of bacteria from clinical samples: Media, incubation condition and colony characteristics are described.

Detection of toxins: *In-vivo* assay for the toxin demonstration is currently not a common practice. Previously lethal activity of the toxin was demonstrated by the mice protection test. The toxin present in the suspected culture filtrate is injected intramuscularly at hind leg (0.2 ml) of the laboratory mice. Tetanus antitoxin is injected two hours earlier in those mice except controls. If there is no death of the mice within stipulated time, it is assumed that the antitoxin neutralizes the toxin. In control mice (without antitoxin), the signs of tetanic spasm are developed at the site of the inoculation.

Molecular biology: A real-time PCR is developed to detect a fragment of the neurotoxin gene of *C. tetani* (TeNT) during investigation of wound infection among illegal drug users in UK. The assay is sensitive, specific and rapid to perform.

Prevention and Control

Proper hygiene, sterile environment and disinfection of the instruments should be maintained during castration, shearing and docking of the animals. Tetanus antitoxin (1500 IU) can provide short-term immunity for 10-15 days. In injured animals the tetanus toxoid can be administered along with the antitoxin preferably at the different site. Rarely the serum hepatitis may be developed in horses receiving the antitoxin.

Formalin-inactivated adjuvinated toxoids are available to provide long-term immunity to the horses and sheep. Cattle are only vaccinated in endemic zone. The toxoid is administered in two doses with 3-6 weeks gap and it can provide the immunity for 1-5 years. Pregnant animals require a booster 5-6 weeks before parturition to transfer the immunity to the offspring through the colostrum.

Clostridium botulinum

Emile van Ermengem (1895) first isolated the bacteria from homemade raw salted ham during investigation of a food borne outbreak in Ellezelles (Belgium). He also established that food borne botulism was intoxication, not an infection, and that the toxin was produced by a spore-forming obligate anaerobic bacterium.

Properties of the genus

1. *Morphology*: *C. botulinum* is gram positive rod measuring 4-6 µm in length and 1 µm in width. It occurs in single, pair or chain. Older cultures are gram negative. They are non-capsulated, sluggishly motile by peritrichous flagella and sporulating. The endospores are oval, situated sub-terminally but sometimes may occur terminally or centrally (Figure 3).
2. *C. botulinum* is a strict anaerobe.
3. *Classification*: *C. botulinum* belongs to the family Clostridiaceae. It consists of four phylogenetically and physiologically distinct groups, known as group I, II, III and IV. Group I (proteolytic) and group II (non-proteolytic) *C. botulinum* are major causes of food borne botulism in human, cattle, horse, and chicken. Group III *C. botulinum* infects waterfowls, cattle, horses, sheep and dogs. Whereas, group IV *C. botulinum* affects human only in Argentina. In some literature, it is renamed as *C. argentinense.*
4. *Resistance*: The spores of *C. botulinum* vary in heat resistance. Group I *C. botulinum* spores require rigorous sterilization. Canned food items are heated at 121°C for 3 minutes to eliminate the group I (proteolytic) spores by a factor of 10^{12} (12 log reduction in numbers of spore). It is known as 'botulinum cook' (12D process). Group II (non-proteolytic) spores are less heat resistant and they can be eliminated by pasteurization (75°C-95°C). The packed food items are targeted to eliminate 10^6 group II spores (6D process). It can be achieved by heating at 90°C for 10 minutes or 85°C for 52 minutes or 80°C for 270 minutes. In pasteurized milk (80°C -85°C for a few minutes), the spores may be heat injured but are not killed. A few (0.1-1%) of these heat injured spores can germinate

with the help of milk lysozyme. Specially, the bovine milk lysozyme is heat stable in nature. The lysozyme enters through the spore coat and degrades the spore peptidoglycan. The water can enter into the spore and induces germination. However, pasteurization of milk by ultra-high temperature (135°C for 1-2 seconds) method can eliminate all kinds of *C. botulinum* spores.

5. *Natural habitat: C. botulinum* is commonly found in soils (majority are A, B toxin producers) of any region of the world and marine sediments. It is present in both cultivated and unproductive lands. In wetlands, the toxin type C, D, E, F, G producers are usually present. It can contaminate raw vegetables, fruits, hay, pastures which are grown or come in contact with the contaminated soil. The spores can also enter and reside the gastro intestinal tract of mammals, birds and fishes. It is less common in adult human intestinal tract due to the presence of *Clostridium* inhibiting bile acids.

6. *Genome:* Proteolytic (group I) *C. botulinum* genome comprises a chromosome (3.76-4.26 Mbp, 3650 coding sequences) and a bacteriocin-encoding plasmid (16.3 kbp, 19 CDSs). The genome (G+C) content is low (28.1-28.5 mol %). The neurotoxin encoding genes are located in the chromosome or a large plasmid. The genome of non-proteolytic *C. botulinum* (group II) is smaller (3.66-3.80 Mbp) than proteolytic *C. botulinum*, and the (G+C) mol% is also slightly lower (27.4– 27.5 mol %). The neurotoxin genes in non-proteolytic *C. botulinum* are located either in the chromosome or in the plasmid. The plasmid is also smaller than the plasmid of proteolytic strains.

Isolation, growth and colony characteristics

Strict anaerobic condition is required for isolation of *C. botulinum*. Proteolytic strains (group I) can grow and produce neurotoxins at as low as 12°C and at as high as 48°C temperature. The non-proteolytic strains (group II) are psychotropic. They can grow and produce neurotoxins at 3°C. Optimum incubation temperature is 25°C. Group III *C. botulinum* can grow between 15-40°C and for group IV *C. botulinum* optimum growth temperature is 37°C. The optimum pH for all types of *C. botulinum* is 7-7.6.

The common bacteriological media (blood agar and RCM) can be used for the isolation of *C. botulinum.*

In blood agar, the colonies are haemolytic, large, semi-transparent with irregular edges. Sometimes, the 'film' like growth is found. The colonies grown deep in the agar are fluffy. In cooked meat media, the proteolytic strains (group I) can produce black colour.

Biochemical characteristics

C. botulinum produces following biochemical reactions

Biochemical test	Expected result			
	Group I	Group II	Group III	Group IV
Catalase	(-ve)	(-ve)	(-ve)	(-ve)
Oxidase	(-ve)	(-ve)	(-ve)	(-ve)
Indole	(-ve)	(-ve)	variable	(-ve)
Casein digestion	(+ve)	(-ve)	(-ve)	(+ve)
Gelatin hydrolysis	(+ve)	(+ve)	(+ve)	(+ve)
Lipase production in egg yolk agar	(+ve)	(+ve)	(+ve)	(-ve)
Carbohydrate fermentation				
Glucose	(+ve)	(+ve)	(+ve)	(-ve)
Lactose	(-ve)	(-ve)	(-ve)	Not detected
Sucrose	(-ve)	(-ve)	(-ve)	(-ve)
Maltose	(+ve)	(+ve)	variable	Not detected

Antigenic characteristics: *C. botulinum* possesses somatic, flagellar and spore antigens. The group II *C. botulinum* are classified into six serotypes on the basis of antigenic variation. The antigen is also shared with *C. sporogenes*. There is no relation between the serotypes and the different types of toxin produced by *C. botulinum*.

Toxins and virulence factors produced

Toxin

C. botulinum produces 'botulinum neurotoxin' (BoNT), botunolysin, C2 and C3 toxins.

Botulinum neurotoxin (BoNT): It is considered as most potent biological toxin (mice lethal dose : < 0.01 ngm). It is heat labile. It is destroyed at 100°C for 20 minutes exposure. There are seven antigenic types of botulinum neurotoxin i.e. A, B, C1, D, E, F and G. Each antigenic type is classified into subtypes based on the toxin sequence variations. The seven types of neurotoxins are produced by different *C. botulinum* groups.

Neurotoxin production by different *C. botulinum* groups

C. botulinum groups	Neurotoxin type
Group-I	A, B, F
Group-II	B, E, F
Group-III	C, D
Group-IV	G

Some other Clostridia like *C. baritii* and *C. butyricum* can also produce F and E toxins, respectively. The neurotoxin is encoded by the bacteriophage. Probably the toxin gene is transferred by transduction to other clostridia.

The BoNT has structural similarity with the tetanus neurotoxin (TeNT). Both are secreated as an inactive precursor from the bacterial cell. The toxins are activated by clostridial protease or the protease present in the intestinal tract of the host animals. Active neurotoxin consists a light chain (50 KDa) and a heavy chain (100 KDa) joined by a disulfide bridge. *C. botulinum* can liberate the toxin in the food items like meat and dairy products kept for a long time. The toxin can enter the host intestine through oral route. Sometimes, the bacteria liberate the neurotoxin in the gut of the animals and birds after multiplication. The toxin undergoes transcytosis across the digestive mucosa. After diffusion into the extracellular fluid and bloodstream the toxins target the motor neuron endings. The toxin has specific receptor on demyelinated nerve endings. Like tetanus neurotoxin (TeNT) receptor, the receptor for BoNT also contains ganglioside associated with a membrane protein, although it varies for the different types of the BoNT. After binding with the receptor, BoNT is directly endocytosed through clathrin coated vesicles which can become acidified (unlike TeNT which enters through non-acidified vesicles during receptor mediated endocytosis). Acidification of the vesicles can cause conformational changes of the toxin and liberate the light chain into the cytosol of the motor neuron in the peripheral somatic and autonomic fibres. It has no direct effect on central nervous system (CNS) or spinal cord. Whereas, tetanus neurotoxin undergoes retrograde axonal transport until it reaches the CNS to enter the target neuron.

The light chain (Zinc mettaloprotease) of BoNT (B/D/F/G types) can cleave the 'synaptobrevin' (vesicular associated membrane protein, VAMP), which is present in the synaptic vesicle membrane and helps in the neurotransmitter release. Whereas, BoNT- A/E and BoNT/ C1 can cleave SNAP 25 (synaptosomal associated protein-25; part of SNARE) and syntaxin (nerve plasmalemma protein) with SNAP 25, respectively. These proteins are conserved for all species and help in 'docking and fusion' events in every cell. The cleavage of these proteins interferes the release of acetylcholine, causing 'flaccid paralysis'.

Botulinum neurotoxins (BoNT) and their receptors

BoNT types	Receptors
BoNT/A	SV2 (membrane protein of synaptic vesicle)
BoNT/B	Synaptotagmin II
BoNT/C	Ganglioside
BoNT/D	Phosphatidyl ethanolamine
BoNT/E	SV 2A and SV2B
BoNT/G	Synaptotagmin I and II

Botunolysin: It is a cholesterol dependent cytolysin like streptolysin-O, listeriolysin-O and other clostridial toxins (perfringolysin, tetanolysin). It has no role in 'botulism' production.

C2 and C3 toxin: The toxins are binary toxin and can cause ADP-ribosylation (like iota toxin of *C. perfringens*). They are produced by *C. botulinum* toxinotype C and D. The C2 toxin induces intestinal haemorrhage and pulmonary emphysema in birds.

Pathogenesis (Botulism)

Transmission

In animals and birds, the 'botulism' is caused by ingestion of botulinum neuro toxin (BoNT) along with the feed.

Cattle

The cattle may obtain the botulinum neurotoxin (BoNT) from different feeds like carcasses of the animals, hay or silage, poultry litter, malt etc. Ingestion of toxin directly is known as 'intoxication'. In phosphorus deficient areas, the cattle may develop an abnormal appetite for unconventional items like bone and flesh (Pica). In these areas, type D toxin producing *C. botulinum* commonly resides in the gut by producing spores. After death of the animals (due to any cause) the spores may germinate into vegetative bacteria and liberate the toxin in the tissues. Ingestion of the flesh along with the toxin produces 'botulism' in cattle; known as 'lamsiekte' (South Africa), 'lame sickness', 'bulbar paralysis' (Australia), 'loin disease' (USA). As it is associated with lameness due to phosphorus deficiency, so it is called 'lame sickness'. The toxin entering through the oral route is more lethal probably due to its activation by rumen microbes.

- Cattle botulism originated from ingestion of hay or silage with type C-botulinum neurotoxin is known as 'forage poisoning'. Contamination of the hay or silages takes place through the carcasses of the animals (cat, wild rodents). The toxin from the decomposed carcass diffuses into the surrounding hay/silage and persists for a long time.
- Poultry litters are used in cattle feed and beddings. The litter contains faeces and carcass remnants, both of which may contain the toxin (type C or D).

Horses and foals: In horses, 'forage poisoning' can occur like the cattle. It is primarily produced by type C or D toxin. In foals (3-8 weeks of age) the bacteria enter the host through the oral route, multiply in the gut and liberate the toxin. It is called 'toxicoinfection'. The foals, originating from the mares maintained in high nutritious diet, are more susceptible to the toxicoinfection.

Poultry: In poultry, the botulism outbreaks occur in backyard as well as organized broiler farms, specially kept on deep litter system. It occurs due to type A and C toxins. The poultry may acquire the toxin through cannibalism of carcasses or ingestion of toxin containing larvae of blowfly and green bottle fly. Sometimes, infection of *C. botulinum* occurs through oral route followed by bacterial multiplication in the intestine and toxin liberation in the caecum.

Wild waterfowls: In wild waterfowl (e.g. ducks), the transmission of botulinum toxin takes place through the invertebrate carcasses. Aquatic and terrestrial invertebrates are killed by receding waters and flooding, respectively. *C. botulinum* can multiply and liberate the toxin in the carcasses (type C toxin) which is taken by the birds during feeding. It is known as 'microenvironment concept' of botulism transmission. After the onset of the outbreak, the dead birds also act as a source of the toxin. The fly larvae can survive on the carcasses. The waterfowls ingest the contaminated maggots and die. The carcass- maggot cycle continues.

Type E toxin producing *C. botulinum* is observed to cause mortality in other wild waterfowls (loon, gull, diving ducks). It occurs due to the ingestion of toxin containing fish carcasses.

Human: In human, ingestion of home preserved food items like fish, vegetables containing the toxin can cause botulism. Spores of the bacteria are heat resistant but the toxin is heat labile. So proper boiling of the food may reduce the chance of intoxication. In infants (less than 6 months old), 'toxicoinfection' may occur through the ingestion of spore contaminated food items (e.g. honey). It is called 'infant botulism' or 'floppy baby syndrome'. Probably the bacteria colonize in the infant gut due to the absence of protective micro flora and *Clostridium* inhibiting bile acids. *C. botulinum* toxin can also enter the human body through the inhalation of the toxin in powder form (used as bioweapon) and intramuscular injection of the toxin for therapy or drug abuse.

Pathogenesis

The toxin can enter the host intestine through oral route (intoxication). Sometimes the bacteria liberate the neurotoxin in the gut of animals and birds after multiplication (toxicoinfection). The toxin undergoes transcytosis across the digestive mucosa. After diffusion into the extracellular fluid and bloodstream the toxins target the motor neuron endings. The toxin interferes the release of acetylcholine (as described earlier) and causes flaccid paralysis..

Disease produced

Bacteria	Host	Disease Produced
Clostridium botulinum	Cattle	Forage poisoning: It is primarily caused by type C-botulinum toxin. It originates from ingestion of contaminated hay or silage. It is characterized by anorexia, incoordination, facial paralysis, difficulty in swallowing, death due to respiratory failure. 'Lamsiekte' (South Africa), lame sickness, bulbar paralysis (Australia), loin disease (USA): It is primarily caused by type D-botulinum toxin. It originates from ingestion of contaminated bone or flesh. Phosphorus deficiency causes abnormal appetite and forces the cattle to take the bone and flesh. It is characterized by drooling of saliva, inability to urinate, dysphagia, lateral recumbancy before death.
	Foals (3-8 weeks of age)	Shaker foal syndrome: It is caused by type C or D-botulinum toxin. It is a kind of toxicoinfection. It is characterized by sudden death of the foals without any symptom. Sometimes stilled gait, tremor and inability to stand for a few minutes followed by dyspnoea, extension of head and neck, tachycardia, respiratory failure before death is observed.
	Horse	Equine Botulism: It is commonly found in European countries. It is caused by type C and D toxin producers. It is characterized by muscle weakness and tremors, reduced tongue tone, slow chewing, salivation and difficulties in swallowing, drooping eyelids, mydriasis. It originates from the ingestion of contaminated fodder (haylage).
	Poultry	'Limberneck'/ 'Western duck sickness': It is caused by type C toxin. It is characterized by paralysis of face, wings, legs, neck and eyelids. 'Limberneck' means 'drooping of head 'or'neck paralyses.
	Wild waterfowls (loon, gull, diving ducks)	Botulism: It is caused by type C and E toxins. Clinical signs are same as 'Limberneck'.
	Human	Botulism: In adults the symptoms appear 18-36 hours after ingestion of the toxin. It is caused by type E toxin. It is characterized by nausea, vomiting, abdominal cramps or diarrhoea. The initial symptoms are dry mouth, blurring of vision and diplopia, followed by ptosis, ophthalmoplegia, dysarthria, and dysphagia. Death occurs due to paralysis of the respiratory muscles. Infant botulism: It occurs in children less than one year old. Constipation for consecutive 3 days is early sign followed by lethargy, difficulty in sucking and swallowing, weak cry, hypotonia, pooled oral secreations and loss of head control.

Immunity : Natural host defences against botulinum neurotoxin do not play any role in protection. The toxin is highly poisonous, so, the lethal dose is very small. Immunizing dose is always higher than the lethal dose. Therefore, before generation of the immunity the animal dies. Some birds like vultures can develop the acquired immunity through the repeated exposure of sub-lethal dose of the toxin.

Diagnosis

Clinical samples

Gastrointestinal contents, liver, wound exudate and serum from recently died animal carcasses or live animals, animal feed, suspected human food items can be collected for the detection of botulinum toxin or the bacteria. Detection of the toxin or the bacteria from the samples of the animal carcasses died long time ago is not valid. The bacterial spores present in the intestine of the animals may germinate after death of the animals and liberate the toxin. Anaerobic condition created in the carcasses favours the germination. So, positive findings cannot be correlated with the etiology.

Laboratory examination

Direct examination: The smear is prepared from the tissues or isolates and is stained by Gram's method. Predominance presence of gram-positive rods with single, pair or chain like arrangement and occasional sub-terminal spores in the microscopic field is observed. It is not confirmatory but aids in diagnosis.

Isolation of bacteria from clinical samples: Feedstuffs are macerated in normal saline and heated at 60-65°C for 30 minutes to destroy the contaminants and to germinate the *C. botulinum* spores. Type E toxin-producers require lysozyme treatment for spore germination.

Media, incubation condition and colony characteristics are described earlier.

Detection of toxins: For demonstration of toxin in feedstuffs it should be treated properly. It is macerated with normal saline and is kept overnight. On the next day it is centrifuged and the supernatant is filtered through 0.45 μm filter. The filtrate (prototoxin) is activated by trypsin. Activated toxin is injected intraperitoneally (0.5 ml) into the laboratory mice or guinea pigs. In positive cases, the characteristic abdominal breathing is observed within few hours to 5 days post inoculation.

Molecular biology: For testing a large number of samples collected during the animal botulism surveillance (type C and type D toxin-producers) a real time multiplex PCR is developed. The test is found 100% selective and accurate. The detection limit is 277 and 580 DNA copies for type C and type D toxin-producers, respectively.

Prevention and Control

Nutritional deficiencies of the livestock should be corrected with supplementation of phosphorus and proteins. Mono or polyvalent botulinum antiserum can be administered to foals (30000 IU) and adult horses (70000 IU) as therapy, but single dose is expensive. Few commercial bivalent toxoids (type B and C; type C and D) are available in different countries according to the prevalence of the toxin types. Vaccination of mares does not always transfer the immunity to the foals.

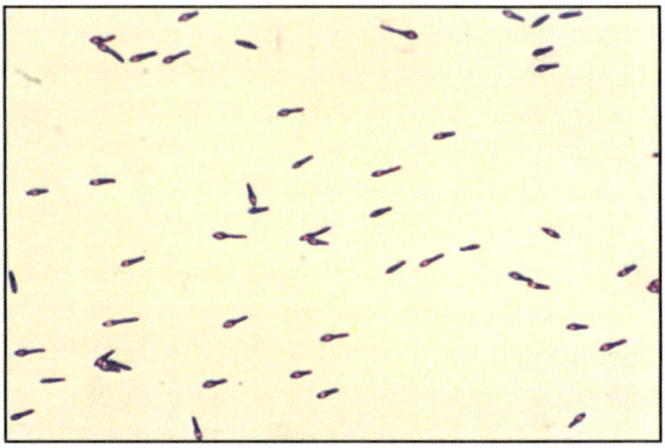

Fig. 3: Gram-positive spore bearing rods of *Clostridium botulinum*
(*Courtesy*: Kristen Catlin, American Society for Microbiology)

Clostridium chauvoei

Clostridium chauvoei is responsible for 'blackleg' (black quarter, Rauschbrand, Gerausch, charbon symptomatique) in cattle. In the middle of the 19th century, blackleg and malignant edema (caused by *Clostridium novyi*) were confused with anthrax. Bollinger (1875) first differentiated the causative organisms of blackleg and anthrax which was confirmed by Feser (1876). Previously the bacterium was named as *Clostridium feseri.* Arloing, Cornevin and Thomas described the blackleg bacterium in detail in 1880. In 1887, Roux first isolated the bacteria in the artificial media. The name *Clostridium chauvoei* was given in honour of the French veterinarian and bacteriologist Auguste Chauveau.

Properties of the genus

1. *Morphology*: *C. chauvoei* are gram positive, straight rods (cigar or lemon shaped) with rounded ends, measuring 3-8 μm in length and 0.5 μm in width. Older cultures may appear as gram negative. They are non-capsulated, motile by peritrichous flagella and sporulating. Oval endospores are found centrally or sub-terminally which may bulge the bacteria producing lemon / citron shape. Granular materials are sometimes found in one or both poles of the bacteria.

2. *C. chauvoei* is a strict anaerobe.
3. *Resistance*: The spores are resistant to desiccation and remain viable in the soil. The spores can also resist alcohol, phenol, quaternary ammonium disinfectants. It can be destroyed by boiling for 2-5 minutes, autoclaving and exposure to 3% formalin and lye for 15 minutes.
4. *Natural habitat:* Animal intestine, liver and other tissues are the major natural habitat of *C. chauvoei*. The spores can survive in the external environment specially in the soil that serves as a major source of infection in the animals. The bacteria also survive in the preserved meat for 10-12 years.
5. *Genome:* The genome of *C. chauvoei* is highly homogeneous. The genome consists of a chromosome (2.8 Mbp) and a cryptic plasmid (5.5 Kbp). The chromosome contains the genes encoding enzymes required for glycolysis, sugar, purine and pyrimidine metabolisms but the genes required for amino acid metabolism (Histidine, Tyrosine, Phenylalanine, and Tryptophan) and citric acid cycle are absent. The bacteria acquire the essential amino acids during host tissue damage by the toxins. The only heterogeneous region in the genome is the 'clustered regularly interspaced short palindromic repeats' (CRISPR) locus, on which the strain differentiation is possible.

Isolation, growth and colony characteristics

C. chauvoei is a strict anaerobe and prefers enriched media like blood agar (Batty and Walker *C. chauvoei* blood agar) and RCM for its growth. Media containing liver extract, glucose, cystine, vitamins enhances the growth. The solid media stored for a long time under aerobic condition may gradually absorb the oxygen that prevents the growth of oxygen sensitive *C. chauvoei*. The freshly prepared blood agar or pre-reduced plates, which are stored at anaerobic condition, are preferred. Optimum incubation temperature is 37°C. The colonies are beta haemolytic, circular, convex or raised, grey, 2-4 mm in diameter, shiny or dull in the blood agar. Sometimes, 'swarming growth' is observed. In RCM, the growth is slow and the meat becomes pink (saccharolytic nature).

Biochemical characteristics

C. chauvoei produces following biochemical reactions

Biochemical test	Expected result
Catalase	(-ve)
Oxidase	(-ve)
Indole	(-ve)
Casein digestion	(-ve)
Gelatin hydrolysis	(+ve)
Carbohydrate fermentation	Acid (butyric and acetic acids) and gas are production]
Glucose	(+ve)
Lactose	(+ve)
Maltose	(+ve)
Mannose	(+ve)
Sucrose	(+ve) [difference with C. septicum]
Salicin	(-ve) [difference with C. septicum]

Antigenic characteristics

C. chauvoei possesses somatic, flagellar and spore antigen. The antigens are referred by Arabic numerals, lower case letters and capital letters, respectively. The somatic antigen is common for all the strains. On the basis of flagellar antigen, the bacteria can be subdivided into two antigenic subgroups. *C. chauvoei* shares a common spore antigen with *C. septicum*.

Toxins and virulence factors produced

Toxins

C. chauvoei possesses four major types of toxins.

Alpha-toxin (α-toxin): C. chauvoei produces alpha-toxin that has a molecular mass of 27 kDa. It is formed as part of a larger 53.5 kDa complex, which is referred as the 'soluble immunizing component'. It is an oxygen stable haemolysin and it lyses sheep erythrocytes. It is lethal and necrotising. It also acts as neurotoxin and may cause dermonecrosis and fibrinolysis.

Beta toxin (β-toxin): It is a heat stable deoxyribonuclease (DNAse), having molecular mass of 45 kDa. The enzyme activity is enhanced by barium or magnesium ions and the activity is inhibited by copper, iron, mercury, zinc or silver ions. It causes destruction of the nuclei in the muscle cells observed in the local lesion. It can be assayed by the acid-congo red-alcohol test, using DNA as the substrate.

Gamma toxin (γ-toxin): The gamma-toxin is a hyaluronidase, an enzyme that hydrolyzes glycosidic bonds between N-acetyl-glucosamine and glucuronic acid residues of hyaluronic acid. This enzyme is readily inactivated by heat treatment. It is activated by calcium, barium and magnesium. The acid-congo red-alcohol test can be used to assay gamma-toxin by using hyaluronic acid as the substrate instead of DNA.

Delta toxin (δ-toxin; chauveolysin): It is an oxygen-labile haemolysin similar to the theta-toxin of *C. perfringens*, tetanolysin of *C. tetani* and delta toxin of *C. septicum* (septicolysin). It is also known as 'chauveolysin'.Cholesterol acts as cellular receptor of the toxin (cholesterol dependent cytolysin). It causes lysis of the cell by pore formation. The haemolytic potency of the toxins is inactivated by oxidizing agents such as hydrogen peroxide and iodine. The inactivation can be reversed by treatment with reducing agents such as sodium thioglycolate and hydrogen sulphide. Haemolysis produced by the delta toxin occurs more rapidly than the alpha toxin.

Pathogenesis (Black leg)

Transmission

1. Ingestion of the contaminated feed is the most common source of the infection. Soil is contaminated with faeces, carcass of the infected animals. The infection is endemic and it occurs repeatedly in the same pasture.
2. Infection through wound may take place during castration, docking, parturition, and injection during vaccination. It is more common in sheep and cattle than the pigs.

Pathogenesis

The disease 'blackleg' occurs due to germination of the dormant *C. chauvoei* spores in the skeletal muscle. The spores are deposited in the muscle from the liver and intestine with the help of the macrophages. Heavy muscles of the gluteal region, loin, shoulders are commonly affected. Bruising of the muscle, additional exercise, indigestion provides favourable environment for the spore germination. After germination, the vegetative bacilli multiply and liberate different exotoxins (α, β, γ, δ), which can result the following consequences.

- A local lesion is developed, which is marked by edema, haemorrhage and myofibrillar necrosis. Center of the lesion is dry and contains gas bubble (emphysema) due to bacterial fermentation of the muscle sugar.
- The periphery of the lesion is edematous and dark in colour. Dark colour is due to the staining of the muscle with haemoglobin released from the lysed erythrocytes. Bacterial haemolysins are responsible for the erythrocyte lysis.

- A typical rancid butter odour of the lesion is found due to the formation of butyric acid as an end product of the bacterial sugar fermentation.

Affected animals may show fever, anorexia, lameness and death due to toxaemia. Some animals may die without showing any syndrome.

Disease produced

Bacteria	Host	Disease Produced
Clostridium chauvoei	Cattle, sheep	**Black leg (Black quarter):** It is found in young calves (6 month- 3 years) maintained in high plane of nutrition. It is characterized by necrotizing emphysematous myositis in hind leg. A crepitating sound is heard during rubbing of the lesion with the fingers. Occasionally diaphragm, myocardium or tongue is affected. Fever, lameness, trembling of the muscle is found. Death occurs within 24 hours, if not treated.

Immunity: The circulating antibodies against the bacterial toxins and cellular components play crucial role in developing immunity.

Diagnosis

Clinical samples: Block of affected tissue from the hind leg may be collected in air free sterile container for isolation of *C. chauvoei*. The swabs taken from the area in ordinary sterile container is not useful. Exposure to atmospheric oxygen is lethal for the bacteria.

Laboratory examinations

Isolation of bacteria from clinical samples: Media, incubation condition and colony characteristics are described earlier.

Immunological test: Fluorescent antibody test (FAT) can detect the bacteria in the acetone fixed smear prepared from the clinical specimen (direct examination). The test can differentiate *C. chauvoei* from *C. septicum*. Fluorescein labelled specific antisera is available against *C. chauvoei*, *C. septicum*, *C. novyi* and *C. sordellii.*

Molecular biology: A single-step PCR system is developed for specific detection of *C. chauvoei* DNA using primers derived from the 16S-23S rDNA spacer region and partial 23S rDNA sequences. It can detect the bacteria from the clinical samples and the bacterial cultures.

Prevention and Control

In cattle, sheep and goats vaccination against black quarter (BQ) is practiced with polyvalent BQ vaccine, formaldehyde killed and adjuvinated BQ vaccine, combined black quarter and haemorrhagic septicaemia vaccine, and combined vaccine against *C. chauvoei*, *C. septicum* and *C. novyi*. It is administered before the prevalent season (monsoon in India) in two doses 15-30 days apart. The vaccination should be done in the calves above 3 months of the age to avoid the interference from maternal antibodies. Annual booster vaccination is recommended in endemic zones.

The carcasses of the diseased animals should be burnt or buried properly to prevent the soil contamination with the bacterial spores.

Clostridium novyi (C. oedematiens)

Novy (1894) first described the bacteria as *Bacillus oedematis maligni,* isolated from a guinea pig suffering with 'malignant edema'. Migula (1900) proposed the name *Bacillus novyi,* later renamed as *Clostridium oedematiens* (*novyi*).

Properties of the genus

1. *Morphology: C. novyi* are gram positive, rods measuring 5-10 µm in length and 1-1.5 µm in width. Type B-*C. novyi* is larger than the other types. Older cultures are gram negative. The bacteria are non-capsulated, motile by peritrichous flagella and sporulating. The endospores are oval, situated centrally or sub-terminally and sometimes wider than the vegetative bacteria. There is little or no swelling of the parent cells due to the presence of endospores.
2. *C. novyi* is one of the strictest anaerobe.
3. *Resistance*: The bacterial spores are destroyed at 120°C for 5 minutes exposure. The spores can resist 5% phenol, 10% formalin and 0.1% merthiolate for 1 hour. *C. novyi* can be destroyed by hypochlorites.
4. *Natural habitat*: *C. novyi* remain viable for a long time in soil (type A) and bones of animal carcasses. Intestinal tract and liver of live animals is another natural habitat for type A and B.
5. *Genome*: *C. novyi* genome is very small and is composed of a single circular chromosome (2,547,720 base pairs).The GC content of the genome is 28.9 mol %.The spores of *C. novyi* contain mRNA which is an exception. Generally the bacterial spores are considered as dormant cells and are unable to express mRNA and proteins. *C. novyi* type-B typically possesses 3-5 plasmids and *C. novyi*-type A contains only one plasmid (alpha-toxin encoding).

Isolation, growth and colony characteristics

Strict anaerobic condition is required for isolation of *C. novyi*. It rapidly dies with exposure to air. The common bacteriological media (blood agar and RCM) can be used for the isolation. Only freshly prepared solid and liquid media can be used for the isolation. The prepared and stored medium can absorb oxygen that inhibits clostridial growth. Incubation for 2-4 days is required under strict anaerobic condition (with 10% CO_2 tension) at 37°C.

In blood agar, the colonies are flat with irregular edges, forming a thin film over the surface. The haemolysis is found only in the sheep blood agar due to the secreation of beta, gamma and delta toxins. On the moist surface of solid media, the 'colonial motility' is developed after 3-4 days of incubation. It is unique and it is different from the bacterial swarming (as observed in *Proteus*). The daughter colonies move in an arc on the surface of the media from the parent colony and again return back to fuse with them. In RCM, slow growth with pink colouration of the meat (saccharolytic) is found.

In egg yolk agar, opaque zones surrounding the colonies are produced due to the lecithinase activities of beta-or gamma toxins. It is like the 'Nagler reaction' produced by *C. perfringens*. A pearly layer associated with the colony surface or its periphery is found in egg yolk agar with strains that produce the epsilon-toxin (lipase).

Biochemical characteristics

Different types of *C. novyi* produce following biochemical reactions

Biochemical test	Expected result			
	Type A	Type B	Type C	Type D (*C. haemolyticum*)
Catalase	(-ve)	(-ve)	(-ve)	(-ve)
Oxidase	(-ve)	(-ve)	(-ve)	(-ve)
Indole	(-ve)	Variable	(+ve)	(+ve)
Casein digestion	(-ve)	(+ve)	(-ve)	(+ve)
Gelatin hydrolysis	(+ve)	(+ve)	(+ve)	(+ve)
Lecithinase production in egg yolk agar	(+ve)	(+ve)	(-ve)	(+ve)
Lipase production in egg yolk agar	(+ve)	(-ve)	(-ve)	(-ve)
Carbohydrate fermentation				
Glucose	(+ve)	(+ve)	(+ve)	(+ve)
Lactose	(-ve)	(-ve)	(-ve)	(-ve)
Sucrose	(-ve)	(-ve)	(-ve)	(-ve)
Maltose	(+ve)	(+ve)	Not detected	(-ve)

Antigenic characteristics: *C. novyi* has somatic and flagellar antigens. The antigens are not used in serotyping of the bacteria.

Toxins and virulence factors

Toxins

C. novyi produces five major toxins (α, β, γ, δ, ε) and three minor toxins (ζ, η, θ). On the basis of the toxin production, it can be divided into three types: A, B and C. The type-D is currently considered as a separate species (*C. haemolyticum*). *C. novyi* toxinotypes and their major and minor toxins are described in the table.

Toxinotype	Major toxins	Minor Toxins
Type-A	α, γ, δ, ε	-
Type-B	α, β	ζ, η, θ
Type-C	-	-
Type-D (C. haemolyticum)	β	η

Alpha toxin (α-toxin, Tcn A): It is a large (200-300 KDa) glucosylating toxin, lethal and necrotizing. It is a single protein chain containing three functional domains. Active part of the toxin consists of a beta strand surrounded by numerous alpha helices. The toxin enters the cells via receptor mediated endocytosis. The toxin catalyses the glucosylation of Rho/ Ras-GTPase cellular proteins. The UDP-N acetylglucosamine acts as co-substrate in the chemical reaction. Glucose is attached with the threonine residue residing in the effector region of the GTPases, i.e., Thr-37 in RhoA and Thr-35 in Rac, Cdc42, Ras. The toxin transfers the N-acetyl-glucosamine moiety to the effector regions and inactivates Rho/Ras-GTPase proteins causing the rounding of the cells. It also causes the loss of actin fibres, disruption of intercellular junction and thus increases the cell barrier permeability. The toxin after intravenous injection can produce edema, hypovolemic shock and death. LD_{50} for mice is 200 ngm/ kg body weight. Alpha toxin of *C. novyi* is encoded by bacteriophage.

Beta toxin (β-toxin): It is a lecithinase (phospholipase C, 32KDa), lethal, necrotizing, and haemolytic. It is heat labile (60°C) and trypsin sensitive. It is not related serologically to *C. perfringens* alpha-toxin or to the gamma-toxin of *C. novyi*.

Gamma toxin (γ-toxin): It is a phospholipsae-D (30KDa). It can hydrolyze lecithin, phosphatidyl inositol and phosphatidyl glycerol.

Delta toxin (δ-toxin): It is an oxygen labile, cholesterol dependent pore forming cytolysin (haemolysin), serologically related to teatanolysin, perfringolysin etc. It is also known as 'novyilysin'.

Epsilon toxin (ε-toxin): It is a lipolytic enzyme (lipase). It causes 'pearly layer' surrounding the colonies in egg yolk agar. It is shared with type C and D toxin producing *C. botulinum* strains.

Zeta toxin (ζ-toxin): It is an oxygen labile haemolysin, serologically unrelated with delta toxin. Its pathogenic role is not clear.

Eta toxin (η-toxin): It is a tropomyosinase. It degrades tropomyosin, myosin and thus it can spoil the infected muscles. The enzyme is activated by sulfhydryl groups present in cysteine, glutathione and thiolactate. It is not inhibited by soybean trypsin inhibitor.

Pathogenesis

Bighead: Type A *C. novyi* primarily causes wound infection in cattle, sheep and other animals. In rams during fighting the animals get injuries in subcutaneous tissue of the head regions. The wounds are invaded by type A *C. novyi*. The bacteria can produce extensive edema (alpha toxin) and subsequent swelling of the wound.

Infectious necrotic hepatitis (Black disease/ German Braxy): In sheep, the spores of *C. novyi* type B normally reside at the liver (in endemic area 17-20% of healthy animals). Damage of liver by migration of immature liver fluke (*Fasciola hepatica*) may trigger the spore germination. The vegetative bacteria are generated with the release of toxin. Alpha toxin is absorbed into the circulation causing systemic effects. Venous congestion produces dark colouration of the skin. So it is known as 'black disease'. A similar condition is also detected in other species like cattle and horses.

Bacillary haemoglobinuria (Red water disease): *C. haemolyticum* (type D *C. novyi*) produces the infection in cattle. Pathogenesis is similar like black disease except the type of the toxin. The spores normally reside at the liver after ingestion of *C. haemolyticum* contaminated feeds. The bacteria germinate during liver damage by the liver flukes. Migration of immature liver flukes damages the arterioles and causes necrosis of the liver tissue. This condition favours hypoxia and triggers the spore germination in the liver cells (kupffer cells). The germinated spores produce numerous vegetative bacteria. The bacteria liberate toxins (primarily beta toxin). The toxin is absorbed into the blood circulation. It causes haemoglobinuria and capillary endothelium damage producing loss of blood into the tissues and serous cavities. Death occurs due to anoxia.

Disease produced

Bacteria	Host	Disease Produced
Clostridium novyi type A	Sheep	**Bighead:** In association with *C. novyi*, *C. sordellii*, and rarely *C. chauvoei* are associated. It is characterized by an edematous swelling of the head, face and neck of young rams. Swelling is non-haemorrhagic and no gas is detected.
Clostridium novyi type B	Sheep (1-4 years old), cattle	**Infectious Necrotic Hepatitis (Black disease/ German Braxy):** It is characterized by sudden death without any symptoms. In the liver yellowish necrotic foci are found that follows the migratory track of the flukes. In cattle sub-acute form is found which is characterized by ruminostasis, serous effusion in peritoneal cavity, blood stained froth coming through the nostrils
Clostridium haemolyticum (Clostridium novyi type D)	Cattle, sheep, dog (rare)	**Bacillary haemoglobinuria (Red water disease):** It is an acute, infectious, toxaemic disease, commonly found in tropical and sub-tropical areas. It occurs in well fed animals having a year or more of age. There is a sudden onset of severe depression, fever, abdominal pain, dyspnoea, dysentery and haemoglobinuria, jaundice, brown faeces. Sometimes the cattle die without signs. Rigor mortis is quick and infarction of liver is found during post mortem. Infarction occurs due to agglutination of blood in the vein. Mortality rate is 95%.

Immunity: Antibodies produced against cellular components of *C. novyi* and circulating antitoxin produce protective immunity against the bacteria.

Diagnosis

Clinical samples

Block of affected tissue may be collected in air free sterile container for isolation of *C. novyi*. The swabs taken from the area in ordinary sterile container may not serve the purpose. Exposure to atmospheric oxygen is lethal for the bacteria.

Laboratory Examinations

Isolation of bacteria from clinical samples: Media, incubation condition and colony characteristics are described earlier.

Immunological test: Fluorescent antibody test (FAT) can detect the bacteria in the acetone fixed smear prepared from the clinical specimen (direct examination). Fluorescein labelled specific antisera is available against *C. chauvoei*, *C. septicum*, *C. novyi* and *C. sordellii.*

Molecular biology: Polymerase chain reaction (PCR) targeting the 16S rRNA and 23S rRNA genes of *Clostridium* species is developed to differentiate pathogenic clostridia like *C. novyi*, *C. chauvoei*, *C. speticum* from gas gangrene cases. A multiplex PCR is also developed based on flagellin gene sequence (*fliC*) to identify rapidly *C. novyi* type A, *C. novyi* type B, *C. haemolyticum* and *C. chauvoei*.

Prevention and control

The alum-precipitated toxoid is used as vaccine against *C. novyi* in sheep in few countries before the prevalent season. The primary dose is followed by a booster 4-6 weeks later and subsequently by annual vaccination. The liver flukes should be controlled by destroying snails at the farm.

The formalin-killed, aluminum hydroxide adsorbed whole culture of *C. haemolyticum* is used as vaccine in cattle. Annual vaccination is recommended in endemic zones.

Clostridium septicum

In 1877, Louis Pasteur and Joubert first described the bacteria observed in the carcasses of the animals died due to anthrax. They observed that due to lack of oxygen in the blood anthrax bacilli disappears. It was replaced with spore forming anaerobes. Pasteur named the bacteria as *Vibrion septique*. In 1881, Robert Koch and Gaffky also described the bacteria as *Bacillus oedematis maligni*. Later, it is recognized as *Clostridium septicum*.

Properties of the genus

1. *Morphology*: *C. septicum* are gram-positive rods with rounded ends, measuring 2-10 μm in length and 0.4-1 μm in width. Older cultures are often gram-negative. Sometimes curved long filamentous form is found. The bacteria are non-capsulated, motile by peritrichous flagella and readily sporulating. The endospores are oval, situated centrally or sub-terminally and the presence of spores often bulges the bacteria.
2. *C. septicum* are strict anaerobe
3. *Resistance*: The spores are resistant to desiccation and remain viable in the soil for years. The spores can resist alcohol, phenol, quaternary ammonium disinfectants. However, it is destroyed by boiling for 2-5 minutes, autoclaving and exposure to 3% formalin and lye for 15 minutes.
4. *Natural habitat:* The soil is the major natural habitat of *C. septicum*. They are present in human and domestic animal intestine. It is a frequent

post-mortem invader from the gut of domestic animals, particularly ruminants.

5. *Genome:* The (G+C) content of the genome is 24 mol%.

Isolation, growth and colony characteristics

The blood agar and RCM are the most commonly used media for isolation. The incubation temperature is 37°C. Strict anaerobic condition is required for the isolation.

The colonies are initially semi transparent and round, later become grey, large with filamentous edges. Sometimes the colonies spread over the surface as a thin film. Beta-haemolysis is observed in horse blood agar.

In RCM, pink colour and rancid odour is produced (saccharolytic nature).

Biochemical characteristics

C. septicum produces following biochemical reactions

Biochemical test	Expected result
Catalase	(-ve)
Oxidase	(-ve)
Indole	(-ve)
Casein digestion	(+ve)
Gelatin hydrolysis	(+ve)
Carbohydrate fermentation	Acid (butyric and acetic acids) and
Glucose	gas are production]
Lactose	(+ve)
Maltose	(+ve)
Sucrose	(+ve)
Salicin	(-ve)
	(+ve)
Litmus milk	(+ve) [acid and gas production, no marked 'stormy fermentation']

Antigenic characteristics: *C. septicum* possesses somatic, flagellar and spore antigens. Six serotypes are found on the basis of the two kinds of somatic and five kinds of flagellar antigens. The bacteria share a common spore antigen with *C. chauvoei.*

Toxins and virulence factors produced

Toxins

Alpha-toxin (α-toxin): It is a cationic (pI, 8.4), glycosyl phosphatidyl inositol (GPI) anchored protein of about 48 kDa. It acts as an O_2-stable haemolysin with dermonecrotizing and lethal properties. It is structurally related with 'aerolysin' (produced by *Aeromonas hydrophila*) and ε-toxin of *C. perfringens*. It is encoded by *csa* gene. The toxin is secreated as an inactive 'prototoxin'. The prototoxin binds with the GPI anchored membrane protein. Folate receptor, contactin, Thy1 can act as the toxin receptor. The prototoxin is activated by the proteolytic cleavage of N-terminal (4 KDa) by trypsin, proteinase K and furin (cell surface proteinase, major activator *in vivo*). The activated toxin produces pores in the lipid bilayer of the cellular membrane. The diameter of the pore is 1.3-1.6 nm. The formation of pore in the cell membrane causes 'osmotic shock' of the cells. There is release of haemoglobin with potassium ion from the red blood cells. The pore formation is required for cytotoxicity and *in vivo* myonecrosis. The toxin is also responsible for the cardiac muscle and capillary damage. The LD_{50} for mice is 10μgm / kg body weight.

*Beta-toxin (β-toxin):*It is a heat stable deoxyribonuclease (DNAse). Enzyme activity is enhanced by barium or magnesium ions and it is inhibited by copper, iron, mercury, zinc or silver ions.

Gamma toxin (γ-toxin): The gamma-toxin is a hyaluronidase. It is an enzyme that hydrolyzes glycosidic bonds between N-acetyl-glucosamine and glucuronic acid residues of hyaluronic acid. This enzyme is readily inactivated by heat treatment. The gamma-toxin of *C. septicum* is much more sensitive to heat than that of *C. chauvoei*. It is activated by calcium, barium and magnesium. The acid-congo red-alcohol test can be used to assay gamma-toxin by using hyaluronic acid as the substrate.

Delta toxin (δ-toxin): It is an oxygen-labile haemolysin similar to the theta-toxin of *C. perfringens*, tetanolysin of *C. tetani* and delta toxin of *C. chauvoei* (chauveolysin). It is also known as 'septicolysin'. The cholesterol acts as cellular receptor of the toxin (cholesterol dependent cytolysin). It causes lysis of the cell by pore formation. The haemolytic potency of the toxins is inactivated by oxidizing agents such as hydrogen peroxide and iodine. The inactivation can be reversed by treatment with reducing agents such as sodium thioglycolate and hydrogen sulphide. Haemolysis produced by the delta toxin occurs more rapidly than the alpha toxin.

Pathogenesis

Transmission

1. *C. septicum* commonly resides in the intestine of the animals. It can contaminate the soil through the faeces. The wound infection can take place through the contaminated soil.
2. *C. septicum* may also enter the animal hosts from the environment through different life stages of the liver flukes. The bacteria are isolated from the snails, which acts as an intermediate host in the life cycle of the flukes.
3. Iatrogenic infections (through injection syringe, surgical instruments) have also been reported specially in horses.
4. In turkeys, bird to bird transmission can take place via direct contact and ingestion of contaminated feed. Several predisposing factors like overcrowding, poor quality and wet litter, viral immunosuppression (Haemorrhagic enteritis virus), contaminated vaccine and vaccine equipments are associated with the development of the infection ('clostridial dermatitis of turkey').

Pathogenesis

Braxy / Bradsot: It is a kind of necrotizing abomasitis found in sheep. It is associated with sudden multiplication and invasion of the abomasal lining by the bacteria. Ingestion of frozen grass and other feed is the predisposing factor. The chilly feed materials may impair mucosal function and allows entry of the bacteria. After entry, *C. septicum* multiplies locally and disseminates throughout the body. It produces local lesions as well as toxaemia. The abomasal walls including the proximal small intestine are edematous, haemorrhagic and sometimes necrotic. Internal organs show only degenerative changes.

Malignant edema: It occurs in domestic animals during direct contamination of the wound with *C. septicum.* Multiplication of the bacteria and toxin production is required for the myonecrosis. Individual role of each toxin in myonecrosis is not established.

Clostridial dermatitis of turkey (CDT)

a) Damaged intestinal wall is required for the entry of the organism or its toxin into the blood circulation. It is known as 'inside-out' mechanism with unknown details.

b) Moist or abraded skin helps in entry of the organism. It is proposed 'outside in' mechanism of pathogenesis. The mechanism in details is also not studied.

Disease produced

Bacteria	Host	Disease Produced
Clostridium septicum	Sheep, lamb	**Braxy (Scots) or Bradsot (In Danish language means 'quick plague'):** It is a necrotizing abomasitis and toxaemia and is characterized by sudden death without any symptoms. Anorexia, grinding of teeth, coma followed by death is observed. The carcasses decompose rapidly. It is commonly found in UK, Ireland, Norway, Iceland, other European countries, Australia, USA. Sometimes, it is also associated with other clostridia like C. chauvoei, C. perfringens, C. novyi, C. sordelli
	Domestic animals	**Malignant edema:** Gas gangrene type of lesion is produced in the wound contaminated with the bacteria. The bacteria are isolated from the cases of post-parturient vulvo-vaginitis and metritis in cattle
	Turkey	**Clostridial dermatitis of turkey (CDT):** Previously it was known as 'cellulitis'. It is often found in 16-18 weeks aged birds. It is characterized by lateral recumbency, weakness, ataxia, anorexia, depression and cyanosis of the head. Blisters along with broken feather follicles are found at the tail base ('bubbly-tail'). Mortality rate is few birds per day to 2-3% per week. The carcasses decompose rapidly

Immunity: Antibodies against the bacterial toxins play crucial role in developing resistance.

Diagnosis

Clinical samples: Exudates, skin part (turkey) may be collected for isolation of *C. septicum*. The post mortem materials (block of affected tissues) should be collected immediately after death. *C. septicum* is a frequent contaminant found in the post mortem materials.

Laboratory examinations

Direct examination: The smear is prepared from the exudate, skin part (impression smear) and is stained by Gram's method. Predominance presence of gram positive rods with other characteristics in the microscopic field is required to establish the bacteria as a major causative agent.

Isolation of bacteria from clinical samples: Necrotic tissue, exudates are heated at 80°C for 20 minutes and inoculated into the suitable media. Media, incubation condition and colony characteristics are described earlier.

Immunological test: Fluorescent antibody test (FAT) can detect the bacteria in the acetone fixed smear prepared from the clinical specimen (direct examination). The test can differentiate *C. chauvoei* from *C. septicum*. Fluorescein labelled specific antisera is available against *C. chauvoei*, *C. septicum*, *C. novyi* and *C. sordellii.*

Molecular Biology: A single-step PCR system is developed for specific detection of *C. septicum* alpha toxin gene (*csa*) from the cases of malignant edema. Real time PCR is developed for rapid differentiation of *C. septicum* from *C. chauvoei* based on *TP1* and *spo* genes.

Prevention and control

Frosted pasture should be avoided for grazing of the sheep. In few countries, vaccination with formalin-killed whole culture of *C. septicum* is practiced.

Clostridium sordellii

Clostridium sordellii was first isolated in 1922 by the Argentinean microbiologist Alfredo Sordelli. He named it *Bacillus oedematis sporogenes* on the basis of its morphology and the production of edema. In 1927, the bacteria were renamed as *Bacillus sordellii*. In 1929, it was shown to be related with *Clostridium* genus and the name *Clostridium sordellii* was accepted.

Previously it was known as a subgroup of *Clostridium bifermentans*. On the basis of urease and major lethal toxin production the separate species status is assigned.

Properties of the genus

1. *Morphology*: *C. sordellii* are gram-positive rods, measuring 2-5 µm in length and 0.5-1 µm in width. The bacteria are non-capsulated, motile by peritrichous flagella and sporulating. The endospores are oval, situated centrally, sub-terminally and do not bulge the vegetative bacteria.
2. *C. sordellii* are strict anaerobe
3. *Resistance*: The resistance is almost similar with other clostridial species.
4. *Natural habitat*: The bacteria are commonly found in the soil and healthy intestine of animals and human (0.5%).

Isolation, growth and colony characteristics

Common bacteriological media (blood agar and RCM) can be used for isolation of *C. sordellii.* Some strains prefer to grow in stiff blood agar (agar concentration 3%). The colonies appear translucent to opaque with small zones of β- haemolysis on sheep or rabbit blood agar. Margins of the colonies are lobate or entire. The colonies become white after ageing. In cooked medium, meat particles first become red followed by black colouration with partial digestion.

Biochemical characteristics

C. sordellii produces following biochemical reactions

Biochemical test	Expected result
Catalase	(-ve)
Oxidase	(-ve)
Indole	(+ve)
Casein digestion	(+ve)
Gelatin hydrolysis	(+ve)
Carbohydrate fermentation	
Glucose	(+ve)
Lactose	(-ve)
Maltose	(+ve)
Sucrose	(-ve)
Lecithinase production in egg yolk agar	(+ve)
Lipase production in egg yolk agar	(-ve)

Antigenic characteristics: Antigenically *C. sordellii* are homogenous. It possesses some species specific antigen (previously designated as 'spore-agglutinogen'). *C. sordellii* shares antigen with C. *bifermentans.*

Toxins and virulence factors produced

Toxins

Major toxin: *C. sordellii* produces major lethal toxin responsible for edema and haemorrhage. Previously it was known as 'beta toxin'. The toxin has two parts i.e. lethal toxin (TcsL) and haemorrhagic toxin (TcsH). Both lethal and haemorrhagic toxins are large glucosylating toxins. The lethal toxin is a protein of 250 KDa and it is serologically related to toxin B of *C. difficile*. The lethal toxin glucosylates Ras, Rac, Ral, and Rap proteins present in the host cells. The haemorrhagic toxin is 525 KDa protein and it glucosylates Rho, Rac, cdc42 proteins present in the host cells. It is lethal for mice, cytotoxic and enterotoxic. It can accumulate fluid in the ligated rabbit ileal loop like other enteric toxins. It is serologically related with toxin A of *C. difficile.*

Minor toxins: *C. sordellii* produces few minor toxins having structural similarity with the toxin produced by *C. bifermentans.* The toxins are lecithinase, oxygen-labile haemolysin (sordellilysin), DNAse and a fibrinolysin. The lecithinase is a phospholipase C, serologically related to the alpha-toxin of *C. perfringens* as evidenced by the positive Nagler reaction. It is non-toxic for the mice. Deoxyribonuclease (DNAse) plays a role in pathogenesis by destruction of the cell nucleus.

Pathogenesis

Ingestion of the contaminated feed and drinking water is the major route of transmission. Lethal toxin plays significant role in production of clinical signs and death. The precise pathway of pathogenesis in animals is not established.

Disease produced

Bacteria	Host	Disease Produced
Clostridium sordellii	Cattle, sheep, horse	**Sudden death syndrome:** It is characterized by death without clinical signs, muscle myositis and edema of subcutaneous tissues and fascial planes surrounding the muscles. Sub-endocardial haemorrhage in the ventricles and septicaemia before death is found
	Horse	**Pasture myodystrophy (Equine Atypical Myopathy):** It is an acute disease with signs of rhabdomyolysis and mortality rate over 90%. It affects grazing horses under frosty, windy and rainy conditions. Lethal toxin (TcsL) plays significant role in muscle dystrophy. It is characterized by acute degeneration of muscle fibres leading to sudden death due to collapse of the respiratory system
	Cattle	Gas gangrene (myositis), black leg (black quarter)
	Cattle, foal	Enterotoxaemia
	Chicken and turkey	**Gangrenous dermatitis (Clostridial dermatitis):** *C. sordellii* is an occasional cause along with C. septicum and C. perfringens type A. The infection is characterized by subcutaneous emphysema, skin vesicles specially in the breast, moist dark wrinkled skin including the tail area
	Human	It rarely causes human infection. Spontaneous endocarditis, post-operative infection, septic shock, pneumonitis, ear infection are sometimes reported

Diagnosis

Clinical samples: Block of affected tissue may be collected for isolation of *C. sordellii*.

Laboratory examinations

Isolation of bacteria from clinical samples: Media, incubation condition and colony characteristics are described earlier.

Immunological test: Fluorescent antibody test (FAT) can detect the organism in the acetone fixed smear prepared from the clinical specimen (direct examination). The test can differentiate *C. chauvoei* from *C. septicum*. Fluorescein labelled specific antisera is available against *C. chauvoei*, *C. septicum*, *C. novyi* and *C. sordellii.*

Molecular biology: The polymerase chain reaction (PCR) using common primers designed from the 16S rRNA and 23S rRNA genes of *Clostridium* species is developed to identify pathogenic clostridia associated with gas gangrene (myonecrosis). It can differentiate *C. sordellii* from *C. chauvoei, C. septicum,* and *C. novyi*.

Clostridium difficile

The bacterium was first isolated from the newborn baby's intestinal flora by Hall and O'Toole (1935). It was described as *Bacillus difficilis* due to the 'difficulty' they faced in its isolation. A small number of reports are available in the next 40 years about its pathogenic significance. Bartlett (1978) and his colleagues identified *C. difficile* as the primary cause of pseudomembranous colitis in human.

Properties of the genus

1. *Morphology*: *C. difficile* are gram-positive rods, measuring 3-5 µm in length and 0.5 µm in width. Older cultures may appear as gram-negative. The bacteria are capsulated, motile by peritrichous flagella and sporulating. Some strains also contain S-layer. The spores are produced in artificial cultures after 72 hours incubation during decline phase of the growth. The spores are oval, sub-terminal or terminal in position and presence of spores do not bulge the bacterial cells. Some strains may contain fimbriae, 6 µm in length and polar.
2. *C. difficile* are strict anaerobe
3. *Resistance*: The spores are highly resistant to the environmental stress like heat, alcohol, enzymes, detergents, disinfectants, ultraviolet light and ionising radiation. Vegetative bacteria rapidly die during exposure to oxygen.
4. *Natural habitat*: *C. difficile* are commonly found in the soil, sand, river, lake, swimming pools, human hospitals, veterinary clinics, marine sediments, river bank mud, raw vegetables, and floor swabs of private houses. It is found as a part of the normal flora of human intestine (2-4% in young adults). The isolation rate increases with the age of the human (10-20% in elderly persons). In animals, the bacteria are isolated from the faeces of cattle, horse, donkey, domestic birds, ducks, geese, dogs and cats. However, it is not known as zoonotic.
5. *Genome*: The complete whole genome sequence is available for *C. tetani, C. perfringens, C. botulinum* and *C. difficile*. The GC content of the genome is 29 mol%. Plasmids are detected in the genome with molecular weights ranging from 2.7×10^6 to 100×10^6.

Isolation, growth and colony characteristics

C. difficile is a strict anaerobe and prefers enriched media like blood agar for its growth. Selective medium is cycloserine cefoxitin fructose agar (CCFA), cefoxitin mannitol agar (CMA), and cefoxitin mannitol blood agar (CMBA).

The colonies in blood agar are 3-5 mm in diameter with an irregular, lobate edge, grey in colour, non-haemolytic. Some strains may produce greenish alpha haemolysis. Young colonies produce yellow-green colour under long wavelength ultraviolet illumination (365 nm). After 48-72 hours incubation, grey or white coloured centre develops in the middle of the colonies. The centre sometimes rises from its surrounding and produces a 'fried egg' appearance (like *Mycoplasma*). The centre formation is associated with the sporulation in the artificial media.

Colonies in CCFA are 4 mm in diameter, yellow or ground glass like with filamentous edges. Colonies have typical 'horse manure' like smell.

Biochemical characteristics

C. difficile produces following biochemical reactions

Biochemical test	Expected result
Catalase	(-ve)
Oxidase	(-ve)
Indole	(-ve)
Casein digestion	(-ve)
Gelatin hydrolysis	(+ve)
Carbohydrate fermentation	
Glucose	(+ve)
Lactose	(-ve)
Maltose	(-ve)
Sucrose	(-ve)

Antigenic characteristics : S-layer protein is the major antigen of *C. difficile* used in the typing. The bacteria express two kinds of S-layer proteins, high molecular weight (HMW) and low molecular weight (LMW) proteins. Both the proteins are encoded by *slpA* and are produced by post transitional cleavage of a single precursor. At present, *C. difficile* comprises 14 serogroups.

Serologically it can cross react with other clostridia like *C. sordellii, C. bifermentans* and *C. glycolicum*.

Toxins and virulence factors produced

Major toxin: *C. difficile* produces two large glycosylating toxins known as TcdA (308 KDa) and TcdB (270 KDa). The toxins are considered as largest bacterial toxins reported so far. The toxins are glucosyl transferases, which inactivate Rho, Rac, and Cdc42 within target cells like the toxins of *C. novyi* (Tcnα) and *C. sordellii* (TcsL). Former one (TcdA) acts as enterotoxin causing accumulation of fluid in the intestine and later one (TcdB) is a potent cytotoxin. On the basis of sequence variations of the toxins, there are 22 toxinotypes of the bacterium. The toxinotypes are designated by roman numerical (I-XXII).

The genes encoding the toxins (*tcdA*, *tcdB*) are located in a pathogenicity island (19.6 Kb) within the chromosome. The toxins are expressed efficiently during the late log and stationary phases of bacterial growth in response to a variety of environmental stimuli. The two toxin genes are closely situated. There are three other genes (*tcdC*, *tcdD*, *tcdE*) found within the same pathogenicity island. These additional proteins (TcdC, TcdD, TcdE) regulate the toxin expression (regulatory proteins). The TcdC and TcdD may function as a negative and positive regulator of the toxin production, respectively. The TcdE protein helps in release of the toxins by increasing the cell wall permeability.

The production of the toxins is correlated with the environment. The stress conditions (including antibiotics) and 'catabolite repression' (a mechanism, by which the bacteria only produce those enzymes that can hydrolyze a particular carbohydrate available in the surroundings, not the others) may enhance the toxin production. The starvation (deficiency in amino acids) may cause the production of only one toxin, not the both. However, the toxin production is not related with the sporulation like other clostridia.

Mechanism of action: The toxins enter the cell via receptor mediated endocytosis. Unusually the receptor for the toxin is a carbohydrate, not a protein. The receptor for TcdA is a disaccharide (Galβ1-4GlcNac) which is present in a variety of cells. After binding with the receptor, the acidified endosomes are required for the translocation of the toxin into the cytosol. Within the cell, TcdB glucosylates RhoA, Rac and cdc42 protein via transfer of a sugar moiety to Thr-37 of the GTPase with UDP-glucose as a co-substrate. TcdA can also glucosylate RhoA protein in a similar way (less active than TcdB). Thus, both of the toxins inactivate small GTPases within the cell. It results cellular actin filament condensation, consequent rounding of the cells, membrane blebbing and apoptosis of the target cell. It can cause severe inflammation in mammalian intestine with epithelial cell necrosis and infiltration with inflammatory cells.

Minor toxin

C. difficile transferase (CDT): It is a binary toxin (43 KDa) like *C. botulinum* C2 toxin, *C. perfringens* iota toxin etc. It has two components i.e. enzymatic and binding part. The enzymatic part ADP ribosylates monomeric actin and causes depolymerization of all the actin filaments. It is not cytotoxic. The exact role in pathogenesis is not established.

Virulence factors: Pilli, capsule and degradative enzymes may act as additional virulence factors. Enzymes like hyaluronidase, neuraminidase, chondroitin-4-sulphatase and heparinase are detected. The hyaluronidase plays major role in degradation of connective tissues.

Pathogenesis

C. difficile infection (CDI) is associated with the absence of microflora in the gut in animals and humans. Protective microflora is destroyed by prolonged antibiotic therapy in adults. In neonates and germ free animals (experimental animals born and maintained under sterile conditions) the flora is yet to be developed. Sometimes, in adult animals, dietary changes may disrupt the normal flora. The gut microflora prevents the colonization of *C. difficile* with the intestinal epithelium ('colonization resistance'). So its absence is an important factor for adherence of the bacteria. Additional factors like competitive ability for nutrients, toxin production, adhering property with the colon and number of the bacteria influence the infection. After establishment, the bacteria multiply and liberate toxins. The toxins degranulate the mucosal mast cells and release inflammatory mediators causing an invasion of granulocytes. It causes the distinct pathological lesions by substantial tissue damage and clinical signs.

Disease produced

Bacteria	Host	Disease
Clostridium difficile	Horse	**Haemorrhagic necrotizing enterocolitis (neonatal foals):** It is characterized by colic, weakness, diarrhoea, dehydration followed by death within 24 hours. Surface of the necrotic villi are lined by numerous gram positive rods. Diarrhoea and typhilitis in adult horses
	Piglets (0-7 days old)	**Neonatal necrotizing colitis:** Signs include respiratory distress, diarrhoea soon after birth. Mesocolonic edema, yellowish contents in the colon, hydrothorax and ascites are observed. Erosion of the epithelial surface of colon is found. Through this eroded part there is exudation of neutrophils and fibrin into the lumen. The condition leads to 'volcano lesion'. However, no lesion is found in the small intestine. Morbidity rate is 97-100%. Mortality is low. Weight loss is encountered after recovery
	Dogs	Chronic diarrhoea
	Hamsters	Typhilitis
	Mice, rabbit, guinea pigs	Antibiotic associated diarrhoea

Immunity: Role of antibodies against *C. difficile* is not established.

Diagnosis

Clinical samples: Faeces, rectal swabs, tissues may be collected for isolation of *C. difficile*.

Laboratory examinations

Isolation of bacteria from clinical samples: Media, incubation condition and colony characteristics are described earlier.

Detection of toxin: Toxin in the processed samples (tissue, rectal swabs) can be detected by cell culture or enzyme immunoassays. Cell culture in Chinese hamster ovary (CHO) cell line is suitable for detection of *C. difficile* toxin from faecal samples. It is based on the finding of cytotoxic activity as noted by rounding of the cells and neutralization of the toxin by *C. djficile* antitoxin. The test is considered as 'gold standard' for *C. difficile* diagnosis as it can correlate with the infection. Among the enzyme immunoassays, counter immune electrophoresis (CIE), latex agglutination test and ELISA can be performed. CIE can cross-react with *C. sordellii*, *C. bifermentans* and gives false-positive results. Latex agglutination test is not specific for toxin producing (tox+) *C. difficile* isolates. It can detect tox (-ve) isolates as well as *C. sporogenes* and other bacteria. ELISA is specific and sensitive.

Molecular Biology

Detection of C. difficile: PCR is developed for the toxin gene detection of the bacteria from the isolates of the equine faecal samples. TaqMan real-time PCR (TMrtPCR) assay targeting the *TcdA* and *TcdB* genes is developed for direct detection from the faeces of symptomatic and asymptomatic animals.

Typing of C. difficile: Typing of the isolates can be performed by different molecular tools like PCR ribotyping, multilocus variable number tandem repeat analysis (MLVA), restriction enzyme analysis (REA) etc. PCR ribotyping is based on the differences in the spacer regions of 16S and 23S ribosomal RNA. MLVA is the method of counting the numbers of repeat alleles in the genome. It produces a particular numerical score for a strain. However, it requires expensive equipment.

Prevention and control

Strict hygienic measures should be followed in animal farms. The premises after parturition should be disinfected with sporicidal chemicals.

Clostridium histolyticum

It is motile, proteolytic, and sporulating *Clostridium*. Spores are oval and sub terminal. It is aerotolerant like *C. perfringens*. It produces five major toxins (α, β, γ, δ, ε). Alpha toxin is lethal and necrotizing, beta is a collagenase, gamma and delta are proteinase and epsilon is haemolytic. The bacteria are associated with 'gas gangrene' in human.

Clostridium fallax

It can cause 'malignant edema' (gas edema) in horses. Rarely the bacteria are isolated from septicaemia in human also.

Clostridium colinum

C. colinum resides in soil. The GC content of the genome (43%) is higher than other clostridia. It causes 'Quail Disease' in Bobwhite Quail and other domestic and wild birds. The chicken are little resistant to the infection. It can only take place during stress conditions produced by viral infection, coccidiosis and aplastic anaemia. The infection is characterized by intestinal wall ulcers and necrosis of liver and spleen. Sudden death of the birds is found. The mortality rate is 100% for quails, whereas, only 10-30% for the chicken.

Clostridium spiroforme

It appears as spiral, loosely coiled *Clostridium* in a smear prepared from isolates in the artificial medium. In faeces or caecum, it appears as semi-circular. It is sporulating and the spores are terminal.

It liberates a binary exotoxin identical with the iota toxin of *C. perfringens*. The toxin is dermonecrotic for guinea pigs and lethal for mice. The toxin has ADP ribolysating property on monomeric actin causing destruction of the cellular microfilaments.

Clostridium spiroforme causes 'mucoid enteritis' in rabbits, enterocolitis in pigs and foals.

Clostridium piliforme (previously *Bacillus piliformis*)

It cannot be isolated in the artificial bacteriological media. In laboratory, it is grown in mice embryo fibroblast cell line.

It causes Tyzzer's disease in rabbits, mice, rats, guinea pigs, dogs, foals, calves and other animals. The birds are apparently resistant. Acute infection in rabbits is manifested with profuse diarrhoea and sudden death. Mortality rate is 15-50%. Chronically infected animals show depression, anorexia, cachexia and weight loss. Arabian foals suffering from severe combined immunodeficiency (SCID) are more susceptible to the infection. In dogs, it occurs primarily in young animals, rarely in immunocompromised older dogs. The infection is characterized by hepatitis, myocarditis and enterocolitis in dogs.

15

Actinomyces

Cohn (1875) first observed and described a branching filamentous micro-organism in the 'concretions' (coagulated mass) taken from a lacrimal canal, later identified as *Actinomyces israelii*. Bollinger first reported the yellow granules in jaw tissues of the cattle in 1877 and established the significance of the bacteria as the etiological agent. In 1878, Israel described the first human case. In 1879, Hartz observed the microscopic appearance of granules of *Actinomyces* and suggested the name *Actinomyces bovis*. Mosselman & Lihnaux (1890) and Wolf & Israel (1891) first isolated the bacteria in artificial laboratory media from lumpy jaw cases of cattle and human actinomycosis, respectively.

Properties of genus

1. *Morphology: Actinomyces* are gram positive filamentous organisms with branching rods (Figure 1). In artificial media, short bacilli or cocci forms are also observed. During infection, the bacteria can produce yellow coloured granules (sulphur granule), commonly found in the pus as 'opaque speck' and are visible under naked eye (1-2 mm in diameter). The granules are usually soft and easily broken under light pressure, but the granules may occasionally be tough or even calcified. The granules are composed of club shaped bodies, arranged radially with their narrow ends towards the centre. So, the bacteria are also known as 'ray fungus'. In the centre of the club, filamentous masses of gram positive bacteria with some bacilli or cocci form are found. Together the club like processes and bacterial masses are known as 'rosette' (Figure 2.) The club is composed of calcium phosphate and inflammatory debris. The club represents encapsulation of the bacteria by layers of the calcium phosphate-protein complex. It occurs as a result of the bacterial phosphatase activity in response to inflammation. However, the clubs are more prominently observed in tissue section than the granules. During gram staining of the crushed granules, the clubs stain as gram-negative, whereas the bacteria appear as gram-positive. *Actinomyces* are non-motile, non-sporing and non-acid fast.

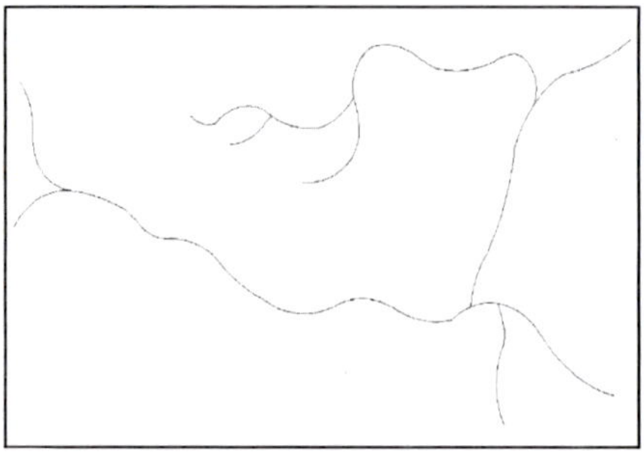

Fig. 1: Branching filaments of *Actinomyces* (schematic)

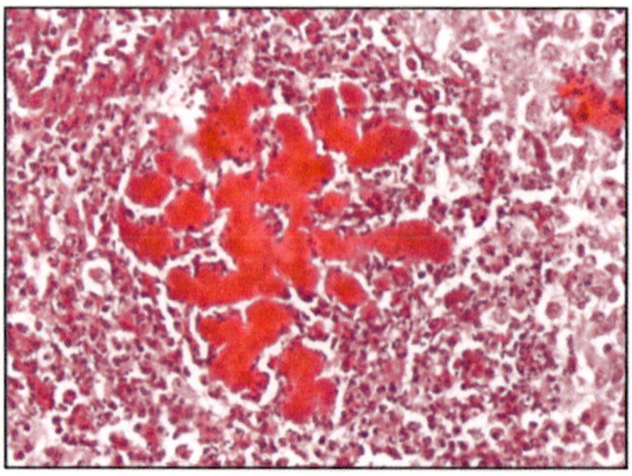

Fig. 2: Club shaped body arranged radially produced by *Actinomyces*
(*Courtesy*: Gauri Chandratre, Department of Veterinary Pathology, Lala Lajpat Rai University of Veterinary and Animal Sciences, Hisar, India)

2. *Actinomyces* are facultative anaerobic and capnophilic (require CO_2 for growth) in nature

3. *Classification*: The family Actinomycetes contains several genera like *Actinomyces, Nocardia, Corynebacterium, Mycobacterium, Arcanobacterium, Dermatophilus, Propionibacterium, Actinomadura, Gordonia, Rhodococcus, Sreptomyces, Rothia, Nocardiopsis* etc. Veterinary important genera are *Actinomyces, Nocardia, Corynebacterium, Mycobacterium, Arcanobacterium, Dermatophilus* and *Rhodococcus.*

   The genus *Actinomyces* contains more than 30 species like *A. bovis, A. viscosus, A. suis, A. israelii, A. hyovaginalis, A. howelli, A. naeslundii, A. bowdenii.* Among the species, *A. bovis* and *A. israelii* are the most common pathogens in animals and human, respectively.

4. *Resistance:* 60°C temperature for 20 minute exposure and autoclaving (120°C for 15 minute) is lethal to *Actinomyces*. *A. israelii* is easily killed by moderate heating (62-64°C for 3-10 minutes). The granules in the actinomycotic pus remain viable after being air-dried in test tubes for 18-22 days.The bacteria are susceptible to common disinfectants like phenol, cresol etc. Cultures in artificial media require frequent passage for their survival.

5. *Natural habitat:* Most of the *Actinomyces* are obligate parasites on the mucous membrane of mouth, pharynx, tonsils, teeth surface and alimentary tract of different animal and human reservoirs. Most of the infections are endogenous in origin. The bacteria do not survive in the environment for a long time.

Isolation, growth and colony characteristics

Actinomyces can be isolated in the media enriched with blood (chocolate blood agar) or serum. Specific media are Garrod's media, brain heart infusion agar with or without sheep blood (10%), *Brucella* blood agar with haemin and vitamin K1, phenylethyl alcohol or mupirocin-metronidazole blood agar. No growth is observed in Sabouraud's dextrose agar at room temperature. To isolate the bacteria from the clinical samples, sulfur granules are picked from the pus and transferred into a tube of sterile distilled water. The tube is shaken vigorously and the granules are allowed to settle at the bottom, and the supernatant liquid is withdrawn with a sterile pipette. The washing procedure is repeated at least twice. After the final washing, the granules are ground up in the residual fluid with a sterile glass rod. The homogenate is then streaked into the isolation media.

The incubation is performed at 37°C for 4-6 days with 5% CO_2 tension. Under aerobic condition, most of the colonies appear in the sub-surface layer of the media, where oxygen tension is low. The colonies of *A. bovis* are non-haemolytic, round, flat, pale yellow in colour, 1 mm in diameter, non-filamentous or filamentous with irregular edges. Colonies can adhere with the solid medium.

Early growth of *A. viscosus* after 24 hour of incubation is a microscopic meshwork of filaments, known as 'spider colony'. Later the colonies develop ridges, known as 'molar tooth colony'. Both of the colonies are non-haemolytic. Typical clubs within granules are absent.

A. suis produces brown, small, smooth or rough granular colonies with filamentous extension.

In the liquid medium (thioglycollate broth), the growth is settled at the bottom. It is either mucoid i.e. forming spiraling viscous ropes when the contents of the tubes are swirled, or granular or flaky.

Biochemical characteristics

Actinomyces bovis produces following biochemical reactions

Biochemical test	Expected result
Catalase	(-ve) [A. viscosus is +ve]
Urease	(-ve)
Nitrate reduction	(-ve)
Carbohydrate fermentation	
Glucose	(+ve) (without gas)
Mannitol	(-ve)
Gelatinase production	(-ve)
CAMP	(-ve)

Antigenic characteristics

Earlier six serogroups (A-F) were detected in *Actinomyces* based on surface antigens, later designated as six different species. Each of the species can be sub-divided into at least two serotypes. The two serotypes of *A. bovis* show little or no cross reaction with each other. Serotype 1 and 2 produce non-filamentous and filamentous colonies, respectively. In *A. viscosus*, serotype 1 is restricted to animals, whereas serotype 2 is typically detected in humans. The two serotypes (1 and 2) are serologically distinct.

Toxins and virulence factors produced

Toxins: No true exotoxins are produced by *Actinomyces*. Trauma and break in the host defense are required for establishment of the endogenous infection. Sometimes other bacteria (companion bacteria) are also recovered from the actinomycotic lesion, possibly having a role in the infection process.

Virulence factors

Virulence factors	Function
Fimbriae	Two types of fimbriae are observed in A. viscosus. Type-1 fimbriae help in adherence of the bacteria with the teeth surface (stratherin protein) and salivary proline-rich protein in human. Type-2 fimbriae help in binding with certain oral streptococci (co-aggregation) or buccal epithelial cells of human. In animals, role of fimbriae in disease production is not established.

Pathogenesis

Transmission

Actinomycosis in animals and human is an endogenous infection. The bacteria have natural habitat in the mucous membrane of mouth, pharynx, tonsils and teeth surface. The bacteria can enter the underlying deeper tissues either through dental alveoli or through the damaged mucosa by thorny feed, foreign bodies, accidental trauma, and injury. Rarely animal bite is another way of transmission in susceptible animals and human.

Pathogenesis

A. bovis

After entry into the deeper tissues of the buccal cavity, *A. bovis* grows in the tongue, pharynx, and subcutaneous tissues of the head and neck. The areas of suppuration are produced containing bacteria and neutrophils in the center, which is surrounded by granulation, fibrosis and infiltration of mononuclear cells. Neutrophils accumulate at the site due to secreation of chemotactic molecules by *Actinomyces.* Suppurative necrosis is observed in the esophagus and reticulum with the production of thick green / yellow coloured pus. Sometimes excess pus may overflow the surface through the sinus or fistula. Infection may disseminate into the lungs, lymph nodes, liver, vertebrae and bones through the blood. Osteomyelitis develops and bones become porous (honeycombed) with pus filled sinuses. Old bones are replaced with new bones. Mandibular fractures are also observed. Animals cannot chew properly. However, in other tissues after dissemination infection does not establish.

Disease produced

Bacteria	Host	Disease produced
Actinomyces bovis	Cattle, buffalo	**Lumpy Jaw (Bovine actinomycosis):** It is characterized by the swelling with suppurating osteomyelitis in the cheek, lower jaw, submaxillary region and other parts of the head and neck. The lesions hamper the mastication and movement of the jaw
	Horses	Poll evil and fistulous withers. The infection can occur in association with Brucella sp.
Actinomyces suis	Pigs	**Pyrogranulomatous mastitis:** It is characterized by the formation of more granulation tissues and enlargement of the mammary gland. Pus secreating from the gland contains sulphur granules.
Actinomyces viscosus	Dogs	**Canine actinomycosis:** It is characterized by localized cutaneous granulomatous abscess and granulomas in the thoracic cavity
	Human	Cervicofacial actinomycosis, thoracic actinomycosis, actinomycosis of the abdomen and pelvis
Actinomyces israelii	Human	Cervicofacial actinomycosis, thoracic actinomycosis, actinomycosis of the abdomen and pelvis.

Immunity: During the course of the infection, circulating antibodies are produced. However, it offers no protection against the disease.

Diagnosis

Clinical samples: Pus, aspirates from the unopened lesion preferably with sulphur granules can be collected as ante-mortem samples (Figure 3). Fine needle aspiration biopsy (FNAB) can be carried out from the depth of the suspected actinomycotic growth and also from the mandibular lymph node with the help of the long needle. Tissue biopsies are collected in 10% formalin for histopathology.

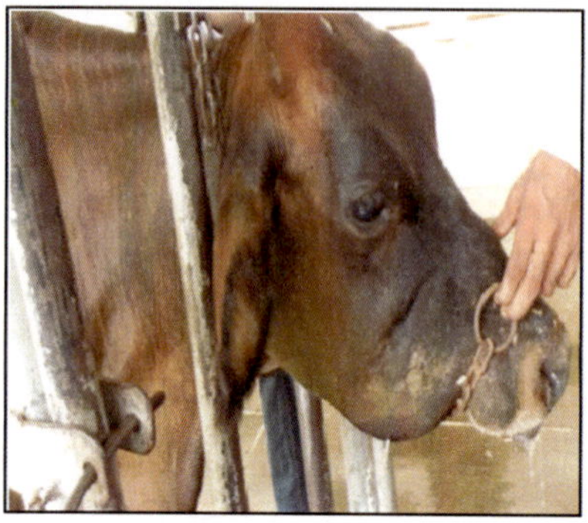

Fig. 3: Lumpy jaw of a buffalo showing swelling at mandibular region and salivation (*Courtesy*: Ankit Kumar, Department of Veterinary Medicine, Lala Lajpat Rai University of Veterinary and Animal Sciences, Hisar, India)

Laboratory examinations

Direct examination: For direct examination of the bacteria in clinical sample, the following method is adopted.

Yellow coloured 'sulphur granules' are observed in the pus/ exudate

↓

Granules are washed with distilled water in a sterile petri dish\

↓

Granules are placed in one drop of 10% KOH in a glass slide

↓

Granules are gently crushed with cover slip and observed under low power of light microscope

↓

'Club shaped' bacterial micro-colonies (like actinobacillosis) are found. If gram stained, at the centre of the colony, gram-positive rods with branching filaments are observed. Other pleomorphic forms like cocci, diptheroidal form, spirals are also found. The club colony is more common in the tissue section than the pus samples.

Isolation of bacteria from clinical samples: Media, incubation condition and colony characteristics are described earlier.

Serological tests: Immunodiffusion, fluorescent antibody test (FAT) can be performed for the detection of *A. Bovis*.

Prevention and control

Isolation or disposal of animals with oral lesions and salivation is effective control measure for animal actinomycosis.

16

Nocardia

Edmond Nocard (French veterinarian) first isolated filamentous aerobic bacteria from clinical cases of 'bovine farcy' in 1888. In 1889, the genus *Nocardia* was formed by Trevisan and the bacterium originally described by Nocard was named as *Nocardia farcinica*. In 1891, another similar bacterium (*Nocardia asteroides*) was isolated by Eppinger from a human brain abscess. Initially it was thought that they are the same bacteria. On the basis of the genetic differences the separate entity was established later.

The re-examination of Nocard's original isolate revealed the existence of two different filamentous bacteria i.e. *Mycobacterium* and *Nocardia*. The cause of 'bovine farcy' has been subsequently attributed to *Mycobacterium*. Later, it is proved that *Mycobacterium farcinogenes* is the actual causative agent of 'bovine farcy'.

Properties of genus

1. *Morphology:* *Nocardia* are gram positive, long filamentous, branching rods like *Actinomyces* and *Streptomyces*. In artificial media, the bacteria may appear as bacilli or cocci. In tissues, the bacteria appear as weak gram-positive and the filaments show discontinuous (uneven) stained branches like the string of beads (beaded filament) (Figure 1). The branches appear at right angle of both the sides of the filament. The beaded filaments are generally not found in *Actinomyces* and *Streptomyces*.

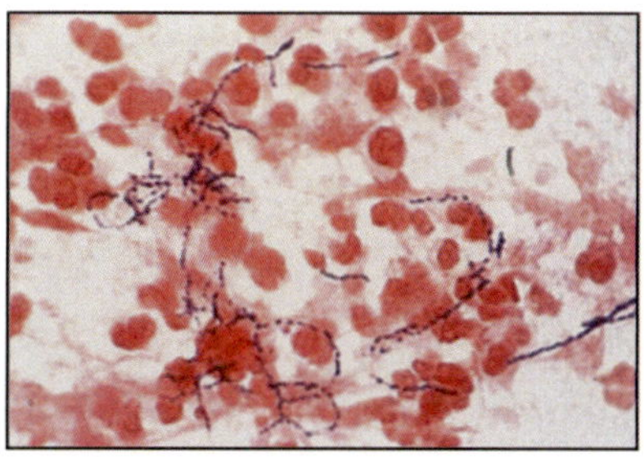

Fig. 1: Branching, gram-positive, beaded filamentous *Nocardia asteroides* (*Courtesy*: Rebecca Buxton, American Society for Microbiology)

Like other members of 'Coryneform' bacteria (*Corynebacteium, Mycobacterium, Rhodococcus*) the cell wall of *Nocardia* contains mycolic acids (short chain, 40-60 carbon atoms).The cell wall also contains peptidoglycan composed of meso-DAP, arabinose and galactose. Some strains of *N. asteroides* are partially acid-fast. The strains can retain carbol-fuchsin in modified Ziehl Neelsen's (Z-N) staining method where 1% sulphuric acid is used for decolourization instead of acid-alcohol.

All the species of *Nocardia* are non-motile. In human, a cell wall deficient morphological form (L-phase variant) is detected within lungs. The L-phase variant is associated with pathogenesis and persistence of the infection.

2. *Nocardia* is obligate aerobe
3. *Classification*: *Nocardia* belongs to the family Actinomycetes. As per the recent classification of 'List of prokaryotic names with standing in the literature' (LPSN, http://www.bacterio.net/index.html), there are 92 species under the genus *Nocardia* of which 54 species have clinical significance. Major veterinary important species are *N. asteroides, N. farcinica,* and *N. nova* (*N. asteroides* complex), *N. brasiliensis*, and *N. otitidis-caviarum*. In human, *Nocardia farcinica* is the most virulent species, intrinsically resistant to various antibiotics. Other major pathogenic species are *N. cyriacigeorgica*, *N. nova*, and *N. pseudobrasiliensis*.
4. *Resistance: Nocardia* are heat resistant. *N. asteroides* can tolerate 60°C for several hours. The bacteria can be destroyed by chlorine (100 ppm for 5 minutes) and benzalkonium chloride (100 ppm for 10 minutes).
5. *Natural habitat: Nocardia* is saprophyte, commonly found in the soil, vegetables, compost, fresh and saline water and animal faeces.

Isolation, growth and colony characteristics

Nocardia can be isolated in blood agar or Sabouraud's dextrose agar. The plates are incubated at 25-37°C for 4-5 days. The cultures develop a 'wet dirt' type of odour.

In blood agar, initial colonies after 48 hours of incubation are small. Later the colonies adhere to the surface of the media with their peripheral edges embedded into the agar. The colonies of *N. asteroides* are non-haemolytic except for few strains which may show haemolysis on sheep blood agar. Matured colonies are several centimetres in diameter, salmon coloured, waxy to powdery to velvety in texture depending on the production of white-pinkish mycelium.

In Sabouraud dextrose agar, the colonies are dry, wrinkled, and yellow and the colonies become deep orange colour with age.

In broth the surface pellicle with little turbidity is found.

Biochemical characteristics

Nocardia spp. produces following biochemical reactions

Biochemical Tests	Expected Results		
	N. asteroides	N. farcinica	N. brasiliensis
Catalase	(+ve)	(+ve)	(+ve)
Urease	(+ve)	(+ve)	(+ve)
Nitrate Reduction	(+ve)	(+ve)	(+ve)
Casein hydrolysis	(-ve)	(-ve)	(+ve)
Carbohydrate fermentation			
Glucose	(+ve)		(+ve)
Glycerol	(+ve)		(+ve)
Lactose	(-ve)		(-ve)

Antigenic characteristics

The polysaccharide antigens are found in cell extracts of *N. asteroides* and *N. brasiliensis*. On the basis of soluble antigen (protein in nature) *N. asteroides* can be classified into seven immunotypes.

Toxins and virulence factors produced

Toxins

Nocardia does not produce exotoxin in true sense. A toxic substance (HS-6) was detected in *N. otitidiscaviarum* isolated from cutaneous nocardiosis. The mouse intraperitoneal LD_{50} value of HS-6 is 1.25 mg/kg.

Virulence factors

Virulence Factors	Role in pathogenesis
Trehalose 6-6' dimycolate (cord factor)	It is present in the nocardial cell wall. It prevents phagosome-lysosome fusion and helps in intracellular survival of the bacteria within phagocytes
Catalase, superoxide dismutase	The enzymes help in intracellular survival of the bacteria within phagocytes and save the bacteria from the phagocytes (neutrophil)
Peptidoglycan	Highly virulent strains of N. asteroides have thicker peptidoglycan (15 nm) layer than weakly virulent strains (5 nm). Increased thickness provides more resistance against phagosomal enzymes specially the lysozyme
Growth phase	Log phase cells of N. asteroides are more virulent than stationary phase probably due to difference in fatty acid and mycolic acid composition. Filamentous forms are also more common in log phase having higher invasiveness than the coccoid form found in the stationary phase

Pathogenesis

Transmission

Nocardia are transmitted by ingestion, inhalation and wound contamination. The soil, fresh and saline waters are the major reservoirs of the infection. Nocardial mastitis in cattle occurs through contaminated hands, personnel and utensils. During dry period the bacteria are introduced with intramammary therapy.

Pathogenesis

After transmission of *Nocardia* within the susceptible host, anatomical barriers like skin, cilia present in the trachea and the phagocytes try to prevent the establishment of the infection. The virulent *Nocardia* survive within the phagocytes by preventing the phago-lysosome fusion through the surface lipid (cord factor). Other virulence factors like catalase, superoxide dismutase, thicker peptidoglycan, log phase of growth also help in intracellular survival of the bacteria. After establishment, generally the infection is localized. Sometimes the bacteria invade blood vessels and spread through the haematogenous route. Osteomyelitis, widespread abscess and encephalitis occur due to the dissemination.

Disease produced

Bacteria	Host	Disease produced
Nocardia asteroides	Cattle, pig	a) Acute and chronic mastitis: It is characterized by sudden onset, fever, anorexia, abnormal milk production. Hot, swollen, painful udder with granulomatous lesion and draining fistulous tracts. Lymphoadenopathy is common. Dissemination of infection into other organs is possible. b) Sporadic abortion
	Dog, cat	Mycetoma, lymphadenitis, nocardial stomatitis, pleuritis, peritonitis, abscess formation in heart, liver, kidney and brain
	Horses	Skin infection, abscess in lymph nodes, sporadic abortion
	Human	Pulmonary infection, 'Nocardia keratitis' associated with trauma, surgery, corticosteroid use and contact lens wear
Nocardia farcinica	Cattle, goat	Mastitis
	Cattle	Sporadic abortion, still-birth
Nocardia nova	Cattle	Mastitis
	Dog	Canine nocardiosis (along with Canine Distemper virus)

Bacteria	Host	Disease produced
Nocardia brasiliensis	Horse	Pneumonia, pleuritis
Nocardia otitidiscaviarum	Cattle Guinea pigs	Mastitis Ear infection

Immunity: Cell mediated immunity plays significant role in development of the protection. Antibodies are irregularly produced in low titres in human patients offering little protection. Nocardiosis is associated with immunosuppression in several species.

Diagnosis

Clinical samples: Mastitic milk, pus, aspirates from the nodules can be collected for detection of nocardiosis. The samples should not be frozen if intended for the isolation of the bacteria. The granules are found (like actinomycosis) in the clinical specimens in *N. brasiliensis* and *N. otitidiscaviarum* infection and rarely in *N. asteroides* infection. Tissues and thin section from granulomas in 10% formalin are collected for histopathology.

Laboratory examinations

Direct examination: A smear is prepared from the clinical sample and stained with Gram's as well as modified Ziehl Neelsen's stain. Gram-positive, partially acid-fast, uneven stained, filaments with branches are observed (Figure 1). Sometimes cocci or coccobacilli are also found. The author has personal experience on its primary identification from clinical cases of bovine mastitis based on typical microscopical appearance.

Isolation of bacteria from clinical samples: Media, incubation condition and colony characteristics are described earlier.

Serological tests: Serological tests for nocardial infection are not sensitive or specific. Nocardial antigen is heterogeneous and produces cross reaction with other bacteria. In humans, ELISA and western blot are used successfully for detection of antibodies.

Molecular biology: PCR is developed for detection of *N. farcinica* from clinical specimens using Nf1 and Nf2 primers generating a single intense 314-bp fragment.

Prevention and control

Hygienic milking, maintenance of personal hygiene of the milkers, cleanliness during intramammary infusion are the measures to prevent nocardial mastitis

17

Streptomyces and *Dermatophilus*

Streptomyces are soil-borne bacteria known for production of several antibiotics, antifungals, antivirals, antitumoral, anti-hypertensives and immunosuppressives.Krainsky (1914) first described *S. griseus* and named the species *Actinomyces griseus*. Waksman and Henrici (1948) changed the name to *Streptomyces griseus*.

Dermatophilus congolensis was first described from clinical case of exudative dermatitis in cattle in Congo by Van Saceghem (1915). It is primarily known as an animal pathogen causing acute, sub acute or chronic skin disease. The first cases of human infection with *D. congolensis* were reported in 1961 in four people who developed skin infection after handling an infected deer in USA.

Properties of genus

1. *Morphology: Streptomyces* are gram-positive filamentous bacteria (Figure 1). It consists of fungus-like mycelium, from which the vegetative and aerial hyphae emerge. The aerial hyphae carry the chain of spores. The aerial hyphae with the spores form a fuzzy layer on the surface of the colony. *Streptomyces* follows a typical growth cycle. In presence of favourable temperature, moisture and nutrients the spores germinate. The germination process involves swelling of the spores, formation of cell polarity and apical growth, which produces germ-tube, later converted into hyphae. The hypha grows by extension of tips and the mycelial network is produced by connecting across the growing branches. The hyphae secreate hydrolytic enzymes to get the nutrients from the polymeric substances. During formation of spores, the basal septum separates the sporogenic cells of aerial hyphae from the underlying cells ('subapical stem'). There is upregulation of FtsZ protein in the sporogenic hyphae which forms Z-rings in a regular interval. The Z-rings are converted later into septa, which divide synchronously the apical cells into a string of unicellular pre-spores. The septa help in separation and release of the individual spores. The spores are not reproductive units like fungus. The spores help in survival of the bacteria

under hostile environment associated with pigment and aroma present in the spores. *Streptomyces* spores are although less resistant to environment than other bacterial spores due to absence of dipicolinic acid (DPA) and small, acid-soluble, DNA-binding proteins (SASP) homologs. The spores and aerial hyphae (not vegetative) are covered with a fibrous sheath which produces the hydrophobic cell surface. The sheath is composed of proteins such as SapB, chaplin, and rodlin. The SapB helps in formation of structure of the spores. The chaplin is associated with formation of sheath over the aerial hyphae. The rodlins help in organization of the chaplins into the rodlet structure. Two systems (ParAB and FtsK) and five genes (*whiA*, *whiB*, *whiG*, *whiH*, and *whiI*) regulate the conversion of aerial hyphae into spores.'

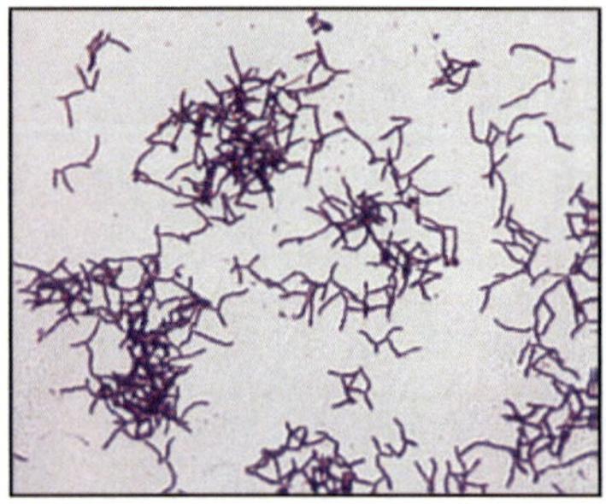

Fig.1: Gram-positive, branched rods of *Streptomyces*
(*Courtesy*: Ann C. Smith, American Society for Microbiology)

Dermatophilus are gram-positive, non-acid fast, unusual bacteria having branched filaments. It follows a life cycle with different morphological features. Young filaments are 0.5 to 1.5 μm in diameter. The filaments expand within epidermis as they produce layers of transverse and longitudinal septations and reach 5 to 8 μm in diameter, surrounded by a mucoid capsule. The septations result in the formation of sporangia (a kind of fungal fruiting body, sac like structure with spores) containing up to eight cocci cells. In the presence of liquid, the cocci are released and converted into flagellated motile zoospores. The motile zoospores are the infective form of the bacteria. The spores can infect the new site in the same animal or a new host. The zoospores become visible in the smear as parallel lines forming a 'railway-track' or 'trum-track' appearance (Figure 2). Under favourable conditions, the zoospores form germ tubes that develop into branching filaments. The filaments are the invasive form of the bacteria and the

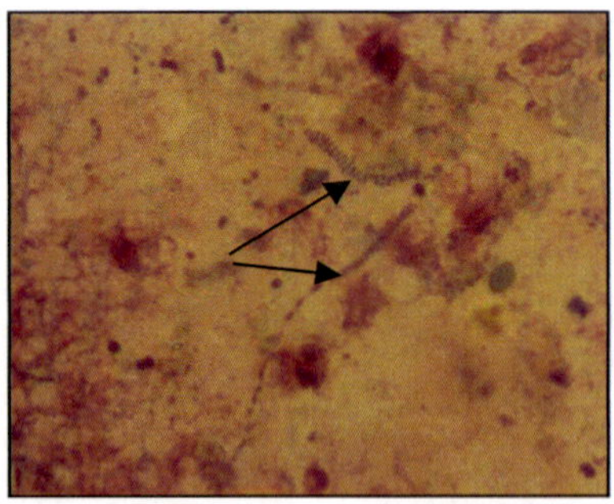

Fig. 2: Typical 'railway-track' or 'trum-track' appearance of *Dermatophilus* in Giemsa stained smear (1000X)
(*Courtesy*: M. Ananda Chitra, Central University Laboratory, Madhavaram Milk Colony, Tamil Nadu Veterinary and Animal Sciences University, Chennai)

cycle is repeated. *Dermatophilus* has cell wall composed of meso-DAP but lacks arabinose, galactose and glycine.

2. *Streptomyces* are aerobic in nature. *Dermatophilus* are facultative anaerobes and capnophilic (prefer 5-10% CO_2 tension for growth).

3. *Classification*: The genera *Streptomyces* and *Dermatophilus* are the members of phylum Actinobacteria and order Actinomycetales. The genera *Streptomyces* and *Dermatophilus* belong to Streptomycetaceae and Dermatophilaceae families, respectively. The genus *Streptomyces* is the sole member of Streptomycetaceae family and it consists of more than 500 species. *Streptomyces venezuelae* is considered as the model species of the genus. Major *Dermatophilus* species are *D. Congolensis* and *D. chelonae*. The second species was isolated from turtles and cobra snake.

4. *Resistance: Streptomyces* are resistant to the antibiotics produced by them and nitric oxide, the natural antimicrobial gas produced by the host immune system. The resistance determinants possessed by *Streptomyces* can be transferred into other soil bacteria and generate the pool of antimicrobial resistance genes ('resistome'). Enterococci acquire vancomycin resistance genes from the soil dwelling *Streptomyces*.

   D. congolensis can resist desiccation in exudative crust for several days. The bacteria are sensitive to pH and osmotic changes. The bacteria cannot survive or multiply in the environment for a long time and are susceptible to phenol, chlorhexidine, and benzalkonium chloride.

5. *Natural habitat*: *Streptomyces* are common in soil (40% of soil bacteria), water, rhizopshere (surrounding area of plant root) and other natural environments. The 'earthy' smell of the soil is attributed to the geosmin ('earth smell'), the secondary metabolite produced by the bacteria. *Streptomyces* also produces symbioses with plants and invertebrates (beewolf solitary digger wasps, ants etc.). The plants or insects provide nutrients to the bacteria and the bacteria protect them from other pathogens by producing antibiotics.

   Environment like soil is not an important source of *D. congolensis*. Infected animals such as cattle, sheep, goat, horses act as common reservoir. It is found throughout the world but is most prevalent in tropical and subtropical regions and has a broad host range.

6. *Genome*: *Streptomyces* genome is 8.1-1193 Mbp and is GC-rich (70 mol %). Recent analysis revealed the presence of 20-40 cryptic secondary metabolite biosynthetic gene clusters in a single genome. *S. coelicolor* is the most widely used species in genetic studies. The genome of *S.*

coelicolor encodes large numbers of enzymes such as proteases, chitinases / chitosanases, cellulases / endoglucanases, amylases, and pactato lyases. The antibiotics produced by different species of *Streptomyces* originate as signal molecules, which can alter the expression of certain genes, not associated with the stress response.

Isolation, growth and colony characteristics

Isolation of *Streptomyces* from soil samples requires serial 10-fold dilution of the sample. The isolation media includes *Streptomyces* agar, starch casein Agar (SCA), and international *Streptomyces* project 2 (ISP2) specific media. The malt extract present in the media provides acidic environment and nutrients. Calcium carbonate is the source of essential cations for growth. The plates after inoculation are incubated at 25°C-30°C for 4-5 days. Luxuriant colonies are detected after the incubation.

Commonly used media for the isolation of *Dermatophilus* is blood agar. It is incubated at 37°C with 5-10% CO_2 tension for 24-48 hours. The bacteria do not grow in Sabouraud dextrose agar. The colonies are rough, haemolytic, grayish-yellow, about 1 mm in diameter. The colonies can pit the media after 24 hours. Initially the rough colonies are formed by the branching filaments, but prolonged incubation stimulates the production of the cocci that produces yellowish colonies.

Biochemical characteristics

D. congolensis produce following biochemical reactions. It is not routinely practiced for identification of the bacteria

Biochemical Tests	Expected Results
Catalase	(+ve)
Indole	(-ve)
Urease	(+ve)
Nitrate reduction	(-ve)
Carbohydrate fermentation	
Glucose	(+ve)
Fructose	(+ve)
Maltose	(+ve)
Sucrose	(-ve)
Lactose	(-ve)
Mannitol	(-ve)

Antigenic characteristics

Streptomyces cells and the surface of spores contain protein antigens.

D. congolensis possesses somatic and flagellar antigens. The somatic antigen is shared by all the strains of the bacteria, whereas, the flagellar antigen is strain specific. It has antigenic relationship with *Nocardia*.

Toxins and virulence factors produced

Toxins

Plant pathogenic *Streptomyces* produces phytotoxin thaxtomin A and thaxtomin B, encoded by *txtA* and *txtB* genes. The thaxtomins inhibit cellulose synthesis in plant tissues. Cellobiose and suberin can activate the thaxtomin toxin.

No true exotoxin is produced by *D. congolensis.*

Virulence factors

Virulence factors	Function
Tomatinase (encoded by tomA)	Produced by *Streptomyces* which can inactivate antimicrobial saponin α-tomatine
Transcriptional regulator (txtR)	Regulates the expression of thaxtomin in *Streptomyces*
Serine protease, lipase	It helps in skin penetration of *Dermatophilus*. As well as they have role in nutrient acquisition and hydrolysis of cytokines and other immune effector molecules. Serine protease acts better in alkaline pH. Normal bovine skin pH is 5.6 but it becomes alkaline during inflammation. Trauma, injury, skin damage by biting flies may initiate the inflammatory response

Pathogenesis

Transmission

Pathogenic *Streptomyces* strains causing mycetoma can be transmitted to the susceptible humans and animals through penetrating trauma, puncture or lacerating wound.

Transmission of *D. congolensis* occurs by direct or indirect contact. Trauma, injury, skin damage by biting flies and ticks may help in creating portals for inoculation of the bacteria. The ticks (*Amblyomma variegatum*) causing immunosuppression, rainfall (tropical area), and malnutrition may predispose the infection. Ticks do not act as a vector. Infection begins at the skin if it is damaged and the skin defence is compromised. Heavy rainfall can also cause the skin damage by maceration of the epidermis. The damp weather facilitates the release of zoospores and their transmission from affected to healthy skin.

Pathogenesis

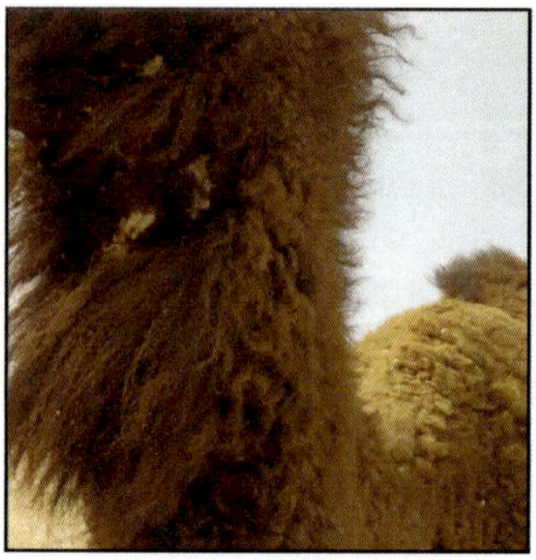
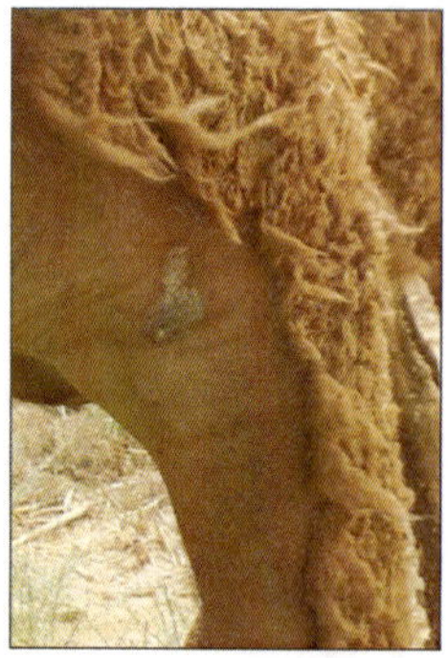

Fig. 3,4: Dermatophilosis in camel showing dry scab (*Courtesy*: Munaa Tawfeeq Abd, Veterinary Medicine College, Al-Muthanna University, Iraq)

D. congolensis infection begins with the entry of the zoospores through the damaged (soaked or injured) skin. Initially the zoospores are deposited into the deeper part of the skin. The spores chemotactically respond to the CO_2. After germination, the germ tubes and filaments are formed that invade the epidermis. Different enzymes produced by *D. congolensis* help in establishment of the infection by inhibiting the host defense. Neutrophils are found as an inflammatory response beneath the infected epidermis. Scab is formed composed of keratinocytes, branching filaments and infiltrated neutrophils (Figure 3, Figure 4). The filaments are restricted in the epidermis. Sometimes non-epidermal tissues like tongue, urinary bladder, lymph nodes are also affected specially in cats.

Disease produced

Bacteria	Host	Disease produced
Streptomyces somaliensis, S. griseus	Humans and animals	Mycetoma: It is a chronic pyrogranulomatous infection of the skin and subcutaneous tissues caused by bacteria or fungi
Streptomyces scabies	Plants	Potato scab
Dermatophilus congolensis	Cattle, sheep, horse, goat, camel, dog, cat, reptiles, human (occasional)	Dermatophilosis (Sterptothrichosis)/ 'lumpy wool'/ 'Strawberry footrot'/ 'Grease Heel'/'Rain rot': Exudative pustular dermatitis which is characterized by formation of dense hard scab. Sometimes lesions are moist with folded skin specially in horses. The dermatitis of wool covered skin in sheep is known as 'lumpy wool'. Ulcerative dermatitis of lower leg and feet in sheep is called 'Strawberry footrot' and in horses it is known as 'grease heel'. Lesions produced in the back after soaking in the heavy rainfall is known as 'rain rot' or 'rain scald' in horses
	Cattle	Associated with 'ulcerative lymphangitis'
Dermatophilus cheloniae	Crocodile (Australia), turtles, cobra snake	Skin infection

Dermatophilosis causes great economic losses in African countries due to poorer wool and leather quality, death and culling and decreased milk production. The disease also has zoonotic importance and can be transmitted to human.

Diagnosis

Clinical samples: Clinical samples are scab and exudate from the lesion.

Laboratory examination

Direct examination: Impression smear is prepared from the moist concave under surface of the freshly removed scab by gentle press. The smear can also be prepared by emulsifying the scab into sterile distilled water. The smear is air dried, fixed with methanol and stained with Gram's stain or methylene blue or Giemsa (30 minutes exposure). Gram positive branched filaments or the coccal zoospores having 'railway track' appearance are characteristically found. Giemsa is the better stain for this railway track appearance than Gram's stain. Sometimes the scab is found to have secondary infection. In thee scabs intact gram positive filaments or railway track is not observed. The cocci are found which cannot be distinguished from other coccus shaped bacteria.

Isolation of bacteria from clinical samples: Media, incubation condition and colony characteristics are described earlier.

Immunological tests: The presence of *D. congolensis* in the scabs with secondary invasion is identified by Immunofluorescence staining. Thin, heat-fixed smears of scab emulsions or impression smears are stained. Polyclonal antibodies against *D. congolensis* are used. Sometimes it produces cross reaction with *Nocardia.*

Serological tests: Serological tests are not routinely practised for diagnosis of *D. congolensis*. Counter immune electrophoresis and ELISA can be performed. Antibody titer is found in healthy animals also. Sometimes cross reaction is found with *Nocardia.*

Molecular biology: PCR can be used for diagnosis of *D. congolensis* using primers for amplification of 16SrRNA gene or alkaline ceramidase gene. The RAPD and PFGE are used for molecular typing of the *D. congolensis* isolates.

Prevention and control

The animals should be protected from rain water to prevent dermatophilosis. The animal sheds should be repaired before the onset of monsoon season. Infected animals should be kept in a separate shed. Tick control is required to prevent dermatophilosis in cattle. In sheep farms dipping is done periodically with bactericide (0.5-1% zinc sulphate, 1% alum) and insecticide. No vaccine is available to prevent the infection.

18

Enterobacteriaceae

The family Enterobacteriaceae belongs to the order Enterobacteriales. The family comprises 25 genera such as *Escherichia, Salmonella, Klebsiella, Yersinia, Proteus, Providencia, Shigella, Enterobacter, Morganella, Edwardsiella, Budvicia, Cedecea, Citrobacter, Ewingella, Hafnia, Kluyvera, Leclercia, Leminorella, Moellerella, Pantoea, Rahnella, Tatumella, Trabulsiella, Serratia* and *Yokenella*, out of which the first 10 genera are consistent pathogenic in humans, animals and birds.

Escherichia coli

Escherichia coli were first isolated by Theodor Escherich in 1885 from the faeces of infants. It was named in honour of the German pediatrician and its major natural habitat (colon). Previously it was also known as *Bacillus coli* or *Bacterium coli* (*B. coli*).

Properties of genus

1. *Morphology: E. coli* are gram-negative, short rods, 0.5µm × 1-3 µm varying form coccoid to long filamentous shape (Figure 1). The bacteria occur singly, in pair or in short chain. The bacteria are non-spore forming and mostly motile by peritrichous flagella. However, the motility may not be observed in some strains due to absence of flagella. The strains, those are adapted outside the intestine are encapsulated producing mucoid type of colonies in the solid media. The capsules are polysaccharide in nature and important virulence determinants, which enable the pathogenic strains to evade or counteract the unspecific host defense during the early phase of the infection. The bacteria interfere with the function of complement and phagocytes. The capsules are divided into two groups (group I and group II), which differ in chemistry and genetic organization. All capsular polysaccharides are chromosomally determined.
2. *E. coli* is aerobe or facultative anaerobe
3. *Classification:* The genus *Escherichia* is classified under the family

Enterobacteriaceae that belongs to the order Enterobacteriales. There are currently 8 numbers of species under the genus *Escherichia* such as *E. coli, E. albertii, E. blattae, E. fergusonii, E. hermannii, E. vulneris, E. marmotae* and *E. adecarboxylata*. Among them, *E. coli* are the important pathogen.

4. *Resistance:* 60°C temperature for 20 minute exposure and autoclaving (120°C for 15 minute) is lethal to *E. coli*. The bacteria may survive for months in dust, water, poultry houses and faeces of animals or humans. The bacteria are susceptible to drying and common disinfectants like phenol, cresol etc.
5. *Natural habitat:* The intestine of all vertebrates including humans is the most common natural habitat of *E. coli*. After birth, the sterile intestine is gradually inhabited by the bacteria from dam or the environment. Throughout the life it remains as major flora of the gastrointestinal tract. Majority of the bacteria are harmless, rather beneficial. Few pathogenic strains may produce the infection after rapid increase in numbers during stress condition of the host or immunosuppression (opportunistic pathogen). The bacteria are excreted through the faeces of animals and humans, which contaminate the environment.
6. *Genome: E. coli* has a larger genome of 4.6 Mbp in size containing approximately 4288 genes. Several DNA binding proteins (HU, H1) are found in the genome like eukaryotes. The HU protein condenses DNA and helps in its replication. Apart from genomic DNA, *E. coli* also has a variety of plasmids including those associated with virulence (compatibility family type IncF). Different pathotypes of *E. coli* possess the virulence plasmids encoding toxins, adhesins, colonization factors etc.

Isolation, growth and colony characteristics

Blood agar, MacConkey's agar are choice of the media for isolation. After producing characteristic growth in MacConkey's agar specific colonies may be transferred into eosine methylene blue (EMB) agar for further observation. Another selective and differential medium is 'sorbitol MacConkey agar (SMA)' that is used to isolate EHEC serotype O157:H7. The plates are incubated at 37°C for 24 hours. However, the bacteria can grow at 15-45°C and at pH 7.

In blood agar, *E. coli* colonies are smooth or rough, 2-3 mm in diameter, convex, moist, shiny and entire. Haemolysis depends on the strains. In MacConkey's agar, the colonies are pink in colour (Figure 2). The bacteria ferment the lactose sugar, present in the medium and make the medium acidic. The neutral red, present in the media as a pH indicator, produces pink colour in the acidic pH. Bile salts of the medium prevent the growth of the gram-positive bacteria. Lactose non-fermenters (*Salmonella, Proteus, Shigella*) produce pale or colourless colonies in MacConkey's agar due to production of basic pH by peptide digestion.

In EMB agar *E. coli* produces characteristic 'green-metallic sheen' that appears on the surface of the bacterial colonies (Figure 3). The dyes in EMB agar, eosin Y and methylene blue are pH indicators and inhibitors of gram-positive bacteria. The lactose present in the media, are fermented by the bacteria and at an acidic pH both the dyes combine to form a green-metallic precipitate (sheen).

In SMA, colourless colonies are produced as O157 cannot ferment the sorbitol.

Biochemical characteristics

E. coli produces following biochemical reactions

Biochemical test	Expected result
Catalase	(+ve)
Oxidase	(-ve)
Indole	(+ve)
Methyl red	(+ve)
Voges- Proskauer	(-ve)
Citrate	(-ve)
Urease	(-ve) [except some STEC strains]
H_2S production	(-ve)
Carbohydrate fermentation:	
Glucose	acid with gas
Lactose	acid with gas
Maltose	acid with gas
Galactose	acid with gas
Mannitol	acid with gas
Sucrose	Variable
Glycerol	Variable
Inositol	(-ve)
Dextrin	(-ve)
Gelatin hydrolysis	(-ve)
Lysin decarboxylase	(+ve)

The characteristic result of IMVC (Indole-Methyl Red- Voges Proskauer-Citrate) i.e. (+, +, -, -) helps is identification of *E. coli.*

Antigenic characteristics

E. coli can be classified into several serotypes on the basis of three major antigens i.e. somatic (O-antigen), capsular (K-antigen) and flagellar (H-antigen). Approximately, 173 O, 80 K and 56 H antigens have identified and numbered accordingly. Antigenically distinct groups can be formed by each of the antigen (O, H, and K) known as 'serogroup' (for e.g. O-serogroup). The antigenically distinct entity formed by all the three/ two major antigens is known as 'serotype' (for e.g. O140: K 56:H7). It means the isolate belongs to 'O-140' serogroup having capsular and flagellar antigen 56th and 7th, respectively.

O-antigen is the extracellular whisker like part of the gram-negative bacterial lipopolysaccharide (LPS). It is polysaccharide in nature and heat stable (not destroyed at 100°C). The sequence variability in the repeat structure of the O-antigen is the basis of the O-serogroup formation.

K-antigen is heat labile capsular polysaccharide produced by some *E. coli* strains. Majority of the strains produce microcapsule. O-serogroups 8, 9, 20, 64, and 101 produce abundant capsule like *Klebsiella*. Presence of K-antigen hinders the O-antigen agglutination with its homologous serum. In few strains, the capsules are poorly immunogenic *in vivo* due to the structural relationship with host cellular polysaccharides. The strains with such capsules (K1 or K5) are very virulent.

H- antigen are flagellar antigens present in motile *E. coli*. It is protein in nature. It acts as virulence marker for some strains. *E. coli* O157: H7 is highly virulent causing haemolytic uraemic syndrome (HUS) in human. Whereas, *E. coli* O157: NM (non-motile) is avirulent in nature. The bacteria can be passed through semisolid agar to increase H-antigen synthesis.

In addition to the major antigens, the strains of *E. coli* also possess fimbrial antigens like other members of Enterobacteriaceae family. It helps in adhesion of bacteria with the host cells (K88 / F4 and K99/F5 pilli). The antigens are not type or group-specific.

Many members of the Enterobacteriaceae family including *E. coli* O14, O56, O124, and O144, *Salmonella*, and *Shigella* share a common heat stable antigen known as 'enterobacterial common antigen (ECA)' or 'Kunin antigen'. The family specificity of ECA can be used for taxonomic and diagnostic purposes. ECA is located in the outer leaflet of the outer membrane. It is a glycol-phospholipid built up by an amino sugar heteropolymer linked to an L-glycerophosphatidyl residue. The genetical determination of ECA is closely related to that of lipopolysaccharide (LPS).

Toxins and virulence factors produced

Pathogenic *E. coli* strains have divided into different pathotypes based upon the diseases that they cause, the virulence factors and toxins that they possess and secreate, and their host of isolation. The types of infections caused by *E. coli* are grossly classified as being either intestinal or extra-intestinal. The infections are produced by two major pathogroups i.e. intestinal and extra-intestinal pathogenic *E. coli* (ExPEC). The pathogroups comprise of several pathotypes as mentioned below.

A. Intestinal pathotypes

i) *Avian pathogenic E. coli* (APEC): The pathotype causes systemic infection in poultry ('avian colibacillosis') and comprises of mainly O1, O2 and O78 serogroups.

ii) *Shiga-toxin-producing E. coli* (STEC): The pathotype produces shiga toxins (stx 1 and stx2) as major virulence factors. Approximately, 380 O-serogroups are isolated as STEC from human and animals. Among them, O 26, 91,103,111,113,121,145 and 157 are most frequently observed.

iii) *Enterotoxigenic E. coli* (ETEC): It produces enterotoxins (LT and ST) as major virulence factors. Serotypes like O8:K25, O8: K85, O9:K30, O9:K35, O101:K28 are considered as bovine ETEC.

iv) *Enteroinvasive E. coli* (EIEC): The bacteria can invade HeLa cells *in vitro* and M-cells, macrophages, and intestinal epithelial cells *in vivo* after attachment with colon mucosa.

v) *Attaching and effacing E. coli* (AEEC): The pathotype can produce characteristic 'attaching-effacing (AE)' lesion in the intestinal mucosa after intimate attachment. It has two following sub-types.

   a) *Enteropathogenic E. coli* (EPEC): It contains the pathogenicity island 'locus for enterocyte effacement (LEE)', which can encode 'intimin' protein, responsible for AE lesion.

   b) *Enterohaemorrhagic E. coli* (EHEC): It produces 'intimin' protein along with shiga toxins (stx1 and stx2) as major virulence factors. It comprises O157, O26, O111, O103, O145 serogroups.

vi) *Enteroaggregative E. coli* (EAEC): The pathotype produces distinct 'aggregative adherence' phenotype, which is seen as a brick-like pattern when the bacteria adhere to cultured HEp-2 cells.

vii) *Diffusely adherent E. coli* (DAEC): The pathotype produces 'diffuse adherence (DA)' pattern on cultured epithelial HEp-2 and HeLa cells. The pathotype appears to form a heterogeneous group.

B. *Extra intestinal pathogenic E. coli* (ExPEC) are a broad group of pathogens that colonize the extra intestinal compartment of animal and human hosts resulting urinary tract infections(UTIs), meningitis, peritonitis etc. The following pathotypes are coming under the pathogroup.

i) *Uropathogenic E. coli* (UPEC): Strains of UPEC are the primary cause of urinary tract infection like cystitis and pyelonephritis. It comprises of O2, 4, 6 and 83 serogroups.

ii) *Mastitic E. coli*: As the name suggests it is mastitis causing pathotype and comprises a wide range of serogroups.

iii) *Septicaemic E. coli*: The bacteria are responsible for septicaemic conditions in calves, pigs and dogs. The group comprises of O15, 35, 78, 115, 117 and 137 serogroups.

C. *Necrotoxigenic E. coli* (NTEC): NTEC strains are responsible for various infections of humans and animals including UTI, septicaemia and diarrhoea. The NTEC strains are both intestinal and extra-intestinal pathogens. It comprises of two major groups i.e. NTEC-1 and NTEC-2. The NTEC-1 is associated with human, cattle, pig, horse, dog and cat, whereas, NTEC-2 is mainly found in cattle and sheep.

The pathotypes produce several toxins and possess different virulence factors as mentioned in following table.

Major toxins

a) *Enterotoxins*: Two classes of enterotoxins are produced by *E. coli*. They are heat labile enterotoxin (LT) and heat stable enterotoxin (ST). Both of the toxins are responsible for diarrhoea production in different ways.

Heat labile enterotoxin (LT): Human and porcine strains of ETEC produce heat labile enterotoxins. LT is a large protein molecule (88KDa) having structural similarity with cholera toxin. Each molecule of toxin has one 'A' and 5 'B' subunits. The 'B' subunit helps in adherence of the toxin with enterocytes having ganglioside (GM1) receptors or intestinal brush borders having glycoprotein receptors. Active site of 'A' subunit is 'A_1'. After adherence, this 'A_1' enters the host cell. It activates adenylate cyclase system located near the basal membrane region of the cell. The system converts adenosine tri-phosphate (ATP) into cyclic adenosine mono-phosphate (cAMP) by the enzyme adenylate cyclase.

'A_1' toxin is adenosine diphosphate ribosyl transferase that causes ADP ribosylation of the regulatory protein of the adenylate cyclase system. The system is active when it is complexed with guanosine tri-phosphate (GTP) and regulatory proteins. It becomes inactive during when the GTP is converted into guanosine di-phosphate (GDP) by GTPase. Ribosylation of regulatory protein inhibits this GTPase. So the system remains in permanently active form.

Activation of the system results elevated level of cAMP. In turn, it increases the efflux of the ions (Na^+ and Cl^-) which enhances the osmotic pressure of the intestinal lumen. The enhanced osmotic pressure removes more amount of water from intestinal cells into the lumen. It results in increased volume of the lumen contents causing diarrhoea.

Heat stable enterotoxin (ST): The heat stable enterotoxins are low molecular weight toxins having two major types STa (STI) and STb (STII).

STa (STI): Bovine, porcine and human ETEC strains produce STa. The toxin is resistant to acidic pH and protease enzyme. It is encoded by a gene present in the transposon. The receptor for the toxin is glycoprotein in nature and is present in the enterocytes. Receptors in younger and weaned pigs are more active in toxin binding than adults and unweaned pigs. The toxin activates guanylate cyclase in the intestinal cells. The guanylate cyclase itself can act as receptor also. The enzyme enhances the cGMP activity and produces diacyl glycerol, inositol 1, 4, 5 tri phosphate and C-kinase from phosphatidyl inositol present in the intestinal villi border. The three products are responsible for Ca^{++} mobilization from intracellular compartments into the villi and the Ca^{++} impairs the absorption of Na^+ and Cl^- from the villi as well as stimulates the secreation of Cl^- from crypts. Thus the toxin acts as anti-absorptive, and more amount of fluid is accumulated into the intestinal lumen causing diarrhoea.

STb (ST II): Porcine ETEC strains produce STb. The gene encoding the toxin is present in the plasmid. The toxin stimulates the production of prostaglandin (PGE2) in the intestinal mucosal cells causing diarrhoea.

b) *Verotoxin / Shiga-like toxin/ Shiga toxin:* It is a heat labile toxin and protein in nature. It produces cytopathic effect in Vero cells and previously it was known as 'Verotoxin'. Later it is observed that it has structural and functional similarity with the toxin produced by *Shigella dysenteriae*. So it is designated as 'shiga-like toxin' or 'shiga toxin'. The strains of *E. coli* producing the toxin are known as shiga toxin-producing *E. coli* (STEC). Like labile toxin (LT) it is a heterohexamer, in which, one 'A' subunit (32 kDa) is non-covalently associated with a pentamer of 'B' subunits (7.7 kDa each) (A1B5). The 'B' subunits help in adherence of the toxin with the cell membrane ceramide receptor. Activated 'A_1' enters the cell and acts as N-glycosidase on 28S rRNA.

The enzymatic action prevents the binding of amino acyl t-RNA with the ribosome and prevents protein synthesis of the cell. Thus it causes cell death.

The shiga toxins are subdivided into two major groups, shiga toxin 1 (stx1) and shiga toxin 2 (stx2). Stx1 is a homologous group in which three variants (stx1, stx1c and stx1d) have been described. The stx2 group is more heterogeneous and is comprised of several subtypes (stx2, stx2c, stx2d, stx2e, stx2f, stx2g and activatable stx2d).

c) *Haemolysin:* Three types of haemolysins are produced by different strains of *E. coli.*

i) *Alpha-haemolysin*: Porcine strains causing diarrhoea produce alpha haemolysin. The genes are encoded by plasmid.

ii) *Enterohaemolysin*: Bovine or human STEC strains produce the weak enterohaemolysin. Its haemolytic activity is only demonstrated in washed red blood cells. The genes are encoded by a bacteriophage.

iii) *Contact haemolysin*: EIEC strains produce this type of haemolysin. It is encoded by virulence plasmid of the bacteria. It helps in lysis of endocytic vacuoles to escape the bacteria into the cytoplasm of colonic epithelial cells.

d) *Cytolethal distending toxin (CDT)*: Cytolethal distending toxin is a bacterial toxin produced by some strains of *E. coli, Salmonella, Shigella, Campylobacter* etc. It causes eukaryotic cell cycle block at the G2 stage prior to mitosis. The functional toxin is composed of three proteins i.e. CdtA, CdtB and CdtC. The CdtA and CdtC function as dimeric subunits, which carry the CdtB subunit and deliver it into the mammalian cells. The CdtB enters the nucleus and exhibits a DNase I-like activity that results DNA double-strand breaks and it causes cell cycle arrest, cellular distension and cell death._

e) *Cytotoxic necrotizing factor (CNF)*: The toxin has two types i.e. CNF1 and CNF2 (previously known as 'Vir' toxin).The toxins are 115 KDa and 110 KDa proteins, respectively and immunologically related. Both of the toxins cause multinucleation of cells in the culture and skin necrosis in rabbits. The toxins are produced by necrotoxigenic *E. coli* (NTEC). However CNF is also associated with *E. coli* strains causing diarrhoea and urinary tract infections in pigs, calves, and human.

Toxins and other virulence factors produced by different *E. coli* pathotypes

E. coli pathotype	Toxins produced	Role in pathogenesis	Virulence factors possessed	Role in pathogenesis
Avian Pathogenic E. coli (APEC)	a) Heat labile enterotoxin (LT)	As discussed	A) Fimbriae i) mannose binding type I fimbriae (F1)	Helps in adhesion of bacteria with host intestinal cells
	b) Homolog of the heat stable enterotoxin	As discussed	ii) Pap/ Prs fimbriae	Helps in adhesion of bacteria with chicken tissues and organs other than trachea.
	c) enterohaemolysin	As discussed	iii) Avian E. coli 1 (AC/1) fimbriae	It mediates adherence to avian epithelial tissues
	d) cytotoxic necrotising factor 1 (CNF 1)	As discussed	iv) Type IV pilli	
	e) cytolethal distending toxin	As discussed	B) Adhesins: i)afa-8 gene Cluster	Acts as adhesin
	f) cytotoxin designated as VT2y		ii) Curli (coiled surface structure)	Binds fibronectin and helps in adhesion
	g) vacuolating autotransporter toxin (encoded by VAT-PAI pathogenicity island)	Exact role is not established	iii) temperature-sensitive haemagglutinin (Tsh)	It helps at the early stages of infection including colonization of air sacs but not subsequent generalized infection.
			C) Invasin i) ibeA gene cluster	Helps in adhesion of bacteria with chicken tissues and organs other than trachea.
			ii) homologue of the 25 kDa 'Tia' protein	It mediates adherence to avian epithelial tissues
			D) Iron acquisition systems i) aerobactin system ii) salmochelin siderophore system (encoded by the iroBCDEN locus). iii) sitABC iron transport systems iv) putative iron transport system novel to APEC (eit)	It helps to sequester iron from body fluids
			E) outer membrane proteins encoded by traT and iss genes present in ColV plasmid	Resists complement deposition (C3), phagocytosis and offers serum resistance.

E. coli pathotype	Toxins produced	Role in pathogenesis	Virulence factors possessed	Role in pathogenesis
Shiga toxin producing *E. coli* (STEC)	a) Shiga toxins (Stx_1 and stx_2) These toxins are encoded by stx_1 and stx_2 genes.	As discussed	a) Non- LEE-encoded effectors (Nles): 32 molecules are distributed among 20 families encoded by prophages. Examples are NleA, NleB, NleC, NleD,,NleE, NleF, NleG.	It helps in pathogenesis
	b) enterohaemolysin (encoded by hlyA)	As discussed	b) F18 fimbriae	It is produced by porcine STEC causing 'edema disease' in pigs.
Enterotoxigenic *E. coli* (ETEC)	a) Heat labile enterotoxin (LT) b)Heat stable enterotoxin (ST)	As discussed	a)K99 / F5 fimbriae	It mediates bacterial binding to the small intestinal glycolipid ganglioside of newborn pigs and helps in production of newborn diarrhoea
			b)987P / F6 fimbriae	It mediates bacterial attachment with intestinal cells
			c)K88 / F4 fimbriae	It is produced by porcine ETEC causing post weaning diarrhoea in piglets. It helps in adherence of the bacteria with the epithelial mucosa.
			d) F18 fimbriae	It is also produced by porcine ETEC causing post weaning diarrhoea in piglets. It helps in adherence of the bacteria with the epithelial mucosa. F18 is the most important factor for adhesion of E. coli with porcine epithelial cells
Enteroinvasive *E. coli* (EIEC)			Inv plasmid	Encodes the protein acting as 'adhesin'
Enteropathogenic *E. coli* (EPEC)			'Intimin' encoded by eae gene present in the Locus for enterocyte effacement (LEE)	It helps in intimate adhesion of the bacteria with host cells and other products of this locus produces characteristic 'attaching-effacing' lesion

E. coli pathotype	Toxins produced	Role in pathogenesis	Virulence factors possessed	Role in pathogenesis
Enterohaemorrhagic *E. coli* (EHEC)	Shiga toxins like STEC	As discussed	'Intimin' encoded by eae gene present in the Locus for enterocyte effacement (LEE)	As discussed
Enteroaggregative *E. coli* (EAEC)	Heat stable toxin-1 (EAST-1) (encoded by high molecular weight virulence plasmid)	It activates guanylate cyclase, resulting in ion secreation into the intestinal lumen. It increases the osmotic pressure of the lumen responsible for accumulation of fluid and diarrhoea.	aggregative adherence fimbriae I and II (AAF/I and AAF/II)	Helps in adhesion of the bacteria
	Plasmid encoded toxin (Pet) (Encoded by high molecular weight virulence plasmid)	It belongs to serine protease autotrans-porter family and confers cytoskeletal rearrangements		
Diffusely adherent *E. coli* (DAEC)			Afa/Dr adhesins (produced by Afa/Dr DAEC)	Acts as bacterial adhesin
			adhesin involved in diffuse adherence (AIDA-I). It is produced along with EspA, EspB, and EspD protein homologues.	Acts as adhesion. Homolog proteins help in production of AE lesion.

E. coli pathotype	Toxins produced	Role in pathogenesis	Virulence factors possessed	Role in pathogenesis
Uropathogenic *E. coli* (UPEC) [O1, O2, O4, O6,O7, O8, O16, O18, O25 and O75]	Alpha haemolysin	At high concentrations, HlyA inserts into the membrane of target host cells and promotes their lysis	A.Fimbriae: i)Type I (encoded by fim) ii) P (Pap) iii)S (sfa) iv)F1C (foc)	They help in adhesion of bacteria with host cells
	Vacuolating auto transporter toxin (VAT) / Secreated auto transporter toxin (SAT)	It induces vacuolation and other cytopathic effects, leading to host tissue damage	B. Iron acquisition system: i) enterobactinsiderophore (ent) ii) salmochelin siderophore (chu) (hemin uptake system) (iro) iii)iron/manganese transport (Sit) iv) aerobactin siderophore (iutA) v) yersiniabactin siderophore (fyuA)	It helps to sequester iron from body fluids
	CNF 1	As discussed		
Mastitic *E. coli*	Endotoxin (LPS)		Capsule, serum resisatnce	
Septicaemic *E. coli* (O1, O2, O78:K80)	Endotoxin (LPS)		Serum resistance	
			Iron acquisition system	It helps to sequester iron from body fluids
Necrotoxigenic *E. coli* (NTEC)	CNF1, CNF2	As discussed		

Pathogenesis

Transmission

In a farm, *E. coli* is mainly transmitted through feed, drinking water, aerosols, fomites and carrier animals. The stress associated with transport, dietary change and extreme climate helps to establish the infection. Specially in piglets after dietary change during weaning with increased protein and less fiber may cause excessive multiplication of ETEC / STEC. Young animals or birds are more susceptible to the infection as their immune system is underdeveloped and some receptors for *E. coli* adhesins are only expressed in young animals.

Neonatal infection of chicks can occur horizontally, from the environment, or vertically, from the hen. A laying hen suffering from *E. coli*-induced oophoritis (inflammation of ovaries) or salpingitis may infect the internal egg before shell formation. Faecal contamination of the eggshell is possible during the passage of the egg through the cloaca and also after laying. The latter possibility is considered as the major route of infection for the eggs.

Pathogenesis

a) ETEC: After reaching small intestine ETEC adheres to the epithelial cells of the intestine with different fimbrial adhesins like F4, F5, F6 and F18. Capsular polysaccharide of some ETEC strains helps in formation of bacterial micro-colonies in the epithelium after adhesion. The polysaccharide increases the bonding between bacteria and the epithelium. After micro-colony formation, the bacteria start multiplication and liberate enterotoxins (LT and ST), which are responsible for diarrhoea.

b) STEC / EHEC / EPEC: After entry within the host, the bacteria require two conditions to establish an infection such as colonization in the intestinal mucosa and production of shiga toxins or other virulence factors. The colonization is mediated through bacterial 'intimin' protein, encoded by eae present in the locus for enterocyte effacement (LEE), a pathogenicity island. The LEE also encodes intimin receptor, known as translocated intimin receptor (Tir, previously Hp90). The process begins with the delivery of the receptor within the cells to make an efficient attachment with the intimin. The attachment produces characteristic 'attaching-effacing (AE)' lesion in the intestinal mucosa. The AE lesion is characterized by intimate adhesion of the bacterium to the epithelial cell membrane, with an intervening gap of approximately 10 nm, accompanied by effacement of enterocyte micro-villi.

Strains without the LEE (STEC) may adhere with the intestinal mucosa through another adhesin protein known as 'STEC autoagglutinating adhesin' (encoded by *saa*).

After colonization, STEC / EHEC start to multiply and produce shiga toxins that are responsible for distinct clinical syndrome.

The EPEC strains do not produce any toxin. It can increase the intracellular calcium level of enterocytes, which in turn inhibits sodium and chloride absorption and stimulates chloride secretion by enterocytes. More amount of fluid is accumulated in the intestinal lumen causing diarrhoea.

c) *UPEC:* Majority of the UPEC strains are opportunistic and remain within the intestine. The favourable conditions help to express the virulence factors like adhesins of different types to adhere and infect the urinary tract. Once inside the urinary tract, UPEC preferentially colonizes the bladder and causes cystitis, but can also ascend through the ureters into the kidneys, causing pyelonephritis. In the bladder, type-I fimbriae of bacteria helps in attachment with the uroepithelial cells. The adhesion should bc firm cnough to withstand the outflow of the urine. After invading the bladder-epithelial cells, the bacteria start to multiply and form intracellular biofilm like communities. The bacterial community activates specific cell signal of the infected uroepithelial cells to exfoliate or slough. Exfoliation is a process by which host can clear more number of bacteria through the outflow of urine. This process leaves the underlying layers of immature bladder epithelial cells exposed and more susceptible to infection. UPEC also liberate different toxins like alpha-haemolysin, VAT/SAT, CNF causing cellular damage. The cellular damage results local inflammatory reaction and cystitis/ pyelonephritis follows.

d) *Mastitic E. coli:* The bacteria enter through the teat canal and establish a local infection within udder. Antiphagocytic capsule and serum resistance property of the bacteria help in establishment of the infection. Bacterial endotoxin plays major role in inflammatory response in the udder and toxaemia.

e) *Septicaemic E. coli:* The bacteria enters bloodstream of young calves (a week age) through the nasopharyngeal area, intestine and umbilicus. Serum resistance property and iron acquisition system from serum helps in bacterial survival. The endotoxin liberated by the bacteria produces characteristic syndrome. Lack of sufficient colostrum feeding is predisposing cause of the infection. It is associated with agammaglobulinemia or hypogammaglobulinemia. Probably a specific factor present in gammaglobulin helps in resistance against this pathotype of *E. coli*.

Disease produced

Bacteria	Host	Disease produced
APEC	Poultry	Avian colibacillosis: It is characterized by perihepatitis, airsacculitis, pericarditis, although other syndromes such as egg peritonitis, salpingitis, omphlitis (mushy-yolk disease), cellulitis and osteomyelitis/ arthritis are also observed. The coligranuloma (Hjarre's disease) occurs following colisepticaemia that is characterized by nodular lesions in liver and intestine. In chickens, swollen head syndrome often results from synergistic infection of turkey rhinotracheitis virus and E. coli
	Turkey	Osteomyelitis complex
STEC	Calves (O5, 26, 103, 111 serogroups)	Haemorrhagic colitis In India, the author with the team first reported isolation and characterization of STEC from diarrhoeic calves and lambs, buffaloes, poultry and free flying pigeons, goats, rabbit and yak
	Pig (after weaning) serogroups like O138, 139, 141 are mostly involved	Edema disease (gut edema/ bowel edema): It is caused by STEC strains specially those can produce stx_{2e} subtype of toxin. The toxin is absorbed from the intestine and it damages the vasculature particularly in the cerebellum. The infection is characterized by edema in different body parts, ataxia, convulsion, paralysis and sudden death.
ETEC	Mammals	Neonatal diarrhoea (watery diarrhoea)
	Pig	Post weaning diarrhoea
	Human	Traveller's diarrhoea
EIEC	Human	Bacillary dysentery
EPEC	Cattle, sheep, goat, dog , cat	Mucoid and chronic diarrhoea
EHEC	Human	EHEC causes haemorrhagic colitis, haemolytic uraemic syndrome (HUS) in human. In India, O157 is reported from diarrhoeic patients but their clinical significance is not established
	Calves	Diarrhoea
EAEC	human	Children diarrhoea, Traveller's diarrhoea

Bacteria	Host	Disease produced
DAEC (Afa/Dr DAEC)	human	Urinary tract infections (pyelonephritis, cystitis and asymptomatic bacteriuria)
DAEC [adhesin involved in diffuse adherence (AIDA-I) producing DAEC]	Children	Infantile diarrhoea
UPEC	Dog, cat	Cystitis, pyometra
Mastitic *E. coli*	Cattle	Coliform mastitis
Septicaemic *E. coli*	Calves	Colisepticaemia (white scours): Diarrhoea occurs in less than 1 week old calves, specifically those are colostrum deprived. Faeces is watery at first, later becomes white paste around the rectum. Animals become dehydrated and emaciated. Death occurs within 7 days, if untreated.
Necrotoxigenic *E. coli*	Cattle, sheep, pig, horse, dogs, cat	Diarrhoea, urinary tract infection, septicaemia
E. coli	Dogs	Canine chronic enteropathy (inflammatory bowel disease): During inflammatory response to bacterial or food antigens, oxygen tension of the intestine is reduced, anaerobe concentration decreases and E. coli flares up. Anorexia, chronic vomition, diarrhoea and weight loss persists for 3 weeks. Extra-intestinal diseases, parasitic infestation, neoplastic disease are ruled out. Few animals respond to dietary changes and are referred to as having dietary-responsive enteropathy

Immunity: The defense mechanisms against *E. coli* depend on production of specific antibodies which can either prevent the bacterial attachment with the host cell or neutralize the bacterial toxin or itself. These antibodies are maternal in origin and transferred from dam to offspring through colostrum.

Diagnosis

Clinical samples

The clinical samples include faeces, urine, mastitic milk, vaginal exudates, cardiac blood and affected tissues like liver, spleen, pericardium or bone marrow. The specimens should be collected from fresh carcasses as the bacteria readily invade the tissues after death.

Laboratory examinations

Direct examination: A smear can be prepared from centrifuged deposit of collected milk and urine or exudate samples or tissues and stained by Gram's Method. *E. coli* appears as gram negative small rod arranged in a pair or short chain (Figure 1).

Isolation of bacteria from clinical samples: Media, incubation condition and colony characteristics are described earlier.

Pathogenicity of *E. coli* isolates from clinical samples should be confirmed as the bacteria are present as normal flora. Pathogenicity can be ascertained by ligated loop assay, cell culture cytotoxicity assay, typing of the isolates and detection of toxin by serological or DNA based methods.

a) *Ligated loop assay*: Sambhu Nath De (1959), Professor of Pathology at Nilratan Sircar Medical College in Kolkata discovered the simple technique to study the toxins of *Vibrio cholerae*. The toxins of *E. coli* such as LT/ STb, CNF-2 toxins can be assayed in rabbit or weaned pig ligated ileal loop. The six-inch segments of small intestine, in which, no feed is present are cut off and both the ends are ligated with silk. The segment is inoculated with the suspected bacterial culture via a 22-gauge needle. A part of the same intestine is inoculated in similar way with tryptic soya broth inoculation. It serves as control. After 24 hours, distension of the inoculated portion with fluid is found in positive case. The fluid in the loop is turbid, very mucinous, and often sanguineous and usually contains clots of precipitated mucus. Occasionally there is edema of the associated mesentery. The degree of distension varies. Fluid weight per gut length of the loop can be calculated to measure the intensity of toxin action. The control shows no distension with fluid.

b) *Cell culture cytotoxicity assay*: Profound cytotoxicity of Vero cells by shiga toxins are 'gold standard' method for detection of STEC/EHEC. The test involves treatment of vero cell monolayer with test bacterial extract and examining cells for cytopathic effect (like virus) after 48-72 hours of incubation. The specificity of the assay can be improved by the addition of shiga toxin specific antisera. HeLa cells can also be used instead of Vero, however, they are less sensitive. Other *E. coli* like EAEC / DAEC/NTEC can be detected by Hep-2 or HeLa cell line adherence test. Effect of LT can be assayed in the Vero cell monolayer.

c) *Greater wax moth (Galleria mellonella) infection model*: Hamilton syringe (10 μl) is used to inject 5 μl aliquots of test *E. coli* suspension into *G. mellonella* larvae through the hindmost left proleg. The larvae are placed in a static incubator in the dark at 30°C. For 50% lethal dose (LD_{50}) experiments, a series of 10-fold serial dilutions of *E. coli* suspension containing from 10^6 to 0 bacteria in 10 mM $MgSO_4$ with 1.2 mg/ml ampicillin are injected into *G. mellonella* larvae. The control larvae are injected with 5 μl of only $MgSO_4$ with ampicillin to detect any lethal effect of the physical injection process. Ten larvae are injected at each dilution. The larvae are scored as dead or alive 48 and 72 hours post infection. The larvae are considered dead when they displayed no movement in response to shaking of the petri dish or touch with a pipette tip.

d) *Serological tests*: Latex agglutination test and ELISA are developed for detection of APEC whole bacterial antigen (O2, O78) or fimbrial antigen. For detection of STEC/ EHEC antigens (stx toxins), the sandwich ELISA, affinity purified polyclonal antibodies, immobilized monoclonal antibody or Gb3 receptors as capture system are developed. Shiga toxin antigens can be detected in culture supernatant, bacterial extract or directly in the faecal sample as well as in saliva. Reverse passive latex agglutination test, colony blot are also developed for detection of STEC/ EHEC.

e) *Histopathology*: Histopathological slide of the intestine (ileum) showing characteristic attaching effacing (AE) lesion helps in diagnosis of AEEC.

f) *Typing methods*: Typing and subtyping of strains is a valuable aid to identify outbreaks. Serotyping can be performed with specific antisera against *E. coli* O, H and K antigens in tube or plate agglutination tests. However it cannot be used for all *E. coli* pathotypes. The EAEC strains auto-agglutinate due to 'aggregative phenotype' and are often described as 'untypeable (UT)' or 'rough' in serotyping report. In India, O-serogrouping of *E. coli* isolates is routinely performed by National *Salmonella* and *Escherichia* Centre (NSEC), Central Research Institute, Kasauli, Himachal Pradesh.

Modern methods of typing or subtyping of *E. coli* isolates include phage-typing, pulsed field gel electrophoresis (PFGE) and multiple-locus variable number tandem repeat analysis (MLVA).

g) *Molecular biology*: DNA based assay for STEC detection includes colony hybridization with polynucleotide probe and PCR. In PCR based detection, crude lysate or DNA extract from single colony, mixed broth cultures, colony sweeps, direct extract of faeces or food can be used as template. Originally the multiplex PCR was developed by Paton and Paton (1998) for detection of stx genes (stx_1, stx_2) along with *eaeA* and *hly*. The author and his team has personal experience in detection of STEC isolates from diverse animal and bird sources in West Bengal and Jammu & Kashmir state of India using the multiplex PCR successfully. Later, several modified PCR methods have developed that can detect shiga toxins and their variants. The problems may arise during use of PCR with direct faecal sample as it contains PCR inhibitory substances producing false negative results. Sometimes false positive result is found for detection of 'cryptic gene' (free *stx* encoding phages or presence of defective *stx* gene in bacteria).

For detection of other pathotypes like EAEC, multiplex PCR targeting three different genes i.e. anti-aggregation protein transporter gene, EAST gene and a chromosomal gene present in the pheU pathogenicity island is designed. The toxin genes of ETEC (encoding LT /ST) can be detected by PCR using specific primers against them.

Prevention and control

Prevention of colibacillosis in poultry and dairy farms is difficult as the bacteria are part of the commensal flora. The following measures can reduce *E. coli* transmission in poultry and animal farms.

a) Strict biosecurity measures should be followed in the poultry farms to reduce the numbers of *E. coli* entering the birds through feed, water, air, soil, and rodents. The farms should have rodent control program to reduce the transmission of *E. coli* and other infections. Feeding with mash can be replaced with pellet (prepared by hot pelleting) to reduce bacterial transmission. Addition of egg-yolk powder (5-10%) into the feed and chlorination of drinking water can reduce *E. coli* numbers. Proper ventilation of the farm can also reduce exposure to the bacteria and endotoxin, and ammonia mediated damage of the respiratory tract. Drying of the wet litter is an effective way for reducing bacterial transmission in poultry farms.

b) Immunosuppression due to concurrent viral infection of the animals or birds should be checked as it favours the replication of *E. coli*.

c) The hatching eggs are another common route of *E. coli* transmission between the flocks. Collection of eggs immediately after hatching, fumigation or disinfecting eggs, discarding the soiled and cracked eggs, daily cleaning and disinfection of hatchery unit can reduce *E. coli* transmission.

d) Pathogenic *E. coli* strains in the gut of the poultry and animals can be omitted by replacing the flora with the intestinal contents of resistant birds or animals, commercial 'competitive exclusion products' consisting of *Bacillus subtilis*, *Lactobacillus* etc.

e) No commercial vaccine against *E. coli* is used extensively in poultry farms. In European Union, a commercial vaccine is available against avian colibacillosis consists of fimbrial (papA) and flagellar antigen (FT). Inactivated vaccine is available against *E. coli* O2 and O78 serotypes. Few experimental vaccines such as live vaccine prepared from non-pathogenic *E. coli* strain (BT-7), vaccine prepared from *carAB* mutant strain of a virulent O2 serotype, and the strain O78 mutants with deletions of *galE*, *purA*, and *aroA* genes are also prepared which produced varied level of protection against avian colibacillosis.

f) Strict biosecurity measures should be maintained to prevent colibacillosis in calves. No commercial vaccine is available.

g) To control post weaning diarrhoea in piglets, intestinal acidification, application of antimicrobials in drinking water and feed, competitive exclusion with probiotics, administration of binding agents such as eggs, milk and zinc oxide are applied. No commercial vaccine is available.

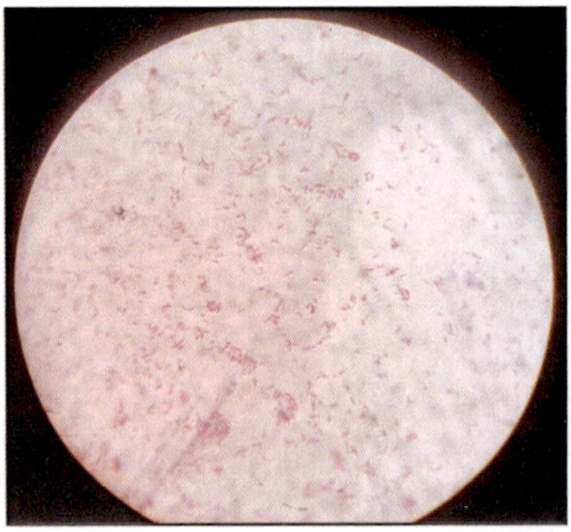

Fig. 1: Gram-stained smear of *E. coli* isolated from birds in India (*Courtesy*: Pratik Ghosh, Department of Veterinary Microbiology, West Bengal University of Animal and Fishery Sciences, Kolkata, India)

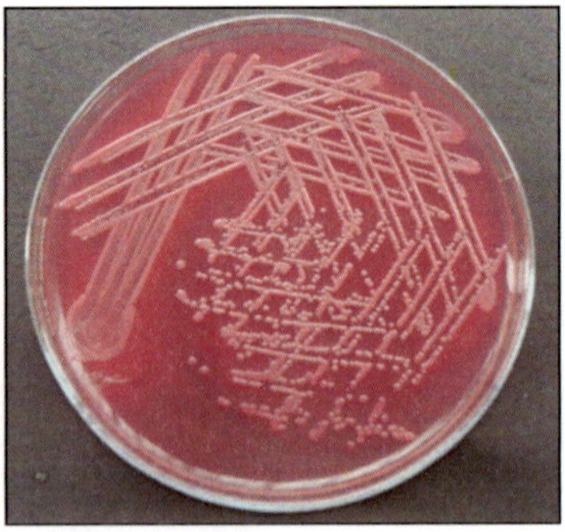

Fig. 2: MacConkey's agar plate showing the typical lactose-fermenting pink-cloured of *E. coli* (*Courtsey*: Achintya Mahanti, Department of Veterinary Microbiology, West Bengal Univertsity of Animal and Fishery Sciences, Kolkata, India)

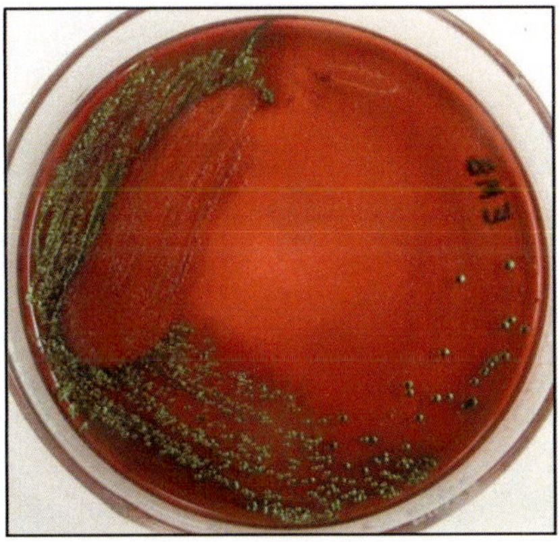

Fig. 3: EMB agar plate inoculated with a mixed culture of *E. coli* and Pseudomonas aeruginosa. The greenish metallic-sheen is produced by *E. coli* and the pinkish colonies are produced by *Pseudomonas aeruginosa* (*Courtesy*: Archana Lal, American Society for Microbiology)

Klebsiella

In 1883, Friedlander first isolated the bacteria from a case of lobar pneumonia in human. The case was later referred as 'Friedlander's pneumonia' and the causative bacteria as *Klebsiella pneumoniae* or 'Friedlander bacillus'.

Properties of genus

1. *Morphology: Klebsiella* are gram-negative thick rods, 1-3 × 0.5-1 µm in measurement. The bacteria occur singly or in pair. The bacteria possess polysaccharide capsule both *in vivo* and *in vitro*. The bacteria are non-spore forming and non-motile. Some strains are fimbriated.

The capsule can be demonstrated by India ink / nigrosin stain or Hiss method (gentian violet and copper sulphate) of staining. This method of staining with India ink / nigrosin is called 'negative staining'. In this technique, instead of staining the bacteria itself, only their background is stained. The capsule is visualized as a clear unstained halo surrounding the bacterial cell. Sometimes crystal violet / methylene blue are used to stain the bacterial cell to differentiate it from the black coloured background (Figure 4).

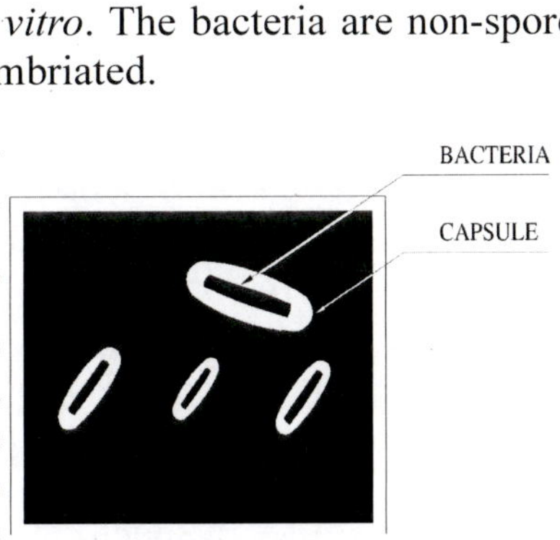

Fig. 4: Negative staining with India Ink demonstrates the *Klebsiella* capsule (schematic)

2. *Klebsiella* is aerobe or facultative anaerobe

3. *Classification:* The genus *Klebsiella* is classified under the family Enterobacteriaceae that belongs to the order Enterobacteriales. There are currently total 23 species and 3 sub-species under the genus *Klebsiella*. The important species are *K. pneumoniae, K. oxytoca, K. granulomatis, K. terrigena, K. planticola (K. trevisanii), K. ornithinolytica. Klebsiella pneumoniae* has three subspecies such as *pneumoniae, ozaenae,* and *rhinoscleromatis.* Among them, *K. pneumoniae* ssp. *pneumoniae* and *K. oxytoca* are animal pathogens.

4. *Resistance:* 60°C temperature for 20 minutes exposure and autoclaving (120°C for 15 minute) are lethal to *Klebsiella*. The bacteria may survive for months in dust, water, faeces of animal and poultry houses. The bacteria are susceptible to drying and common disinfectants like phenol, cresol etc.

Antibiotic resistance: Klebsiella belongs to 'ESKAPE' group of pathogens which are capable of 'escaping' the lethal action of antimicrobial agents and responsible for most of the nosocomial infections. The 'ESKAPE' group is composed of *Enterococcus faecium, Staphylococcus aureus, Klebsiella pneumoniae, Acinetobacter baumannii, Pseudomonas aeruginosa, and Enterobacter* spp. Resistance to beta-lactam group of antibiotics are developed in the bacteria through the production of β-lactamase enzyme that lyses the beta-lactam ring present in these antibiotics. Later, extended spectrum of these antibiotics is developed (cephalosporins) which are resistant to the beta-lactamase enzyme. Unfortunately, this time also the bacteria started to produce a new class of enzyme named as 'extended-spectrum beta-lactamases (ESBLs)' that can lyse cephalosporins (ceftazidime, cefotaxime, and ceftriaxone), monobactams (aztreonam) as well as penicillins. The presence of an ESBL-producing organism in a clinical infection can result in treatment failure if one of the above classes of drugs is used. First described in Germany (1983) and France (1985) among *Klebsiella* spp, ESBLs exist in every region of the world and in most genera of Enterobacteriaceae family. At present, there are three types of ESBL i.e. TEM, SHV and CTX-M. Plasmid borne TEM was first recognized in 1965 among the strains of *E. coli* isolated from a patient in Greece (the designation 'TEM' came from the patient's name, Temoniera). Likewise, another plasmid-mediated β-lactamase, known as 'SHV-1' (sulfhydryl variable), was first identified in *Klebsiella pneumoniae* and *E. coli.* Third variety i.e. CTX-M was first identified in *E. coli* isolated from otitis of a child in Munich (Germany, 1990). The enzyme can hydrolyse specifically cefotaxime and accordingly it was named as 'CTX (cefotaximase)-M (Munich)'.New Delhi metallo-beta-lactamase (NDM) is a kind of carbapenemase enzyme (28 KDa) produced by some members of Enterobacteriaceae family. The carbapenemase enzyme can lyse carbapenem group of antibiotics, active against gram-negative bacteria particularly those producing ESBLs. The NDM-1 was first detected in *Klebsiella pneumoniae,* isolated from a Swedish patient having Indian exposure (New Delhi based hospital). It is encoded by $bla_{NDM\text{-}1}$ gene, carried by an integron. The NDM-1 was also detected in *E. coli, Citrobacter, Morganella.* The treatment of such bacteria is difficult as it shows resistance to most of the antibiotics.

5. *Natural habitat:* Majority of the bacteria are found in soil, surface water, sewage and plants as saprophytes. In animal sheds, it is commonly found in the sawdust beddings. Some strains of *Klebsiella* can live in respiratory, intestinal tract, penis exterior (stallion) of healthy animals and may cause infection during alteration of normal bacterial flora (opportunistic pathogen). In human, the rate of carrier state varies from 1% (respiratory tract) to 38% (faeces).

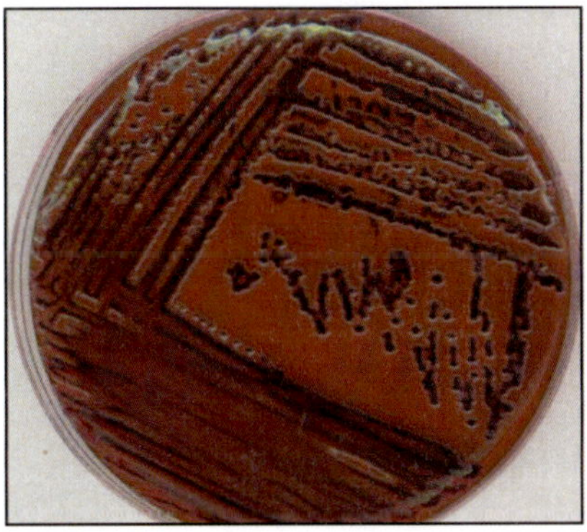

Fig. 5: EMB agar plate inoculated with *Klebsiella pneumoniae* showing brown, dark-centered, mucoid colonies (*Courtesy*: Naowarat Cheeptham, American Society for Microbiology)

Isolation, growth and colony characteristics

Klebsiella can grow in ordinary isolation media like blood agar, MacConkey's agar and EMB agar. The incubation requires 37°C temperature for 24 hours.

The colonies in blood agar, after 24 hour growth are 2-3 mm in diameter, non-haemolytic, mucoid, and viscous. Large mucoid, sometimes dome shaped colonies are formed due to abundant capsule production. It can distinguish *Klebsiella* from other members of Enterobacteriaceae. The capsules are lost after subculture, and small colonies are formed. In MacConkey's agar, the lactose fermenting pink coloured colonies are found. In EMB agar, *K. pneumoniae* produces brown, dark-centered, mucoid colonies (Figure 5). The bacteria produce magenta coloured colonies in specific medium *Klebsiella* selective agar (Figure 6).

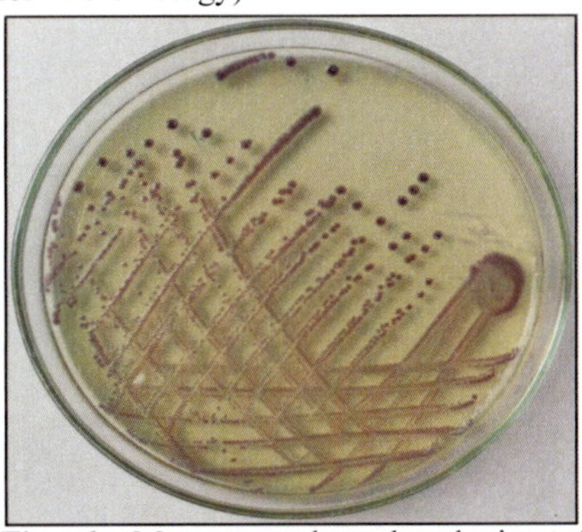

Fig. 6: Magenta coloured colonies of *Klebsiella* sp. in *Klebsiella* selective agar isolated from pigs in India (*Courtesy*: Arindam Samanta, Department of Veterinary Microbiology, West Bengal University of Animal and Fishery Sciences, Kolkata, India)

Certain pathogenic *Klebsiella* (K1 and K2 serotypes of *K. pneumoniae*) produce 'hypermucoviscous phenotype (HMV)' in solid media [encoded by genes like *magA* (mucoviscosity-associated gene A) and *rmpA* (regulator of the mucoid phenotype)]. When a standard bacteriological loop is passed through the colony and it forms a viscous string greater than 5 mm, the strain belongs to HMV phenotype. The isolates with this phenotype is associated with severe clinical syndrome such as primary liver abscess, meningitis and endophthalmitis in human.

Biochemical characteristics

Klebsiella pneumoniae produces following biochemical reactions

Biochemical test	Expected result
Catalase	(+ve)
Oxidase	(-ve)
Indole	(-ve)
Methyl red	(-ve)
Voges- Proskauer	(+ve)
Citrate	(+ve)
Urease	(+ve)
H_2S production	(-ve)
Carbohydrate fermentation:	
Lactose	(+ve)
Maltose	(+ve)
Mannitol	(+ve)
Sucrose	(+ve)
Inositol	(+ve)
Gelatin hydrolysis	(-ve)
Lysin decarboxylase	(+ve)

Antigenic characteristics

Three kinds of antigens are present in *Klebsiella* i.e. somatic (O-antigen), rough (R- antigen) and capsular (K-antigen). There are total 12 and 82 types of somatic and capsular antigens, respectively. The somatic antigens cannot be used for serotyping of the isolates because the detection of somatic antigens is hampered by the heat-stable capsule. The 77 types of capsular antigens form the basis for an internationally recognized capsule typing scheme. The capsule typing shows good reproducibility and is capable of differentiating most clinical isolates. The drawback of the technique is the large numbers of serological cross-reactions that occurs among the 77 capsule types. Thus, individual sera have to be absorbed with the cross-reacting K-antigens. Capsular type K1 and K2 are the major virulent types of *K. pneumoniae*.

Toxins and virulence factors produced

Toxins

a) *Endotoxin (LPS)*: It is responsible for fever, neutropenia, petechiae, shock, pulmonary edema, and vascular collapse.

b) *Enterotoxin*: Some strains of *K. pneumoniae* produce an enterotoxin having structural similarity with stable enterotoxin of *E. coli* (ST). The toxin activates guanylate cyclase of the intestinal epithelial cells causing hyper-secretion of fluid into the intestinal lumen and diarrhoea.

Virulence factors

Virulence factors	Function
Capsule	Antiphagocytic It inhibits the differentiation and functional capacity of macrophages in vitro
Pilli / fimbriae a) Type I pilli b) Type III pilli c) KPF-28 fimbriae	The pilli help in binding of the bacteria to mucus or the epithelial cells of the urogenital, respiratory and intestinal tracts
Adhesins: CF 29K (R-plasmid-encoded) of K. pneumoniae	It mediates adherence to the human intestinal cell lines
Serum resistance and LPS	Serum acts as first line of defense against invading bacteria through complement activation. Most commensal gram-negative bacteria are sensitive to the bactericidal effect of serum, whereas, the pathogenic strains often exhibit serum-resistance. Capsule may hide the bacterial surface and prevent complement activation. In some strains, O-side chain of LPS produces steric hindrance of lytic complement action (MAC formation)
Enterochelin and aerobactin	Acts as siderophore to help in iron acquisition

Pathogenesis

Transmission

1. In cattle, teat canal is the portal of entry of *Klebsiella* into the mammary gland. Coliform infections are usually associated with unhygienic environment. *Klebsiella* are found in bedding materials of cattle shed containing sawdust.

2. In horses, *K. pneumoniae* often utilize venereal route of transmission (coitus, insemination with infected semen and genital manipulations).

3. In humans, the bacteria are frequently acquired in hospitals specially in immunocompromised patients. The principal reservoirs include

gastrointestinal tract of healthy human and hands of the patients. It is estimated that *Klebsiella* species cause 8% of all hospital-acquired infections ('nosocomial infection') in human.

Pathogenesis (mastitis)

Klebsiella enters the udder through the teat canal by unknown mechanism. Unlike to other mastitis causing gram-positive bacteria (*Staphylococcus*), *Klebsiella* and other coliforms (*E. coli*) do not adhere to the epithelial cells or colonize the udder. The coliform can multiply in the udder secreation without attachment with epithelial surfaces. Severity of the infection depends on the multiplication and numbers of coliforms present. The multiplication of the bacteria occurs after effective lactose utilization and survival in nearby anaerobic condition (oxygen tension of the udder interior is low). During dry period bacterial multiplication is decreased due to unavailability of iron. Lactoferrin (iron binding protein) concentration is also increased during dry period, which further decreases iron availability to the bacteria. In this condition, secreation of 'enterochelin' and 'aerobactin' siderophores (iron acquisition system) helps in bacterial survival. *Klebsiella* is found most efficient in establishing udder infection in this unfavourable condition than other coliforms. Coliform mastitis may result in bacteremia as the blood-milk barrier is destroyed.

The host defense system acts by recruiting phagocytes against the infection. Antiphagocytic capsule and serum resistance property of *Klebsiella* helps in evading the immune response. Endotoxin is released from the bacteria at the time of cell death initiating an inflammatory response. It is responsible for certain systemic signs of clinical mastitis like fever and decreased milk production.

Disease produced

Bacteria	Host	Disease produced
Klebsiella pneumoniae ssp. pneumoniae	Cattle, pig, goat	**Acute mastitis (coliform mastitis):** Duration of intramammary infection is 21 days. Infection rate is more in dry period than lactation. During lactation, incidence is highest at calving and decreases as days in milk advances. Systemic signs of clinical mastitis include anorexia, fever, dehydration, diarrhoea and decreased milk production
	Horse	Endometritis, infectious seminal vesiculitis
	Calves, foals, kids	Neonatal septicaemia
	Dog	Pyometra, cystitis, pneumonia, encephalitis, enteritis, mastitis, neonatal septicaemia, otitis
	Poultry	Embryo mortality

	Human	Community acquired bacterial pneumonia: (in alcoholics mortality rate is near 100%)
	Human	**Nosocomial infection:** The bacteria are frequently acquired from hospitals and in immunocompromised patients, it causes respiratory or urinary tract infection.
Klebsiella pneumoniae ssp. *rhinoscleromatis*	Human	**Rhinoscleroma:** It is characterized by a chronic inflammatory process of the nasopharynx. The infection is distributed around the world but is more prevalent in eastern Europe, Latin America, central Africa, and southern Asia
	Human	**Ozena:** a chronic atrophic rhinitis characterized by necrosis of the mucosa and mucopurulent nasal discharge. It has become rare now a day.
K. oxytoca	Horse	Endometritis, infectious seminal vesiculitis
	Companion birds	Septicaemia, respiratory infection, diarrhoea
K. granulomatis	Human	Granuloma inguinale: sexually transmitted disease

Diagnosis

Clinical specimen: Clinical samples for *Klebsiella* detection include mastitic milk, faeces, urine, vaginal exudates, uterine secreations, ear exudates etc. It varies with the species of animals.

Laboratory examinations

Direct examination: A smear can be prepared from centrifuged deposit of collected urine or exudate samples and stained by Gram's Method. *Klebsiella* appears as gram-negative small rods with capsules. The capsule can be demonstrated by India ink/ nigrosin stains.

Isolation of bacteria from clinical samples: Media, incubation condition and colony characteristics are described earlier.

Serological tests: Enzyme linked immunossorbant assay (ELISA) is developed to detect the capsular antigens as well as antibodies against *K. pneumoniae*.

Molecular biology: PCR is developed for detection of *K. pneumoniae* based on identification of 16S-23S internal transcribed spacer. Capsular types K1, K2 and putative virulence factors like *rmpA* (regulator of mucoid phenotype A) are also confirmed by PCR. Molecular biology based typing of *Klebsiella* isolates include plasmid profiling, ribotyping, multilocus enzyme analyses, pulsed-field gel electrophoresis and variable number tandem repeat (VNTR) analysis.

Prevention and control

Coliform mastitis is originated mostly from the contaminated farm environment. Proper sanitation and disinfection of the farm premises, utensils, washing of udder before and after milking, disposal of mastitic milk with 5% phenol, control of fly and insect population can reduce the infection.

Salmonella

Daniel Elmer Salmon (1885), a veterinarian was the first to isolate *Salmonella chloleraesuis* from the infected pigs. It was considered as a cause of 'hog cholera' until the discovery of the actual causative virus. The nomenclature of '*Salmonella*' was done in memory of Salmon. Gartner (1888) first isolated *Salmonella enteritidis* from meat poisoning case in human. In 1889, Klein in UK first isolated *Salmonella gallinarum* from chicken suffering with an infection known as 'fowl typhoid'. Rettger (1899) first described *Salmonella pullorum* from chicken suffering with severe diarrhoea.

Properties of genus

1. *Morphology: Salmonella* are gram-negative short rods, 2-4 µm in length and 0.5 µm in width varying form coccoid shape to long filamentous forms. They are non-spore forming and mostly motile by peritrichous flagella (except *S. Gallinarum, S. Pullorum* due to host adaptation). Although some strains of *S.* Pullorum are motile if grown in special media. Few mucoid colony forming strains produce capsule and some strains are fimbriated.

2. The bacteria are aerobe or facultative anaerobe.

3. *Classification:* The genus *Salmonella* is classified under the family Enterobacteriaceae that belongs to the order Enterobacteriales. The three major species under the genus *Salmonella* are *Salmonella enterica* (2440 serovars), *S. bongori* (20 serovars) and *S. subterranea. Salmonella enterica* is considered as type species of the genus. *S. enterica* has 6 subspecies (ssp) i.e. *salamae, arizonae, diarizonae, houtenae, indica,* and *enterica.*Most of the pathogenic *Salmonella* are designated as 'serovar' under *S. enterica* ssp. *enterica.* The virulent serovars are Typhi, Typhimurium, Dublin, Choleraesuis, Pullorum, Gallinarum, Abortusovis. To avoid confusion between serovars and species, the serovar name is not italicized and starts with a capital letter. The genus name is capitalized and italicized. The species and subspecies name is only italicized. In the beginning of a scientific literature the name of the *Salmonella* serovars are written as *Salmonella enterica* serovar Pullorum. After the first use, the serovar may be used without a species name, e.g., *Salmonella* Pullorum. In India, several new serovars are reported like *S.* Bareilly (cattle,

poultry, fish meal), *S.* Mathura (cattle), *S.* Gokul (pigs), *S.* Brijbhumi (sewage), and *S.* Goverdhan (sewage).

4. *Resistance*: *Salmonella* can be destroyed by exposure to 55°C temperature for 1 hour, 60°C for 20 minutes and autoclaving. Common disinfectants like phenol, cresol and formaldehyde (fumigation) are lethal to the bacteria. The disinfectants are not effective in presence of faeces, mucus, and organic substances. Faecal materials protect the bacteria from desiccation under the direct sunlight. The bacteria can survive freezing.

5. *Natural habitat:* All warm blooded animals and humans, as well as cold blooded animals (snake) can harbour *Salmonella* in the intestinal tract. The faeces are the major source of environmental contamination. The bacteria can survive approximately up to 9 months in moist soil, water, and vegetables.

The carrier animals or birds showing no symptom often shed the bacteria and act as a source of infection. Adults become carrier more frequently than young animals. Different types of *Salmonella* carriers have been detected. i) Active carriers are formed after recovery from the *Salmonella* infection and it can shed the bacteria for several months/ years up to 10^5 cfu / gram of faeces. ii) Passive carriers ingest *Salmonella* from the environment and shed them through the faeces without systemic involvement. They may stop shedding after changing the surrounding environment. iii) Latent carriers harbour the bacteria but do not shed through the faeces. They may become intermittent shedders. Certain stress factors like transportation, parturition, steroid administration, concurrent viral/protozoal infection enhance the shedding.

6. *Genome*: The genome size of *Salmonella* varies from 4659-4686 Mbp. It carries several pseudo- genes. The number of pseudo-genes varies with *Salmonella* serovars.

Salmonella serovars	Number of pseudo-genes
S. Typhi	204
S. Typhimurium	25
S. Gallinarum	309
S. Enteritidis	113

Pathogenicity islands (PI) are genetic elements that carry genes encoding virulence factors, such as adhesin, invasin and toxin genes. The PI is located on the chromosome or on a plasmid. It is flanked by repeat sequences and it has a varied G/C composition compared with the surrounding genome. *Salmonella* has two major PIs i.e. *Salmonella* pathogenicity island-1 (SPI-1) and *Salmonella* pathogenicity island-2 (SPI-2). The two PIs contain type III secreation system (T3SS, a complex of protein that helps in virulence factor transmission into the host cells). Several other PIs are also detected now a day. Among them SPI-7 is the largest genomic island (134 Kb) yet identified in *Salmonella.* It was first discovered as a large insertion in the genome of the human restricted pathogen like *S.* Typhi and *S.* Typhimurium. The 'major pathogenicity island' was renamed as SPI-7 after the discovery of a number of other *S.* Typhi-specific islands.

Recent advancement detects type VI secreation system (T6SS) in many gram-negative bacteria including *Salmonella.* T6SS is associated with biofilm formation, cytotoxicity and survival in the phagocytic cells. It is encoded by the *Salmonella* pathogenicity island 19 (SPI-19), present in serotypes Dublin, Weltevreden, Gallinarum and Enteritidis.

The serovars like Typhimurium, Enteritidis and Choleraesuis are known to harbour virulence plasmids. The virulence plasmids have a genetic region called '*Salmonella* plasmid virulence' (spv), which contains *spvRABCD* genes. The genes help in intracellular bacterial survival and replication. Some of these virulence plasmids contain transfer (*tra*) genes that help in transfer of these plasmids into other compatible bacterial strain by conjugation.

Isolation, growth and colony characteristics

Salmonella do not require blood and serum for growth. However, *Salmonella* are present in the host intestine with lots of other bacteria that can suppress its growth. So use of the enrichment media results better isolation rate. The enrichment media are liquid or semi-solid agar media that contain additives that selectively permit salmonellae to grow while inhibiting the growth of other bacteria. Using selenite-F broth, selenite-cysteine broth, tetrathionate or Muller-Kauffmann Tetrathionate-Brilliant Green broth (MKTBG), Rappaport Vassidialis (RV) broth or semi-solid agar, gram-negative broth (GN) and KIMAN broth can enrich *Salmonella* from clinical or other samples. Selenite, tetrathionate, brilliant green used in the broths prevents the growth of other enteric bacteria. The enrichment varies for different host-adapted *Salmonella* serovars. Poultry or pig adapted serovars (Choleraesuis, Pullorum, Gallinarum) can be better enriched by RV or KIMAN broth. Tetrathionate is inhibitory for some strains of *S.* Pullorum or *S.* Gallinarum. Selenite is toxic for *S.* Choleraesuis, and brilliant green is for *S.* Dublin. Isolation of *Salmonella* from animal/poultry feed samples, pharmaceutical products also requires RV enrichment. The enrichment broth with the samples is incubated at 37°C for overnight. Some laboratories prefer higher temperature (43°C) for specific serovar enrichment.

After enrichment, the aliquot taken from the supernatant of the broth can be inoculated into selective solid media for isolation. Sometimes fresh samples without enrichment are also inoculated into the solid media. The solid selective media includes brilliant green agar (BGA), MacConkey's agar, deoxycholate citrate agar, xylose lysine deoxycholate agar (XLD agar), Hektoen Enteric agar (HE) and *Salmonella* agar (ONOZ). The plates are incubated at 37°C for overnight. However *S.* Pullorum grows slowly and requires incubation for 48 hours.

In selective solid agar, circular, smooth 2-3 mm diameter colonies are produced with characteristic colour reaction from which they can be tentatively identified. Some serovars like *S.* Pullorum, *S.* Choleraesuis grow less in solid media and produce dew drop like colonies. *S.* Gallinarum produces colonies with typical seminal plasma like smell.

In BGA, non-fermentation of lactose by *Salmonella* produces alkaline pH. The phenol red indicator produces red coloured colony in alkaline pH. *Salmonella* produces convex, pale-red and translucent colonies similar to *Citrobacter*. *Proteus* forms pin-point colonies, *Pseudomonas aeruginosa* appears as small red colonies, and lactose fermenters are green. *Salmonella* Pullorum produces small, paler colonies than other salmonellae. BGA is the medium of choice following enrichment.

In MacConkey's agar and deoxycholate (XLD) citrate agar, *Salmonella* produces lactose non-fermenting pale or colourless colonies. MacConkey is the medium of choice for direct plating from tissues. The XLD agar contains bile salt, xylose, lactose, sucrose, lysine and iron salt. The bile salts prevent the growth of gram positive bacteria. *Salmonella* ferments xylose and decarboxylates lysine. Ratio of xylose and lysine is such that the decarboxylation always predominate producing alkaline pH. The phenol red indicator produces red colonies in alkaline pH. The center of the colony is black due to H_2S production that reacts with iron salt to produce iron sulphide (Figure 7).

HE agar contains bile salts, lactose, salicin and iron salt. *Salmonella* does not ferment the sugars and alkaline pH is produced. The bromo-thymol blue indicator produces green coloured colonies in alkaline pH. The center of the colony is black due to H_2S production that reacts with iron salt to produce iron sulphide (Figure 8). All serotypes of *Salmonella* have this appearance on Hektoen enteric agar except for serotype Typhi, which is a weak H_2S producer.

In *Salmonella* agar (ONOZ), yellow coloured colonies are produced. It contains lactose sugar, bile salts, brilliant green and neutral red indicators. The lactose non-fermenters produce alkaline pH by peptide digestion which gives yellow coloured colonies due to the presence of neutral red indicator. The bile salts prevent the growth of gram-positive bacteria.

Biochemical characteristics

Salmonella produces following biochemical reactions

Biochemical test	Expected result
Catalase	(+ve)
Oxidase	(-ve)
Indole	(-ve)
Methyl red	(+ve)
Voges- Proskauer	(-ve)
Citrate	(+ve)
Urease	(-ve)
H_2S production	(+ve)
Triple Sugar Iron Agar	R/Y/H_2S +
Carbohydrate fermentation	
Glucose	acid with gas
Lactose	(-ve)
Maltose	acid production
Mannitol	acid production
Sucrose	(-ve)
Inositol	Variable
Gelatin hydrolysis	(-ve)
Lysin decarboxylase	(+ve)

The characteristic result of IMVC (Indole-Methyl Red- Voges Proskauer-Citrate) i.e. (-, +, -, +) and TSI agar (R/Y, H_2S +) helps is identification of Salmonella.

Antigenic characteristics

Motile *Salmonella* possesses two major types of antigens i.e. somatic (O-side chain of LPS, designated also as O-antigen) and flagellar (flagellin protein, designated as H-antigen). Several numbers of O and H antigens exist in bacterial population due to the variations in the types, numbers, linkage, conformation of sugars present in the O-antigen and variations in the amino acid sequences of flagellin protein. At present, 46 'O' and 114 'H' antigens exist. On the basis of their variations, Kauffman and White (1929) developed a classification system of *Salmonella*, known as 'Kauffman and White scheme'. Each of the O-antigen is designated by numbers like 1, 2, 3 etc. A single strain may possess more than one number of antigens (for e.g. *S.* Choleraesuis contains O-antigens 6, 7). The flagellar antigens have two types i.e. phase 1(H1) and phase 2 (H2), encoded by two types of flagellin genes (*fliC* and *fljB*). Phase I antigens are designated by capital letters of the alphabets (A, B, C, etc.). As the number of antigens has crossed the total number of alphabets (26), later ones are designated as Z1, Z2 and Z3 etc. The phase 2 antigens are represented by numerical (1, 2, etc.). Two flagellar antigens (H1 and H2) are antigenically not related and are produced by two antigenically different types of bacterial cells. It is known as 'phase variation'. It is useful to prevent the antibody mediated attack. The frequency of alternate expression of the two genes (*fliC* and *fljB*) is 10^{23}-10^{25}/ cell/ generation and the switching between the expressions are controlled by fljB operon.

The isolates are identified by serotyping, with more than 2500 serovars. Each serovar is the unique combination of O, H1 and H2 antigens. Most of the serovars are designated by an antigenic formula containing O, H1 and H2 antigens. Each of them is separated by a colon. For e.g. *Salmonella salamae* 9, 46: z: z39. The serotyping of *Salmonella* isolates is routinely performed by National *Salmonella* Centre, Indian veterinary research institute (IVRI), Bareilly, UP, India and Central research institute (CRI), Kasuli, HP, India.

Vi-antigen

It is an additional antigen found in *S.* Typhi, *S.* Paratyphi C, *S.* Hirschfeldii and some strains of *S.* Dublin. Structurally, it is a polymer of N-acetyl aminohexuronic acid. Two genetic loci, *viaA*-locus and *viaB*-locus, are required for the production of Vi antigen in *S.* Typhi and *S.* Paratyphi C. It is associated with virulence of the bacteria in mice. It can also be used for Vi-typing of the isolates possessing the antigen. Currently it is experimentally used in Vi-based vaccine production against *Salmonella.*

Toxins and virulence factors produced

Toxins

Salmonella enterotoxin (Stn): A cholera-toxin (CT) like, heat-labile enterotoxin is produced by *S.* Typhimurium. It is functionally related with cholera toxin, labile toxin (LT) of *E. coli.* It binds with ganglioside receptor of the host cells (G_{M1}). It elevates cAMP level and produces diarrhoea in a similar way of LT/ CT. The toxin can elongate Chinese hamster ovary (CHO) cells in culture and induces fluid secretion in rabbit ligated ileal loop. However, its role in diarrhoea production is not established.

Cytotoxin: The toxin kills target cells through the inhibition of protein synthesis. Death of target cells may hamper absorption or secreation of fluid from intestinal lumen causing diarrhoea. Three kinds of cytotoxins have been detected.

a) Heat labile, trypsin sensitive cytotoxin is detected in several serovars of *Salmonella.* It can produce HeLa and Vero cell cytotoxicity.

b) Low molecular weight cytotoxin (a part of outer membrane protein)

c) Contact haemolysin (26 KDa): It is cytolytic for Vero and other cells

Endotoxin (LPS): The virulence of bacteria depends on length of O-side chain of LPS. Reduced length is associated with low virulence. The LPS produces vascular damage and thrombosis in the intestine through the induction of inflammatory mediators and cytokines. Systemic changes observed in the infection like fever, circulatory collapse, disseminated intravascular coagulation, shock are also attributed to the endotoxin action.

Virulence factors

Virulence factors	Function
Acid tolerance response (ATR) regulatory factors / acid shock proteins (RpoS σ-factor, PhoPQ, and Fur proteins)	RpoS and PhoPQ proteins are important for the regulation of survival in the low pH environment created by inorganic acids, whereas Fur and RpoS are involved in the regulation of organic acid tolerance. Thus the bacteria can survive in the acidic pH of the intestine.
Fimbriae [type 1 fimbriae (Fim), long polar fimbriae (Lpf), thin aggregative or curli fimbriae and plasmid-encoded fimbriae (Pef)]	Fimbriae help in adhesion of the bacteria with host cells. 'Fim-fimbriae' binds α-D-mannose containing receptor in many host cells. 'Lpf' binds to the surface of the Peyer's patches and M cells, 'Pef' binds to the villous intestine, and curli- fimbriae bind to the small intestine.
Salmonella pathogenicity island 1 (SP1) associated type III secretion system (T3SS)	[The T3SS is a complex of proteins that allows the transfer of virulence factors directly into the host cells and is associated with at least 20 structural and regulatory proteins involved in cellular invasion. The base structure of the T3SS complex spans the cell membrane and the cell wall of Salmonella, and a needle like structure protrudes from the base that interacts with the host cells. Within the base and needle structure is an inner rod through which the virulence proteins are transferred.] Major T3SS associated virulence protein is 'SopB'. It causes alteration of ion balance within the cell. It leads to fluid secretion within the intestinal lumen & diarrhoea. Other proteins such as SipA, SopA, SopD, and SopE2 may also play a role in Salmonella-associated gastroenteritis. Other T3SS proteins like 'Salmonella invasion protein' [SipA, SipC; encoded by 'invasin' gene (inv)], as well as SopB interact with the actin cytoskeleton causing cytoskeletal rearrangements leading to membrane ruffling. The organisms are trapped within these ruffles. Later they are up taken by these enterocytes. Membrane ruffling helps in internalization of the bacteria within the cells. Hil-A (hyperinvasion) protein either acts as invasion protein or an activator for expression of an invasion protein.

Virulence factors	Function
Salmonella pathogenicity island 2 (SP2) associated type III secretion system (T3SS)	Invasive Salmonella can express this T3SS associated proteins within 'salmonella containing vacuoles (SCV)' after internalization by the host cell. Major T3SS associated proteins are SifA, SseF, and SseG that interact with microtubule bundles and are involved in the formation of Salmonella-induced filaments (SIF) that extend from SCV. This SIF helps in the bacterial replication. Other protein like SpiC is translocated into the cytosol of host macrophages and disrupts the secreation of antimicrobial products like reactive oxygen intermediates (ROI). So intracellular survival depends on these T3SS proteins. [In poultry adopted serovars (S. Gallinarum) these T3SS proteins are associated with major virulence and persistence of infection]
Salmonella pathogenicity island 3 (SP3) encoded proteins	These proteins also help in intracellular survival and are required for growth in Mg+ deficient conditions.
Salmonella pathogenicity island 4 (SP4) encoded proteins	These proteins help in invasion of host cells
Salmonella pathogenicity island 5 (SP5) encoded proteins	Identified in S. Dublin, required for enteric form of the infection.
Salmonella pathogenicity island 7 (SP7)	Identified in S. Typhi, S. Typhimurium. SP7 is associated with the locus for production and export of Vi antigen (viaB-locus) and a type IV pilli.
Plasmid encoded virulence factors a) Salmonella Plasmid virulence (spv)gene encoded proteins b) 'traT' gene encoded protein c) other genes	a) These proteins help in intracellular bacterial replication specially during extra intestinal infection. b) serum resistance c) intracellular survival & growth, immunosuppression, stimulation of spleenomegaly
Iron acquisition system Enterochelin (enterobactin)	It helps in acquisition of iron required for bacterial growth

Pathogenesis

Transmission

Faeco-oral route is the major transmission route of *Salmonella* in human, animal and birds. Other possible routes include inhalation and conjunctiva. Infected animals, birds act as carrier and excreate the bacteria through the faeces (upto 10^5 cfu/gm), which contaminate the surroundings. Ingestion of contaminated water and feed transmits the infection. Animal and poultry feeds specially prepared from milk, meat, bone or egg contents can act as source of infection. Even fertilizers act as a potent source. However, pelleting of the feeds reduces *Salmonella* transmission.

In human, poultry egg is one of the major sources of *Salmonella* infection (*S.* Enteritidis). The contamination of poultry houses with *Salmonella* occurs through human, sewage, rodents, or any other sources. The bacteria survive and multiply in hen house environment and enter the birds thorough the oral route. The bacteria penetrate the egg shell either after or during oviposition in healthy birds through the faecal contamination. Sometimes, *Salmonella* enter the eggs by direct contamination of yolk, albumen, and egg shell before oviposition due to infection in the reproductive tract. The chances of egg penetration are less before oviposition in healthy laying birds. During laying the reproductive tract of a healthy hen everts the vagina beyond the alimentary tract, which protects the emerging egg from faecal contamination. After laying, from environmental sources the bacteria can penetrate the egg shell, if proper sanitation is not maintained in the hen house. Other than eggs, raw milk, contaminated pasteurized milk, pet turtles also act as source of infection to human. Human to human transmission rarely occurs.

Pathogenesis

After entry through the oral route, *Salmonella* is deposited in the intestine, where they invade enterocytes. In the intestine, low pH, peristalsis, intestinal mucus, lysozyme in secreations and moreover, normal microbial flora try to destabilize the bacterial colonization. Normal microflora in adults prevents the *Salmonella* colonization by occupying the receptors, known as 'competitive exclusion'. Young are more susceptible as their intestinal microflora range is not fully developed like adults. Competitive exclusion is utilized in newly hatched chicks as therapeutic measure to prevent *Salmonella* colonization ('Nurmi concept').

If the infection occurs with *ad libitum* number of *Salmonella,* in spite of all defensive measures few will survive to invade the enterocytes. Bacterial fimbriae, SP-1 T3SS associated proteins (as discussed in virulence factor section) help in adherence with the enterocytes. The interaction between the T3SS proteins (SipA, SipC) with the actin cytoskeleton of enterocytes causes cytoskeletal rearrangements leading to 'membrane ruffling'. The bacteria are trapped within the ruffles. Later, they are taken up by the enterocytes. 'Membrane ruffling' helps in internalization of the bacteria within the cells. Once the *Salmonella* is internalized, the bacteria reside in the membrane bound *Salmonella* containing vacuoles (SCV). As the SCV matures, it migrates from the luminal border of the cell to the basal membrane, where *Salmonella* enter the macrophages associated with Peyer's patches in the sub mucosal space. The SCV never fuse with lysosome within macrophages and thus avoid phagolysosome associated microbial killing mechanism. Other factors like SP-2 T3SS (SipC protein), SP-3 associated proteins also help in intracellular survival. The formation of *Salmonella* induced fibrils (SIF) helps in bacterial replication in an unknown way. The membrane integrity of SCV is associated with SifA, an effector protein translocated by T3SS encoded in *Salmonella* pathogenicity island 2 (SPI-2). The *SifA* mutant *Salmonella* produce defective SCV with damaged membrane. The membrane damage exposes glycan present within the SCV lumen. The glycan is tagged with ubiquitin and is readily recognized by lectins such as galectin-8. The glycan recognition initiates recruitment of autophagy proteins and formation of autophagosome. The autophagy helps in cytosolic replication of the bacteria. The damaged SCV sometimes initiates lysosome recruitment to 'repair' membranes damage, which helps to kill the bacteria. For a transient period of time few *Salmonella* may survive in the cytosol freely before formation of autophagosome or recruitment of lysosome.

The survival and replication in phagocytes helps in dissemination of the bacteria into outside the intestine. The bacteria delivered into the circulation are mostly cleared by reticulo- endothelial cells of liver and spleen. The LPS obtained from the bacteria causes inflammation, shock, fever and death.

Mechanism of Salmonella induced diarrhoea: In true sense no exotoxin produced by *Salmonella* is related with diarrhoea production like other enteric bacteria. There are two proposed hypothesis.

a) Due to infection, there is continuous loss of intestinal epithelial cells causing shortening of villi which leads to less absorption of fluid from the intestinal lumen. It may cause diarrhoea.

b) Major T3SS associated virulence protein (SopB) causes alteration of ion balance within the cell. It leads to fluid secretion within the intestinal lumen and diarrhoea (secreatory diarrhoea).

Disease produced

Bacteria	Host	Disease produced
Salmonella Gallinarum	Poultry, duck, guinea fowl	Fowl typhoid: It is an acute septicaemic infection affecting adult birds (3-6 months). Oral route and conjunctiva are the ways of transmission. The infection is characterized by fever, anorexia, yellow diarrhoea, and bluish comb. From second day of outbreak the death of birds start
Salmonella Pullorum	Poultry, duck, guinea fowl	Bacillary white diarrhoea (BWD): It mainly affects newly hatched chick. The chicks die within 2-7 days without any symptom. In adults, white diarrhoea along with other symptoms like fowl typhoid is observed. Sometimes the bacteria reside in ovary of adults without any symptoms. It may infect the egg contents and newly hatched chicks (transovarian transmission).
Salmonella Dublin	Calves (1-2 week age)	Septicaemia, pneumonia, arthritis, osteomyelitis, encephalitis
	Cattle	Abortion
Salmonella Typhimurium	Calves	Enteritis
	Pig	Enteritis
	Horse	Septicaemia
	Poultry	Fowl paratyphoid ('Keel disease'): Enteritis and septicaemia are observed. Signs are indistinguishable with Pullorum disease. Sometimes birds drink water and keel (upturn) over the backward until death. It is also known as 'keel disease'
	Human	Food poisoning
Salmonella Choleraesuis (Hog Cholera bacillus)	Pig	Systemic secondary infection after swine Fever (Hog cholera)
Salmonella Typhisuis	Pig	Enteritis
Salmonella Abortusovis	Sheep	Abortion
Salmonella Abortusequi	Horse	Abortion
Salmonella Enteritidis	Poultry	Fowl Paratyphoid
	Human	Food poisoning
Salmonella Typhi	Human	Typhoid fever
Salmonella Paratyphi A	Human	Paratyphoid fever
Salmonella Schottmuelleri	Human	Paratyphoid fever
Salmonella Arizonae	Chicken, turkey	Enteritis, septicaemia

Immunity

The humoral and cell mediated immunity play role in protection against *Salmonella*. Humoral immunity is Ig-M mediated. The secreatory Ig-A, found in the intestine, prevents *Salmonella* adhesion with enterocytes. Maternal antibodies can protect the offspring up to 1-2 months after birth. The genetic loci in the host chromosome (mostly found in the autosome of chicken) carrying the genes *TLR4* and *NRAMP1* (natural resistance- associated macrophage protein, now *SLC11A1*), major histocompatibility complex (MHC) and the QTL *SAL1* are found to be associated with *Salmonella* resistance.

Diagnosis

Clinical samples

Clinical samples include faeces, cloacal swabs of birds and affected tissues such as liver, spleen, reproductive tract, caeca etc. In case of a poultry farm, environmental samples, for example naturally pooled faeces, litter, dust, drag, and boot swabs from floor surfaces should be examined in the laboratory to get idea about an outbreak. Specimens should be collected before antibiotic treatment from live animals. After death, the collection should be done immediately from fresh carcasses. In the faecal or environmental samples number of *Salmonella* might be low. For 'pre-enrichment', the swabs should be collected in buffered peptone water to help isolation. Pre-enrichment in buffered peptone water helps in survival of *Salmonella* from freezing, heating and desiccation. However, for host adapted serovars (*S.* Pullorum/Gallinarum), pre-enrichment of faecal samples is not required. It may help in overgrowth of competitive bacteria present in the faeces. The cold chain and care to prevent contamination should be maintained during transportation of the samples to the laboratory.

Laboratory examinations

Direct examination: A smear can be prepared from swab/faecal sample/ tissues and stained by Gram's Method. *Salmonella* appears as gram-negative small rods with no distinct characteristics.

Isolation of bacteria from clinical samples: The media, incubation condition and colony characteristics are described earlier.

Serological tests

a) *Rapid whole blood agglutination test:* It can be used in field condition for rapid detection of *S.* Pullorum/Gallinarum infected poultry birds. It can be tested at any age of chicken, although less than 4 week birds produce positive reaction due to maternal antibodies. Blood is collected from wing vein of the suspected birds. In a clean white tile, a drop of (0.02ml) crystal violet stained or unstained *Salmonella* Pullorum/Gallinarum antigen (available from IVRI, Bareilly, India) is placed. Equal amount of whole blood is gently mixed with a clean glass rod. Tile is agitated gently for 2 minutes and is observed for reading. In positive case, the clumping of antigen is visible within 2 minutes. However it can produce false positive reaction with *S.* Enteritidis, as it shares common antigenic properties with *S.* Gallinarum/Pullorum.

b) *Rapid serum agglutination test:* It is performed in the same way. The blood is substituted with serum.

c) Tube agglutination test

d) Immunodiffusion

e) *ELISA*: Indirect ELISA using LPS antigen is most specific and sensitive for detection of *S.* Pullorum/Gallinarum in a flock. It can be done with sera or egg yolk. Other ELISAs have also developed to detect *S.* Enteritidis and *S.* Typhimurium in egg yolk, *S.* Dublin in bulk milk of cattle, *Salmonella* in sera or tissue fluid samples of pigs.

Molecular biology: For rapid and reliable detection of *Salmonella*, conventional PCR targeting *invA* or other genes are commonly used. Genus and serovar (*S.* Enteritidis and *S.* Typhimurium) specific real-time PCR have also developed.

Prevention and control

Following measures should be taken to prevent salmonellosis in commercial poultry farms

a) Eggs and chicks of the farm should be purchased from *Salmonella*-free breeding flocks

b) Hatching should be done with strict hygienic measures

c) Regular disinfection of poultry houses, utensils, beddings etc.

d) Effective rodent and insect control

e) Pelleted feed should be provided

f) Competitive exclusion products such as probiotics and prebiotics are effective to prevent colonization of *Salmonella* when given with drinking water or by spraying / oral gavage. The strains of *Lactobacillus*, *Bifidobacterium*, *Bacillus subtilis*, *Escherichia*, *Pediococcus*, *Streptococcus*, and *Saccharomyces* act as probiotic. The complex carbohydrates (lactose, glucose, mannose, and fructo-oligosaccharide) can act as prebiotics and provide food to the probiotic bacterial strains. The author has experience in assessment of yeast cell wall extract to reduce *Salmonella* colonization in poultry.

g) Poultry feed supplementation with acids such as formic, propionic, butyric, caprylic, or caproic acid can also reduce *Salmonella* colonization in gut

h) Vaccination of laying hens with adjuvinated bacterin can produce long-lasting immunity. The chicks generated from the vaccinated hen are protected due to presence of maternal antibodies.

In rural and peri-urban India access to poultry meat and eggs largely depends on backyard farming system. The backyard farming is done by marginal farmers as insurance against crop failure, for ready cash and to ensure basic economic returns and the empowerment of women and children. The author developed the ten-point biosecurity strategy for backyard poultry farmers based on the source of microbial infection (*Salmonella*, *E. coli*) and their dissemination through the eggs in backyard flocks kept in West Bengal (India).

a) The feed mixture offered to the birds should be washed with boiled water

b) The potable drinking water preferably boiled should be provided to the birds

c) The utensils for the feed or drinking water should be cleaned with detergent/ash daily

d) The drinking water in the utensil should be changed daily

e) The litter in the poultry house/dried manure under the house should be changed /cleaned frequently

f) The scavenging area of the birds during daytime should be restricted within the house premises. The detergent water (remaining water after cloth washing) may be sprinkled daily in the scavenging area

g) The entry of the wild birds and rodents should be restricted into the house premises

h) Travelling of the farmers to broiler/layer poultry farm or market should be restricted. If travelled, the intruder should enter the poultry house after proper cleaning himself and his dress materials

i) The carcass of the birds should be disposed of through proper way, preferably by garden burial

j) The eggs should be washed with sterile water and preserved at cooling temperature. If the refrigerator is not available, eggs can be stored in a clay pot with a wet cover. The cover should be removed, dipped into water and again placed in the mouth of the pot 5-6 times a day in summer and 2-3 times a day in winter.

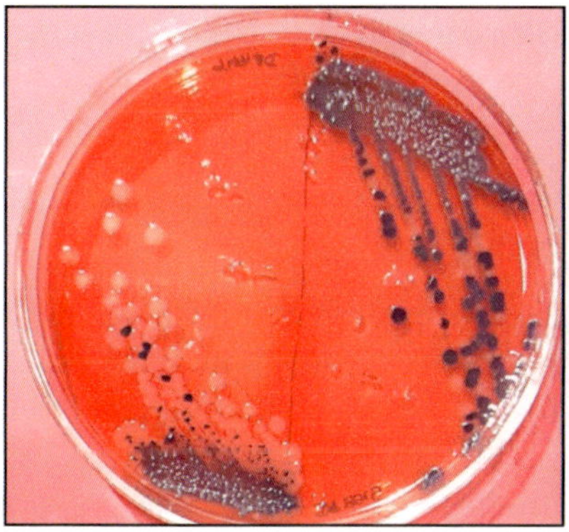

Fig. 7: Black coloured colony of *Salmonella enterica* isolated from poultry in xylose lysine deoxycholate agar (XLD agar) (*Courtesy*: Sneha Bhowmick, Department of Veterinary Microbiology, West Bengal University of Animal and Fishery Sciences, Kolkata, India and ICAR-Central Island Agricultural Research Institute, Port Blair, Andaman and Nicober Islands, India)

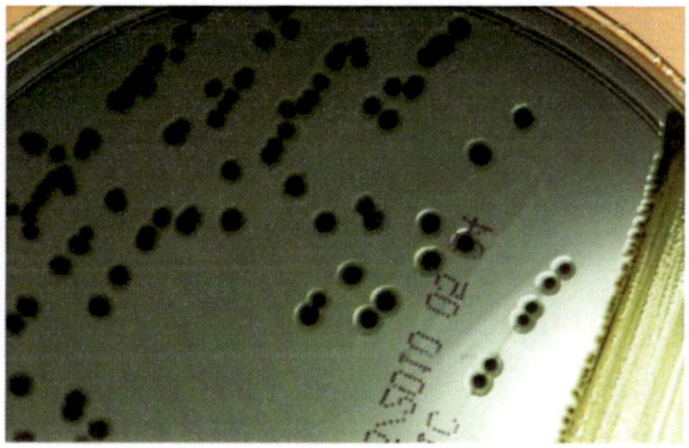

Fig. 8: *Salmonella enterica* on Hektoen enteric agar produces black center of the transparent colonies (*Courtesy*: Jan Hudzicki, American Society for Microbiology)

Yersinia

The plague bacillus (*Yersinia*) was first isolated by Alexandre Yersin in 1894 in Hong Kong. He was sent by Louis Pasteur to investigate about plague outbreak. S. Kitasato (Japan) also independently isolated the bacteria a few days later. Previously, it was known as *Pasteurella pestis* in honour of Pasteur. Yersin also revealed the connection between rat and the disease 'plague'. In memory of this great worker, the bacterium was later renamed as *Yersinia pestis*.

Properties of genus

1. *Morphology: Yersinia* is gram-negative, short rods or coccobacilli, 1.5 µm in length and 0.7 µm in width. The bacteria show bipolar staining characteristics ('safety pin appearance') when stained with Leishman or Wright or Giemsa stain. The appearance is more commonly found in tissue smears. The bacteria are non-spore forming. Most species are flagellated in ambient temperature. Although, *Y. pseudotuberculosis* is

motile at 22°C, not at 37°C. Some mucoid colony forming freshly isolated strains of *Y. pestis* produce capsule which is lost during subculture.

2. The bacteria are aerobe or facultative anaerobe

3. *Classification:* The genus *Yersinia* is classified under the family Enterobacteriaceae that belongs to the order Enterobacteriales. Currently the genus *Yersinia* contains 21 numbers of species. Among them, *Y. pestis, Y. pseudotuberculosis* and *Y. enterocolitica* are zoonotic important.

4. *Resistance:* 55°C temperature for 15 minute exposure is lethal to the bacteria. The bacteria are also killed by common physical and chemical agents like direct sunlight, 0.5% phenol etc.

5. *Natural habitat:* The habitat of *Yersinia* varies with the species. Major reservoir of *Y. pestis* is the rodents. The rodents do not show any clinical symptom and act as the maintenance host. *Y. pestis* is chiefly detected in the soil of burrows of the reservoir rodents. The survival of the bacteria in the soil depends on temperature, humidity and chemical composition of the soil.

   Y. pseudotuberculosis can persist in the environment. As well as, the wild rodents and birds act as the major reservoirs.

   Y. enterocolitica can be isolated from soil, water, vegetables, fruits, as well as human and other warm and cold blooded animals. The pigs specifically can act as carrier for the infection.

6. *Genome:* Most of the *Yersinia* virulence genes such as adhesins, secreation systems and toxins have acquired from other bacteria and viruses. All pathogenic strains of *Yersinia* possess a 70 kbp virulence plasmid (pYV), which harbours genes encoding type III secreation system (T3SS), effector proteins (*Yersinia* outer proteins, Yops) and *Yersinia* adhesin (YadA). The pathogenicity island is present only in highly pathogenic strains of *Yersinia* like *Y. enterocolitica* 1B, *Y. pseudotuberculosis* I and *Y. pestis*, known as 'high-pathogenicity island (HPI)'. The unique feature of HPI is its wide distribution among other members of Enterobacteriaceae family like *E. coli, Klebsiella* and *Citrobacter,* but it was first identified in *Yersinia.*

7. *Y. pestis* is commonly used as a potential bio-warfare agent. It is considered as category 'A' critical biological agent.

Isolation, growth and colony characteristics

Yersinia can grow in blood agar, nutrient agar, MacConkey's agar, brilliant green agar (*Y. enterocolitica).*The growth rate is slower in comparison to other members of Enterobacteriaceae. The incubation temperature is 25°C-37°C. Yersinia selective media is CIN agar [(containing antibiotics cefsulodin (15 mg/lit), irgasin (4 mg/lit) and novobiocin (2.5 mg/lit)].The antibiotics prevent the growth of contaminants. Mannitol present in the media is fermented by *Yersinia*.

'Cold enrichment' method for better isolation like *Listeria* can be followed for primary isolation of *Yersinia pseudotuberculosis* and *Yersinia enterocolitica* from faecal samples. The samples are kept in sterile phosphate buffered saline (PBS) or nutrient broth at 4°C for 3 weeks. Subculture in MacConkey's agar or CIN agar is done in weekly interval.

In blood agar, *Y. pseudotuberculosis* and *Y. enterocolitica* are non-haemolytic. In MacConkey's agar, majority of *Yersinia* produce lactose non-fermenting pale coloured colonies. Whereas, some strains of *Y. enterocolitica* can ferment lactose. In CIN agar, *Y.enterocolitica* produces colonies with dark red center and a transparent periphery (bull's eye colony).

Biochemical characteristics

Yersinia pseudotuberculosis produces following biochemical reactions

Biochemical test	Expected result
Catalase	(+ve)
Oxidase	(-ve)
Indole	(-ve)
Methyl red	(+ve)
Voges- Proskauer	(-ve)
Citrate	(-ve)
Urease	(+ve)
H_2S production	(-ve)
Carbohydrate fermentation	
Glucose	Acid production
Lactose	(-ve)
Maltose	acid production
Mannitol	acid production
Sucrose	(-ve)
Inositol	(-ve)
Gelatin hydrolysis	(-ve)
Lysin decarboxylase	(-ve)

Antigenic characteristics

Yersinia possesses two major types of antigens i.e. somatic (O-antigen) and flagellar (H-antigen). On the basis of antigenic structure, *Y. pseudotuberculosis* is related with *Salmonella* O-antigen and *E. coli*. Whereas, *Y. enterocolitica* is antigenically related with *Brucella*. So, it can produce false positive result in *Brucella* agglutination test.

On the basis of the antigens, *Y. enterocolitica* and *Y. pseudotuberculosis* are classified into 57 and 10 serotypes, respectively. Among them O: 3, O: 5, O: 8, O: 9, O: 27 serotypes of *Y. enterocolitica* are associated with major gastrointestinal tract infection in human and O: 1, O: 2 are associated with animal infections specially in goats.

In addition to the major antigens, *Y. pestis* contains 'fraction 1 (F1) antigen', which is a glycoprotein associated with capsule. It is produced at 37°C, not less than 25°C. It is encoded by plasmid carried *fra* gene. It is antiphagocytic and antibodies against F1 are protective.

Toxins and virulence factors produced

Toxins

Murine toxin: It is produced by *Y. pestis,* protein in nature and lethal for mice (so it is called murine toxin). It is encoded by genes residing on the plasmid (pMT1, 100 Kbp). The toxin has two active parts i.e. toxin A (240 KDa) and toxin B (120 KDa). The toxin acts as beta adrenergic blocker and inhibits the epinephrine. The role of murine toxin in disease production is unclear. The toxin is required for survival of the bacteria in the reservoir host (flea).

Endotoxin (LPS): Endotoxin of *Yersinia* causes different symptoms like fever, vascular damage, disseminated intravascular coagulation, and localized lesions.

Enterotoxin (YST): It is produced by some strains of *Y. enterocolitica.* Structurally and functionally it is related to stable toxin of ETEC (STa). However, YST is produced at 25°C, not 37°C *in vitro*. Its role in disease production is not established.

Yersinia cytotoxic necrotizing factor (CNF-Y): *Y. pseudotuberculosis* produces a homolog of the *E. coli* exotoxin cytotoxic necrotizing factor (CNF). This toxin is named as CNF-Y.

Virulence factors

Virulence factors	Function
Yersinia outer membrane protein (Yop): It is T3SS associated effector protein required for virulence of Yersinia. It is a misnomer and it is not actually outer membrane protein. It has two types: translocator Yop (YopB, YopD, LcrV) and effector Yop (YopE, YopH, YpkA/YopO, YopP/YopJ, YopM, YopT)	Translocator Yops form a pore in host cell membrane, through which the effectors enter the cell
Effetor Yops: a) YopE (GTPase activating protein)	i) Cytotoxin and disrupts actin microfilaments in infected cells. ii) Antiphagocytic (with YopH) iii) It's involved in resealing pores made by the T3SS, thereby preventing the leakage of cellular contents and activation of the host immune system
b) YopH (protein tyrosine phophatase)	One of the most potent phosphatase, it can inhibit phagocytosis by polymorphonuclear neutrophil leukocytes
c) YopM (scaffolding protein)	Exact role in virulence is unclear, may be associated with impairment of gene transcription related with cell cycle & growth
d) YopT (only found in Y. enterocolitica)	It increases the electrophoretic mobility of the small GTPase (RhoA). It is correlated with the disruption of Rho dependent actin structures in the cell. It also causes HeLa cell toxicity.
e) YpkA/YopO	It disrupts the actin cytoskeleton and contributes to the ability of Yersinia to resist phagocytosis by macrophages.
f) YopP/YopJ	i) YopJ blocks cytokine production (TNF α) by inhibiting several signalling pathways in infected cells. ii) It is associated with apoptosis of macrophages.
'Invasin' (Y. enterocolitica and Y. pseudotuberculosis express this chromosomally inv gene encoded outer membrane protein)	It binds with high affinity to β1 integrin receptors. Invasin is thought to trigger the internalization of Yersinia into M-cells
Ail (attachment invasion locus) protein (17 KDa outer membrane protein encoded by chromosomally carried ail gene)	It helps in invasion and internalization of bacteria and serum resistance
pH6 (encoded by chromosomal psaA gene. It is produced at 37°C and pH 6)	It is fibrillar adhesion protein that helps in virulence

Virulence factors	Function
YadA (Yersinia adherence protein encoded by virulence plasmid carried gene)	It acts as adhesin, binds with collagen, fibronectin, intestinal mucosa. It can causes serum resistance
Pesticin (P1) associated virulence factors: [P1 is a peptidoglycan hydrolase. Genes for P1 are found in the plasmid. P1 itself is not a virulence factor, but the genes linked with P1 is associated with virulence]	They act as coagulase and fibrinolysin and help in tissue invasion of the bacteria
Yersiniabactin	It is siderophore and it helps in acquisition of iron.
Absorption of pigment (P): Virulent strains produce pigmented colonies in haemin or congo red containing medium	They use haemin as iron source in siderophore independent way. They can store iron in the form of outer membrane storage complex

Pathogenesis

Transmission

The two major species of *Yersinia* known to be pathogenic for humans and animals (*Y. enterocolitica* and *Y. pseudotuberculosis*) are transmitted by the faecal-oral route.

Y. pestis can survive in the soil of the rodent burrow under favourable conditions. The rat flea (*Xenopsylla cheopis*) can acquire the bacteria during its feeding into the infected rodents. The rodents act as maintenance host of *Y. pestis*. During its death, the fleas are compelled to move to an alternative host like human along with the bacteria. Humans also get the infection from handling infected carcasses of rodents, cats and camels. Infected cat can transmit the infection to its owners through droplets. Human to human transmission can take place via aerosol route or by human flea (*Pulex irritans*). The birds which are making their nests using infected burrow soil can also transmit the bacteria into wider locality.

Pathogenesis

After entry through the oral route, with the help of adhesins (invasin, Ail, YadA) *Y. enterocolitica* and *Y. pseudotuberculosis* adheres with the intestinal epithelium (ileum, colon). Invasin is thought to trigger internalization of yersiniae into the host M-cells. After adherence, the bacteria express type III secreation system (T3SS) that helps in injection of effector proteins known as 'Yops' into the host cell. Interaction between 'Yops' with the actin cytoskeleton of enterocytes causes cytoskeletal rearrangements leading to 'membrane ruffling'. The bacteria are trapped within the ruffles. Later, the bacteria are taken up by enterocytes. The 'membrane ruffling' helps in internalization of the bacteria within the cells.

After internalization, the bacteria encounter phagocytic cells in the mucosa and sub-mucosa. The phagocytes ingest them. The change of temperature (37°C), low Ca^{++} concentration within the cells, gives the signal to the bacteria to induce the expression of effector Yops (YopE, YopH, YpkA/YopO, YopP/YopJ, YopM), which confer resistance phagocyte-mediated lysis. Some bacteria pass through the regional lymph nodes. In both intestinal tissue and lymph node the bacteria and dead tissues form abscess. Sometimes, septicaemia occurs and abscesses are disseminated into different organs like spleen, liver etc.

Mechanism of diarrhoea production by Y. enterocolitica

Due to infection there is continuous loss of intestinal epithelial cells causing shortening of villi which leads to less absorption and as a result accumulation of fluid in the intestinal lumen. It may cause diarrhoea. *In vivo* role of the enterotoxin is not established.

Disease produced

Bacteria	Host	Disease produced
Y. pestis	Human	Plague
	Cat, goat, camel	Plague
	Dog	Suppurative intermandibular lymphadenitis
Y. pseudotuberculosis	Guinea pig, cat, turkey	Pseudotuberculosis: Tuberculosis like nodules are formed in the liver, spleen, lymph nodes
	Cattle, goat	abortion
	Ram	Orchitis, epididymitis
	Human	Abdominal pain, mesenteric lymphadenitis
Y. enterocolitica	Cattle, sheep, goat, dog, horse, pig, birds	enteritis
	Human	Food poisoning (mild diarrhoea): pigs act as carrier for pathogenic strains.
Y. ruckeri	Salmon and trout fish	Red mouth, pink mouth, red/pink throat

Immunity

Cell mediated immunity plays major role in protection of host against plague. The immunity following recovery is excellent but temporary. Disposal of intracellular bacteria depend on activated macrophages.

Y. enterocolitca infection is self-limiting due to innate immune response, phagocytosis, complement activation and lysis of infected epithelial cells.

Diagnosis

Clinical specimen: The specimens for *Y. pestis* are edematous tissues, lymph nodes, nasal swabs, cerebrospinal fluid and blood. For *Y. pseudotuberculosis* and *Y. enterocolitica* major clinical sample is faeces. Post mortem samples include intestine, lymph nodes.

Laboratory examinations

Direct examination: A smear can be prepared from the collected tissues or exudates from abscess and stained by Leishman's or Wright or Giemsa stain. *Yersinia* shows 'bipolar characteristics' (safety-pin appearance). Gram staining reveals gram-negative bipolar coccobacilli.

Isolation of bacteria from clinical samples: Media, incubation condition and colony characteristics are described.

Serological tests: ELISA or passive haemagglutination test in paired sera for detection of anti-F1 antibodies of *Y. pestis* are performed. A titer of equal or more than 1:32 with characteristic syndrome gives conclusive diagnosis of plague in human or animals. Recombinant protein (Ail) is prepared and antiserum is raised against it. Currently the antisera are used in indirect ELISA and Western blot assay for detection of *Y. enterocolitica* in suspected samples.

Molecular biology: Multiplex PCR is used targeting *ail, inv, yadA* and *ystB* genes of *Yersinia enterocolitica* and *Yersinia pseudotuberculosis* for their confirmation. Real time PCR is developed for detection of *Yersinia* in food samples like milk and ground beef. It can detect 10-10^3 CFU/ml in milk and 10^2 - 10^5 CFU/gm in ground beef without any pre-enrichment.

Proteus

'*Proteus*' was named by Hauser (1885) after the name of the character in Homer's Odyssey who 'has the power of assuming different shapes to escape being questioned'. As this bacteria can undergo dramatic morphological and physiological changes in response to growth on surfaces or in viscous environments. Hager and Magath (1925) first isolated the bacteria from a case of human cystitis.

Properties of genus

1. *Morphology: Proteus* is gram-negative rods, measuring 1-3 μm in length and 0.5 μm in width (Figure 9). The shape of the bacteria varies from short, vegetative 'swimmer' cells to elongated, highly flagellated forms, referred as 'swarmer' cells. *Proteus* is thus known as 'dimorphic bacteria.' The 'swimmer' form of the bacteria is found in liquid media, motile by peritrichous flagella (6-10 flagella per cell). When the 'swimmer' form is inoculated into the solid media, they undergo morphogenesis to 'swarmer' cells and swarm over the surface of solid medium. This kind of growth of *Proteus* on solidified medium is called 'swarming phenomenon' (Figure 10). The swarmer cells are 20-80 mm in length, non-septate and

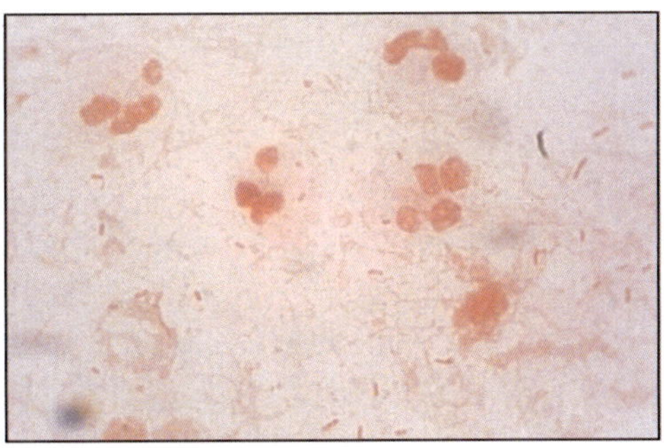

Fig. 9: Gram-stained smear showing *Proteus mirabilis*
(*Courtesy*: Rebecca Buxton, American Society for Microbiology)

multinucleated which is accompanied by 50 to 500 fold increase in the number of flagella. The newly formed flagella are also made of same flagellin protein as found in swimmer cells. There are some structural and biochemical differences between these two kinds of bacterial forms.

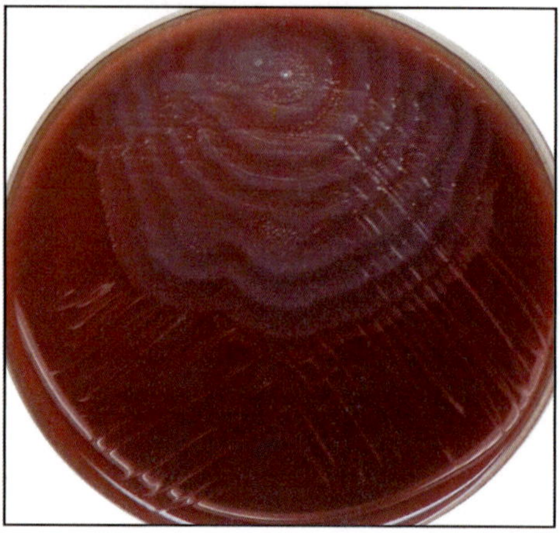

Fig. 10: Distinct rings of 'swarming' growth of *Proteus* originated from 2 isolated colonies (*Courtesy*: Rebecca Buxton, American Society for Microbiology)

Majority of *Proteus* strains produce fimbriae. Types of fimbriae produced by the bacteria include mannose-resistant/*Proteus*-like (MR/P) fimbriae, *P. mirabilis* fimbriae (PMF), uroepithelial cell adhesin (UCA) or nonagglutinating fimbriae (NAF) and ambient-temperature fimbriae (ATF).

Proteus is non-sporing. Some pathogenic strains (*P. mirabilis* O6 and O57 and *P. vulgaris* O19) are capsulated.

2. The bacteria are aerobe or facultative anaerobe

3. *Classification:* The genus *Proteus* is classified under the family Enterobacteriaceae that belongs to the order Enterobacteriales. Currently *Proteus* possesses 15 numbers of species. Among them, *Proteus mirabilis* and *Proteus vulgaris* have pathogenic significance. *P. myxofaciens* is isolated from living and dead larvae of the gypsy moth.

4. *Resistance: Proteus* can be destroyed by exposure to 55°C temperature for 1 hour or 60°C for 20 minutes and autoclaving. Common disinfectants like phenol, cresol, formaldehyde (during fumigation) are lethal to the bacteria.

5. *Natural habitat: Proteus* is widely distributed in the natural environment. The bacteria can be found in polluted water, soil and manure, where the bacteria play an important role in decomposing organic matter of animal origin. It is also common inhabitant of human and animal gastrointestinal tracts. Under favourable conditions, the bacteria can produce serious infections (opportunistic pathogen) in human and animals.

Isolation, growth and colony characteristics

Proteus grows well in common bacteriological media like blood agar and MacConkey's agar. The bacteria are aerobic or facultative anaerobic in nature. Incubation temperature varies from 20°C-40°C, optimum is 37°C.

In solid media like blood agar, *Proteus* growth consists of a characteristic feature, known as 'swarming' (also produced by *Serratia*, *Vibrio*, *Bacillus* and *Clostridium*). Swarming is growth of the bacteria with spreading like a thin film covering the media surface. Often it occurs as wave, producing a series of rings on the surface of the media (Figure 10).The swarming phenomenon is periodic in nature and consists of three phases. At first phase, the 'swimmer' cells are converted into 'swarmer' cells. In the second phase, the 'swarmer' cells migrate away from the colony rapidly and in a co-ordinated manner. It continues until the number of swarmers is reduced either by loss of cells or when the mass of bacteria changes the direction of motion. In the third phase, cessation of swarming movement occurs due to re-conversion of swarmers into short, vegetative swimmer cells. This phase is termed as 'consolidation'. The three phases repeat several times until the whole agar surface is covered with concentric rings. The rings are formed during migration of swarmers from central colony towards the periphery of the plate. A typical smell having similarity with 'burnt chocolate' is often detected in *Proteus* colonies.

In MacConkey's agar, pale / colourless, lactose non-fermenting *Salmonella* like colonies are found.

Biochemical characteristics

Proteus mirabilis produces following biochemical reactions

Biochemical test	Expected result
Catalase	(+ve)
Oxidase	(-ve)
Indole	(-ve)
Methyl red	(+ve)
Voges- Proskauer	(-ve)
Citrate	variable
Urease	(+ve)
H_2S production	(+ve)
Carbohydrate fermentation	
Lactose	(-ve)
Maltose	(-ve)
Mannitol	(-ve)
Sucrose	(-ve)
Inositol	(-ve)
Gelatin hydrolysis	(+ve)
Lysin decarboxylase	(-ve)
swarming	(+ve)

Antigenic characteristics

Proteus is antigenically heterogeneous based on structural differences of its polysaccharide side chain of LPS (O-antigen) and flagellar protein (H-antigen). The serological classification scheme of Kauffman and Perch includes 49 different *P. mirabilis* and *P. vulgaris* O serogroups and 19 serologically distinct H antigens. Penner and Hennessy introduced a separate O-grouping scheme to classify clinical isolates of *P. vulgaris* and *P. mirabilis*. In spite of the efforts, a number of *Proteus* remains unclassified, including strains of *P. penneri*.

The common structural feature of *Proteus* O antigens is the presence of uronic acids, sometimes substituted by amino acids. Besides the typical sugar constituents, widespread in nature, like hexoses, hexosoamines and uronic acids, the bacteria also contain 6-deoxyamino sugars like L-fucosamine, L-quinovosamine, D-quinovoso-3-amine and D-fucoso-3-amine. The amino acids (L- and D-alanine, L-serine, L-threonine, and L-lysine) are attached to the carboxyl group of uronic acids. In *Proteus* O antigens, other unusual acidic components like (*R*)- and (*S*)-lactic acid ethers and (*R*)-hydroxybutyryl, pyruvic, and phosphate groups are found. However, the unusual components do not act as immunodominant antigens.

In addition to O and H antigens, *P. mirabilis* O6, O57 and *P. vulgaris* O19 can synthesize a capsular antigen identical to the O-side chain of their LPS.

Weil-Felix test: O-antigens from *P. vulgaris* OX19 and OX2, as well as *P. mirabilis* OXK serogroups cross-react with antibodies from patients with different Rickettsial infections and are commonly used in the diagnosis of Rickettsial infections. It is known as 'Weil-Felix test'. The LPS from spotted fever group of *Rickettsia* (Thai tick typhus and Katayama strains) share some common structural components with LPS of *P. vulgaris* OX2 [Glc, GlcNAc, QuiNAc (quinovosamine)].

Toxins and virulence factors produced

Toxins

a) *Endotoxin (LPS)*: Exact role of the toxin in *Proteus* urinary tract infection pathogenesis is not clear. However its direct experimental inoculation in dogs produced local nephritis. As well as, it may enhance or inhibit urolith formation (stone) depending on its structure and cation binding ability. The stone formation protects the bacteria from antibiotics and host defence mechanism. The bacteria continue multiplication within the interstices of the urolith.

b) *Haemolysin*: It is a pore forming haemolysin, encoded by *hpmAB*. It causes efflux of sodium ions from eukaryotic cells. The toxin may help in dissemination of infection from bladder to the kidney.

c) *Choleriform thermolabile enterotoxin*: It is a type of enterotoxin produced by some pathogenic strains of *Proteus* causing urinary tract or enteric infection. This toxin can be detected by antisera produced against *E. coli* enterotoxin. It suggests their structural relationship.

Virulence factors

Virulence factors	Function
Fimbriae a) mannose-resistant/Proteus-like (MR/P) fimbriae (encoded by mrpl gene cluster) b) P. mirabilis fimbriae (PMF) [pmf gene cluster] c) uroepithelial cell adhesin (UCA) or nonagglutinating fimbriae (NAF) d) ambient-temperature fimbriae (ATF) [atfA gene]	Adherence of bacteria with epithelial cells a) colonization of bladder & kidney b) colonization of bladder & kidney c) Adhesion to uroepithelial cells in vitro d) association with virulence is not confirmed
Flagella (swarming phenomenon)	Dissemination of bacteria from ureter to the kidneys
Urease (encoded by ure gene cluster)	a) Elevation of pH in the surrounding of bacterial growth resulting in precipitation of soluble ions and urinary calculi (stone) formation ['struvite' (magnesium ammonium phosphate) or 'apatite' (calcium phosphate) crystal]. Within these calculi bacteria are sequestered from host immune effectors & antibacterial and remain viable. The calculi can obstruct the urine flow and is often associated with pyelonephritis. b) Formation of ammonia from urea damages urinary epithelial cells.
IgA proteases (ZapA, metalloprotease)	Disruption of IgA
Amino acid deaminase (encoded by aad gene)	Production of α-keto acids acting as siderophores

Pathogenesis (urinary tract infection)

Most urinary tract infections (UTIs) initiate after the bacteria of faecal origin (*Proteus*) enter the bladder through the urethra. In the bladder, the bacteria can multiply and confine themselves or ascend through the ureters into the kidneys. The route of infection is known as 'ascending route'.

In its primary step of pathogenesis, *Proteus* adheres to the uroepithelial cells through fimbriae (UCA / NAF fimbriae). The adhesion is comparatively less than uropathogenic *E. coli* (UPEC). After adhesion, the parent *Proteus* 'swimmer' cells are differentiated into 'swarmer' cells. The swarmer cells have more numbers of flagella which helps the bacteria to colonize the kidney through ascending route.

In the kidney, MR/P or PMF fimbriae of swarmer cells help in adhesion with renal epithelium. The binding helps in biofilm formation. During this process, urease of bacteria hydrolyzes urea present in the urine causing a rise in local pH. Synergistic action of the urease and bacterial endotoxin forms urinary calculi (stone) followed by epithelial cell necrosis. Haemolysin is responsible for the epithelial cell necrosis. Later, the bacteria may invade renal tubule epithelial cells causing further damage. Sometimes, the bacteria breach this thin barrier and enter the bloodstream.

Disease produced

Bacteria	Host	Disease produced
P. mirabilis and *P. vulgaris*	Human (neonates, preschool girls and sexually active women and men)	Urinary tract infection (cystitis, nosocomial infection from hospital or during catheterization and use of ileal loop, long term urethral catheter)
	Dog and horse	Urinary tract infection
	Dogs and cats	Otitis externa
	Calves, lambs, goats	diarrhoea

Diagnosis

Clinical specimen: Ante-mortem samples for *Proteus* detection include urine, faeces, exudate from ear etc.

Laboratory examinations

Direct examination: A smear can be prepared from centrifuged deposit of collected urine or exudate samples and stained by Gram's Method. *Proteus* appears as gram-negative small rods with no special characteristics under microscope (Figure 9).

Isolation of bacteria from clinical samples: Media, incubation condition and colony characteristics are described earlier.

Serological tests: Enzyme immune assay (EIA) is developed using antisera against *E. coli* enterotoxin for detection of choleriform thermolabile enterotoxin produced by *Proteus*, isolated from patients with purulent inflammatory, urological and enteric infections.

Molecular biology: Genus-specific polymerase chain reaction (PCR) for detection of *Proteus* using primers of bacterial *gyrB* gene is developed. The species-specific PCR for *P. mirabilis* and *P. vulgaris* using 16S rRNA gene as target is being used. Pathogenicity of *Proteus* isolates from urinary calculi can also be confirmed by detection of urease gene through PCR.

19

Pseudomonas and *Burkholderia*

Lucke (1862) first described that the bluish green discolouration of surgical dressing is associated with the presence of small vibrio like organisms. Gessard (1882) first isolated the bacteria as *Pseudomonas*.

Identification of the etiologic agent of glanders was performed in 1882 by isolating a bacterium from the infected liver and spleen of horse. Since its discovery, the pathogen has been classified as *Loefflerella mallei, Pfeifferella mallei, Malleomyces mallei, Actinobacillus mallei, Corynebacterium mallei, Mycobacterium mallei, Pseudomonas mallei*, and currently as *Burkholdria mallei.* The genus *Burkholderia* was created to accommodate former rRNA group II (Pseudomallei group) *Pseudomonas* bacteria. It was based on the 16S rRNA sequences, DNA-DNA homology values, cellular lipid and fatty acid composition.

Properties of genus

1. *Morphology*: *Pseudomonas* is gram-negative straight or curved rod, motile by one or more polar flagella (Figure 1). Usually it is 1.5 μm in length and 0.5 μm in width. Longer filamentous forms are sometimes observed. The bacteria are non- acid fast, non- sporulating and uncapsulated. Pilli on the bacterial surface are detected. Environmental and host associated strains can produce slime. The slime is composed of glycolipoprotein (GLP) and polysaccharide of LPS.

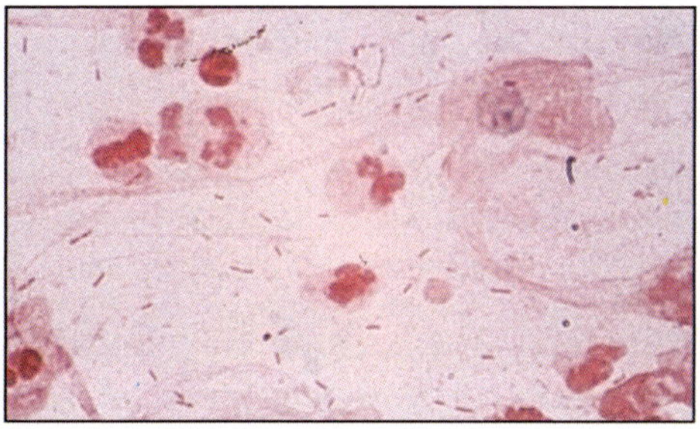

Fig. 1: *Pseudomonas aeruginosa* showing long, slender, gram-negative bacilli (*Courtesy*: Rebecca Buxton, American Society for Microbiology)

Young cultures of *Burkholderia mallei* are gram-negative long slender rods with rounded ends. The bacteria are 2-5 μm long and 0.5 μm width. Older cultures are pleopmorphic showing the variation from coccobacilli to long filamentous. Capsule is present, visible under electron microscope. Spores are not produced. Flagella are absent and the bacteria are non-motile in nature.

Burkholderia pseudomallei are small gram-negative rods with bipolar staining resembling 'safety pins'. Capsule is present. Spores are not produced. Flagella and pilli are present. Previously it was known as 'Whitemore bacillus'.

2. *Pseudomonas* and *Burkholderia* are strict aerobe

3. *Classification*: *Pseudomonas* belongs to order *Pseudomonadales* and family *Pseudomonadaceae*. Previously *Pseudomonas* had two groups of bacteria viz. fluorescent group and pseudomallei group. Recent nomenclature included the pseudomallei group into a new genus known as *Burkholderia*. Currently the genus *Pseudomonas* has 366 species and 21 sub-species. Among them, major pathogenic species are *P. aeruginosa*, *P. fluorescens*, and *P. putida*.

Burkholderia belongs to order *Burkholderiales* and family *Burkholderiaceae*. There are two genera known as *Burkholderia* and *Paraburkholderia*. The genus *Burkholderia* is composed of more than 140 species. Important pathogenic species are *B. mallei*, *B. pseudomallei*, *B. thailandensis*, *B. cepacia* complex and *B. glumae*. *B. pseudomallei* consists of two groups (biovar) based on their capacity to use arabinose. The arabinose users (Ara + biovars) are designated as a new species (*B. thailandensisi*). The group which cannot use arabinose (Ara - biovars) remain as *B. pseudomallei. B. cepacia* complex contains nine closely related species which can cause severe respiratory infections in human suffering from cystic fibrosis or chronic granulomatous disease. *B. glumae* is a plant pathogen causing rot of rice grains and seedlings (panicle blight).

4. *Resistance*: *Pseudomonas* is relatively susceptible to common disinfectants. The bacteria can be destroyed by 55°C temperature for 1 hour exposure. *Pseudomonas* is susceptible to most of the antibiotics except *P. aeruginosa* which is a multi-drug resistant (MDR) bacterium.

Burkholderia mallei can survive damp, cool environment for several months. *B. pseudomallei* are easily destroyed by common disinfectants. It cannot survive the chilling and freezing.

5. *Natural habitat*: *Pseudomonas* is commonly found in soil, water, intestinal tract of man and animals specially in canine ear, uterus of mare, eye of horse, skin and mucous membrane of healthy animals. Wet area with poor ventilation favours the bacterial growth.

Burkholderia is commonly found in diverse ecological niches. The bacteria are isolated from soil, plant rhizosphere, water, insects, fungus, and hospital environments and from infected humans and animals. *B. mallei* bacterium is potent bioweapon as it requires small numbers of bacteria to cause infection through the aerosol route. It was used as bioweapon by Germany during World War I.

6. *Genome*: The size of *Pseudomonas aeruginosa* genome is 5.5-7 Mbp and the GC content is 65-67 mol%. The genome consists of a single circular chromosome and numerous plasmids. The bacteria can utilize varieties of nutrients present in the environment and host due to their metabolic diversity associated with transporters, transcriptional regulators, and two-component regulatory systems present in the genome. The core genome is highly conserved and the variations are detected in accessory genome.

The genome of *Burkholderia mallei* consists of two circular chromosomes. The size of both the chromosomes are 3,510,148 bp (chromosome 1) and 2,325,379 bp (chromosome 2), respectively. The genome can encode approximately 5,500 numbers of proteins. The chromosome 2 mostly consists of essential metabolic genes.

Isolation, growth and colony characteristics

Pseudomonas can be isolated in ordinary bacteriological media like trypticase soya agar with or without blood and MacConkey agar. Incubation temperature is 20°C-42°C. Cetrimide agar and *Pseudomonas* agar are selective media for isolation of *Pseudomonas aeruginosa.* On ordinary agar it produces convex glistening colonies with spreading edges. In blood agar haemolysis is found. It can produce different pigments in the ordinary medium that helps in identification of the bacteria (Figure 2).*Pseudomonas aeruginosa* produces four type of pigments such as pyocyanin (blue), pyoverdin (yellow), pyorubin (red) and pyomelanin (black). First two pigments are water soluble and pyocyanin is soluble in chloroform. Pyoverdin can fluoresce under ultraviolet light, previously known as 'fluorescein'. The cultures also develop a characteristic sweetish odour ('fruity'/'grape like'/'corn taco-like'/'corn tortillas'). *P. fluorescens* does not produce odour but may produce pyoverdin pigment in the artificial culture.

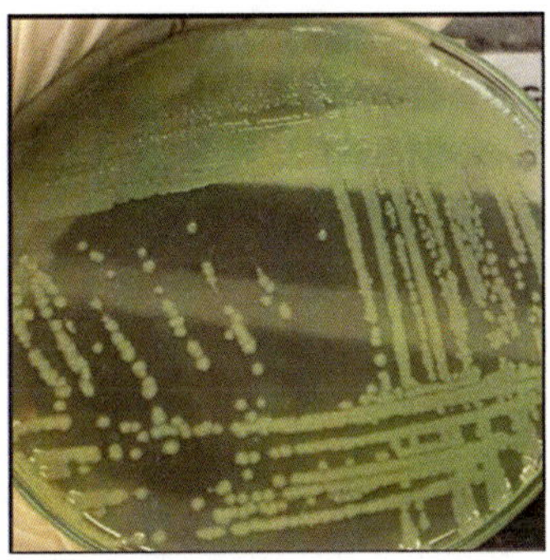

Fig. 2: Appearance of *Pseudomonas aeruginosa* colony in *Pseudomonas* isolation agar (*Courtesy*: Soumen Samanta, Department of Veterinary Microbiology, West Bengal University of Animal and Fishery Sciences, Kolkata, India)

Burkholderia mallei grow slowly in the routine bacteriological media like blood agar, Mac Conkey agar and chocolate agar. Growth is enhanced by the addition of 1% glycerol. *B. pseudomallei* grow more rapidly in the ordinary media even at 42°C. Optimum incubation condition for both is 37°C for 7 days. To avoid the contamination or to isolate from mixed infection, the antibiotics are added into the media.

Bacitracin, polymyxin B, acitidione are added to isolate *B. mallei.* Ashdown's medium, containing gentamicin and crystal violet, is used as selective medium to isolate *B. pseudomallei.* The colonies of *B. mallei* are non-haemolytic, small, round, convex and cream to yellow in colour. Old cultures produce brown coloured hard colonies. Isolation medium containing glycerol produces confluent honey like colonies. *B. pseudomallei* form small smooth colonies after 24-48 hours of incubation, later becomes dry and wrinkled. Pink coloured colonies are produced in Ashdown's medium. In the medium an earthy odour is found during opening the Petri dish.

Biochemical characteristics

Pseudomonas and *Burkholderia* produce following biochemical reactions

Biochemical test	Expected result for *Pseudomonas*	Expected result for *Burkholderia*
Catalase	(+ve)	(+ve)
Oxidase	(+ve)	(+ve)
Indole	(-ve)	(-ve)
Methyl red	(-ve)	-
Voges-Proskauer	(-ve)	-
Urease	(+ve)	(+ve)
Nitrate reduction	(-ve)	(+ve)
H_2S production	(-ve)	-
Carbohydrate fermentation		
Glucose	(+ve)	(+ve)
Arabinose	-	(+ve)
Fructose	-	(+ve)
Galactose	-	(+ve)
Mannose	-	(+ve)
Gelatin liquefaction	(+ve)	-
Arginine hydrolysis	-	(+ve)

Antigenic characteristics

Pseudomonas has two types of antigen i.e. somatic and flagellar. Serotyping can be done using antisera against somatic antigen (O- typing) as well as flagellar antigen (H- typing). Several O-serogroups have described so far. *Pseudomonas aeruginosa* is routinely serotyped in Japan by using the 'Homma scheme'. Other typing schemes like 'Fisher immunotyping scheme' (based on LPS or high molecular weight polysaccharide), 'international antigenic typing system' (IATS) are also practiced worldwide. Currently the pyocin typing is evaluated for epidemiological investigations.

Burkholderia mallei contain two types of antigens i.e. capsular (K- antigen) and somatic (O- antigen, extracellular part of lipopolysaccharide). Serial passages of *B. mallei* cultures in the artificial medium or the animal can produce genome sequence alteration making the bacteria incapable of capsular polysaccharide or lipopolysaccharide (LPS) synthesis. The cultures become less virulent or avirulent. *B. mallei* have antigenic relationship with *B. pseudomallei*. Sequence analysis revealed a 19.9-kb contiguous sequence containing the entire *B. mallei* O- polysaccharide biosynthetic gene cluster. The cluster has 99% similarity at nucleotide level with *B. pseudomallei* O-polysaccharide biosynthetic gene cluster. *B. pseudomallei* are generally considered to be an antigenically homogenous species. The bacteria possess two serotypes based on the differences in the chemical structure of O-polysaccharide (somatic antigen).

Toxins and virulence factors produced

Toxins

a) *Exotoxin A and S*: The toxins can inhibit the protein synthesis by blocking the activity of elongation factor (EF2) like diphtheria toxin, although structurally they are not similar.

b) *Endotoxin (OEP)*: *Pseudomonas* produces a specialized endotoxin, known as original endotoxic protein (OEP). It is structurally composed of lipopolysaccharide (LPS) along with a protein. It can produce protecting antibodies.

c) *Haemolysin: Pseudomonas* produces phospholipase C and glycolipid. The toxins have no direct role in pathogenesis. Phopholipase C helps in secreation of inflammatory mediators from granulocytes. Glycolipid helps in secreation of serotonin and histamine from platelets.

d) *Cytotoxins*: The cytotoxin can damage the cytoplasmic membrane of polymorphonuclear leukocytes of the host.

e) *Bacteriocin*: *Pseudomonas* also produces bacteriocin, known as 'pyocin' which can also inhibit the growth of similar natured bacteria.

f) *Pigment:* Pyocyanin pigment has toxic activity. It can generate reactive oxygen radicals (superoxide) with the exposure to oxygen. The reactive oxygen radicals are toxic to the host cells. The bacteria itself protects from the toxicity by producing catalase and superoxide dismutase that can neutralize the radicals.

The toxins produced by *Burkholderia* include endotoxin, pyocyanin, lecithinase, collagenase and lipase. The pyocyanin interferes terminal electron transfer. Other enzymes cause host cell membrane lysis.

Virulence factors

Pseudomonas produces following virulence factors

Virulence factors	Function
a) Proteases : i) Elastase ii) LasA protein iii) Alkaline protease	i) Elastase is a major virulence factor having strong proteolytic and weak elastolytic activity. It can degrade the proteins like immunoglobulin, complement and causes tissue damage by its attack on elastin ii) LasA also has elastase like activity. It starts the damage of elastin by producing a 'nick' (a type of crack in protein structure) upon which other proteases can act easily
Pyochelins	It is a kind of siderophore. It helps in assimilation of iron from the surrounding media or tissue for the bacterial growth

Burkholderia produces a number of extracellular enzymes like protease, lipase, collagenase, and phospholipase C helping in pathogenesis. Environmental and physiological factors including 'quoram sensing' play role in the enzyme secreation. 'Quorum sensing' is a cell-to-cell communication system used by bacteria in response to environmental conditions to produce a coordinated gene expression for different enzymes. Specific transcriptional regulators are activated. *Burkholderia mallei* produce following virulence factors

Virulence factors	Function antiphagocytic
Capsular polysaccharide	
Type three secretion system (TTSS)	TTSS is required for intracellular survival of the bacteria. TTSS acts like molecular syringe and inject bacterial effector proteins into host cell cytoplasm. The proteins make the cellular processes favourable for survival of the bacteria. B. mallei carries two chromosomal regions encoding for TTSSs: one with similarity to animal-like TTSS and a second TTSS similar to that found in plant pathogens. The animal like TTSS is genetically similar with that of B. pseudomallei, and TTSS of Salmonella (inv/spa/prg) and Shigella (ipa/mxi/spa)
Pili	It helps in bacterial adherence with the host cells.
Extracellular enzymes like lecithinase, lipase, proteases	A centrally located gene (gspC) is essential for exo-production of these enzymes. Their exact role in pathogenesis is till inconclusive
Malleobactin	It is a siderophore, helping iron accumulation. Its synthesis is regulated by mbaA, mbaF genes. It can acquire iron from lactoferrin. As B. pseudomallei initiates infection at the mucosal surface, its ability to take iron from lactoferrin could play an important role in infections. Lactoferrin is found in most secretions bathing mucosal surfaces
Rhamnolipid	It is an extracellular glycolipidic surface-active molecule, toxic for phagocytic cells
Type three secretion system (TTSS), and a range of bacterial effector proteins (BopA, BopB, and BopE).	They help in intracellular survival

Pathogenesis

Transmission

Pseudomonas is opportunistic pathogen. Either it enters the body through damaged mucosa (exogenous infection) or during immunocompromised condition it is activated (endogenous infection).

Burkholderia mallei is transmitted between animals through close contact, inhalation, ingestion of contaminated material. Respiratory tract secreation and skin lesion exudates can act source of infection. The incubation period can range from a few days to many months.

B. pseudomallei is transmitted through ingestion of contaminated materials, inhalation, wound infection and arthropod bite. In human, consumption of infected animal products plays significant role in transmission.

Pathogenesis

Pseudomonas

Adherence to the damaged epithelial cells is the first step of the pathogenesis. Pili and exotoxin S help in adherence. Pili make the first contact with the host cells. Exotoxin S with its receptor in the cell membrane makes the attachment firm. The bacteria start multiplication at the site. Antiphagocytic nature of slime helps in the survival of the bacteria. *Pseudomonas* can also resist complement mediated lysis and survive in low iron concentration (within tissues) due to secreation of siderophores. The infected tissue is damaged by the production of exotoxins like protease, exotoxin A, and phospholipase C. The exotoxin S also helps in spread of the infection throughout the body and the endotoxin (OEP) produces systemic toxicity. In case of persistent infection tissue damage is chiefly immune complex mediated as observed in cystic fibrosis in human.

B. mallei

After entry within body of the host adherence to the intestinal and pharyngeal mucosa is the primary step. The adherence mechanism is not known in details. After adherence with the mucosa, the bacteria are phagocytosed by the macrophages. Within macrophages the bacteria can survive with the help of the TTSS. The bacteria enter regional lymphatic vessel and the blood circulation through the thoracic duct. The bacteria are distributed throughout the body. It colonizes lymphatics of the respiratory tract and the skin. Nodules develop at the point of entry i.e. pharynx, lymph vessels, lung, spleen, liver and skin, which ulcerate to discharge exudates. Nodules are composed of neutrophils, fibrin and red blood cells.

B. pseudomallei

Adherence to the mucosal cells is the initial step. The adherence is temperature sensitive (more effective at 30°C than 37°C) and occurs more in stationary phase cultures than the log phase. Type IV pili present in the bacteria helps in adherence. After adherence of the mucosa, the bacteria are phagocytosed by the macrophages. Within the cell cytoplasm the bacteria escape the endocytic vacuole. It directs the cell to produce a membrane protrusion entering into neighboring cell. The protrusion helps in spread of the bacteria into the neighbouring cells and this process continues. Localization of the bacteria is found in liver, spleen, lung, lymph nodes and joints.

Diseases produced

Bacteria	Host	Disease produced
Pseudomonas aeruginosa	all species of animals and human	Wound infection
	Cattle	Respiratory infection, mastitis, enteritis
	Horse	Abortion, keratitis
	Sheep	Pneumonia, mastitis, fleece rot (inflammation of skin producing poor quality wool characterized by bluish colour due to pigment produced by the organism)
	Dog, cat	Otitis, urinary tract infection, pneumonia
	Poultry	Embryo mortality
	Human	Pseudomonas aeruginosa is a major nosocomial infection (acquired from hospitals). Skin infection after burn is observed. It also causes bacterimia after cystic fibrosis and leukemia
Pseudomonas fluorescens	Cattle	Mastitis
	Poultry	embryo mortality
	Fish	tail rot / fin rot
Pseudomonas putida	Human	It is found in environment specially air of poultry houses. In human it is isolated from cancer patients found to be associated with pneumonia, phlebitis, cellulitis. It also causes different plant diseases. In animal as a specific pathogen it is not yet ascertained
Burkholderia mallei	Horse, Mule, donkeys are major hosts. Cattle, pig are resistant but occasional outbreak is reported in sheep, goat and camel.	Glanders: It was first described by Hippocrates (450 BC) followed by Aristotle in 350 BC when the disease was given the name 'melis'. Although the disease is eradicated from a part of the world, it is still endemic in Asia including India, Africa, Middle East, Central and South America. Glanders has three forms i.e. pulmonary, nasal and cutaneous. Gray coloured nodules are formed in the lungs in the pulmonary form. In the nasal form, the nodules originate in the mucous membrane. It ruptures and discharges purulent exudates. Ruptured nodules become irregularly bordered ulcer. Cutaneous form is known as 'farcy'. Nodules are produced on the skin along the course of lymph vessel between two lymph nodes, specially in the leg of the horse. Prognosis of the animal is poor.
	Human	B. mallei can cause fever, rigors and malaise, pneumonia, bacteremia, pustules and abscesses, leading to death in 7–10 days without treatment. It can be transmitted by direct contact with infected animal or culture. So animal attendants, Veterinarians and laboratory workers are susceptible. Person to person spread is very rare.
Burkholderia pseudomallei	Dog, pig, ruminants and human	Melioidosis: The infection resembles Glanders. Nodules are formed in any tissue and may rupture to generate ulcers. Arthritis, pneumonia, placentitis, metritis are also observed in ruminants. In human, pneumonia is predominant. It is also known as 'Whitemore's disease'

Immunity

Lysis of *P. aeruginosa* depends on phagocytosis by polymorphonuclear leukocytes. Opsonizing antibodies help in phagocytic destruction. However cell mediated immunity plays no major role in offering protection.

Recovered animals are not immune to re-infection with *B. mallei* although both antibody and cell mediated immunity are produced.

Diagnosis

Clinical specimens: *Pseudomonas* is commonly found in the environment, often detected as contaminant in the laboratory. Sometimes its isolation from clinical specimen is inconclusive. It must be correlated with the clinical syndrome. According to site of lesion and symptoms different specimens are collected.

Nodular contents, blood, serum can be collected and sent to the laboratory with precautions. As *B. mallei* is OIE risk group 3 organisms (organisms that can cause severe human or animal disease and may spread in the community and/or animal population but for which there is usually effective prophylaxis and treatment is available), laboratory should have suitable facilities to handle such containment group 3 organisms.

Laboratory examination

Direct examination: A smear can be prepared from collected infected tissues to stain by Gram 's method. *Pseudomonas* is gram-negative medium sized rods with no other distinctive features to identify.

A smear can be prepared from collected samples to stain by Gram's method for diagnosis of glanders. *B. mallei* are long slender gram-negative rods with rounded ends. *Burkholderia pseudomallei* are small gram-negative rods with bipolar staining characteristics.

Isolation of bacteria from clinical samples: Media and incubation condition are described earlier.

Animal inoculation technique: Guinea pig, hamsters are susceptible to *B. mallei* cultures. In male guinea pigs, the culture is inoculated intraperitoneally. In positive case orchitis and peritonitis is developed (Strauss reaction).Five animal inoculations are recommended at once. Strauss reaction is not specific for *B. mallei.* It should be followed by isolation and identification of the bacteria.

Serological test: No serological test can differentiate *B. mallei* from *B. pseudomallei* due to their cross reacting nature.

a) Mallein test

A tuberculin like test is used for diagnosis of Glanders in horses.'Mallein' is a filtrate of bacterial extract, water soluble protein in nature. Mallein can be inoculated into the suspected horse through three different routes i.e. intradermo palpebral, ophthalmic and subcutaneous.

Test procedure

i) Intradermo palpebral route is the most sensitive and reliable than other two routes. 0.1 ml of mallein is injected intradermally into the lower eyelid.

ii) In ophthalmic route, few drops of mallein are instilled into the eye at the canthus.

iii) In subcutaneous route, mallein is injected subcutaneously into the skin of the middle neck region. A 10-15 cm patch of the skin is selected, hair is clipped and disinfected. Mallein (2.5 ml) is injected subcutaneously.

Results

Intradermo palpebral test: a positive result shows edematous swelling of the eyelid, purulent discharge from the inner canthus or conjunctiva. This is usually accompanied by a rise in temperature. With a negative response, there is no reaction or only a little swelling of the lower eyelid.

Ophthalmic test: a positive result shows swelling of eyelids and the side of the face with a little discharge from the eye.

Subcutaneous test: In positive case, fever with above 104°F or more temperature is developed during the first 15 hours, followed by a firm painful swelling with raised edges within next 24 hours at the injection site. In negative cases, there is no or minimal local swelling. Doubtful cases may be re-tested after 14 days using a double dose of mallein.

b) *Complement fixation test (CFT)*: It is less sensitive than mallein test, but 90-95% accurate. It can detect the antibody in the serum collected from suspected horses even 1 week after initiation of the infection. Bacterial crude cell wall preparation is used as antigen. So it can produce false positive reaction by detecting other cross reacting bacteria. Healthy horses can also produce false positive reaction following mallein intradermal test. Mallein and CFT are prescribed by OIE for detection of glanders.

c) Enzyme linked immunossorbent assay (ELISA): Both plate and dot-ELISA is used for diagnosis of glanders.

d) Rose Bengal plate agglutination test: The test is similar as used in diagnosis of *Brucella*.

Molecular biology: Polymerase chain reaction (PCR) is developed to detect *P. aeruginosa* from cystic fibrosis cases of human patients using primers for *groES* and *groEL* genes. It can detect those patients having no previous history of *Pseudomonas* infection or those who appear to be transiently colonized by this organism.

PCR and real time-PCR are developed to detect *B. mallei* and *B. pseudomallei* using primers for *flip* gene as target. However, depending on the sample material a house keeping gene targeting PCR may be used additionally or as an alternative.

Prevention and control

No vaccine is currently available to prevent glanders in horses. The stable and utensils should be disinfected regularly. Introduction of the new animal should be done after quarantine and testing with mallein. The positive reactors should be discarded. The clinically infected horses should be removed from the stable and the remaining horses should be tested with mallein at intervals of 3 weeks.

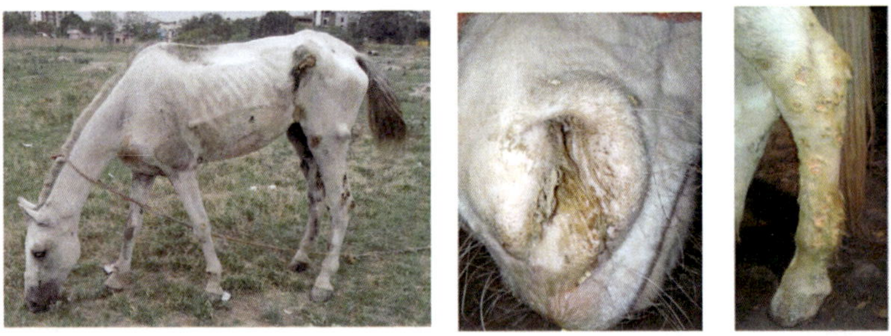

A B C

Fig. 3: A. Horse affected with glanders **B.** Mucopurulent nasal discharge (nasal form) **C.** Ulceration and nodules along the lymphatic vessels of the hind limb (cutaneous form) (*Courtesy*: Hari Sankar Singha, ICAR-National Research Centre on Equines, Hisar, India)

In India, Glanders is a notifiable disease under Prevention and Control of Infectious and Contagious Diseases in Animals act, 2009. The State Government should declare the glanders outbreak if the etiological bacteria are isolated successfully. The culling of the infected animals is done under the supervision of qualified veterinarian and after providing compensation to the farmers. The carcasses should be disposed of either by burial or burning. The site of the burial should be away from river, canal or streams. The pit should be of minimum 8 feet and after putting the carcass into the pit, it should be covered with lime and soil. The area should be fenced properly.

All contaminated farm equipments should be disinfected properly. The animal attendants and veterinarians should follow the personal hygiene strictly during handing of the infected animals. Movement of the animals should be restricted and no animal fare is permitted near the outbreak area. After the outbreak the contact animals should be tested clinically and with CFT for at least two months. The positive reactors should be eliminated.

20

Pasteurella and *Mannheimia*

Louis Pasteur (1881) first isolated the bacterium from fowl cholera outbreak and attenuated the bacteria to develop a vaccine for the chicken. Trevisan (1887) coined the generic name '*Pasteurella*' in honour of Louis Pasteur. Lignieres (1900) proposed the name of the species according to the animals acted as the major hosts such as *Pasteurella aviseptica* for fowls, *P. suiseptica* for pigs, *P. boviseptica* for bovines, *P. oviseptica* for *ovines* and *P. leptiseptica* for rabbits. Rosenbuch and Merchant (1939) proposed the name of single species *Pasteurella multocida* which is in use till date.

Mannheimia is an exclusive animal pathogen and is associated with 'shipping fever' or bovine respiratory disease (BRD) in cattle. Kitt (1885) first described the bacterium as *Bacterium bipolare multocidum* isolated from shipping fever in cattle. The nomenclature was further changed into *Bacillus boviseptica* and finally into *Pasteurella haemolytica*. Based on fermentation capability of arabinose and trehalose, *P. haemolytica* was subdivided into two biotypes (A and T) and several capsular serotypes. The biotype A (with 12 capsular serotypes) was classified under a new genus *Mannheimia* due to disparities in 16S rDNA sequence, cultural and pathological characteristics.

Properties of genus

1. *Morphology*: *P. multocida* are non motile, non spore-forming short rods or coccobacilli, 0.2-0.4 by 0.6-2.5 µm in size. Repeated laboratory subcultures of old cultures or cultures grown under unfavourable conditions tend to be pleomorphic and longer rods or filamentous forms appear. In tissues, exudates and recently isolated cultures, the bacteria show the coccobacillary forms. It gives typical bipolar staining ('safety-pin' appearance), particularly with Leishman or methylene blue stain in fresh cultures and animal tissues (Figure 1).

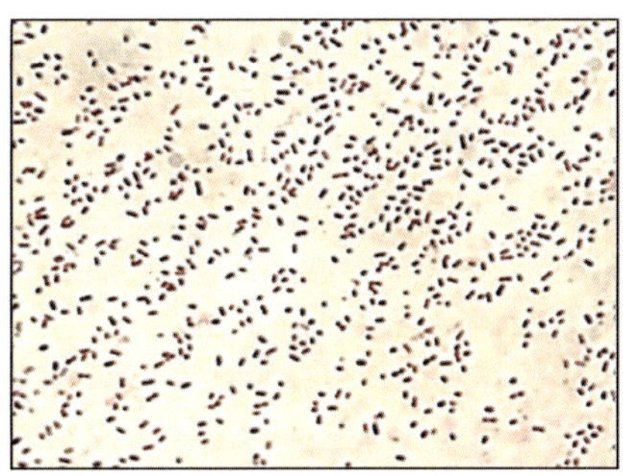

Fig. 1: *Pasteurella* as gram-negative, short, bipolar coccobacilli under 100X magnification (*Courtesy*: Abdulkarim Jafar Karim, College of Veterinary Medicine, University of Baghdad, Iraq)

Mannheimia haemolytica is a small, non-motile, non spore-forming bacillus, often showing coccobacillary forms with occasional bipolar staining (Figure 2).

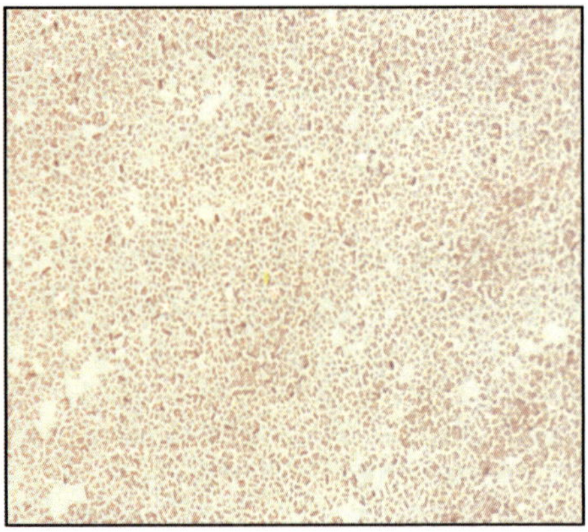

Fig. 2: *Mannheimia haemolytica* as gram-negative, short, bipolar coccobacilli under 100X magnification (Courtesy: Swati Sahay and Rajeswari Shome, Bacteriology Laboratory, ICAR-National Institute of Veterinary Epidemiology and Disease Informatics, Bangalore, India)

2. *Pasteurella* and *Mannheimia* are aerobic or facultative anaerobic in nature

3. *Classification*: The family *Pasteurellaceae* (order *Pasteurellales*, class *Gammaproteobacteria*) is currently comprised of 25 genera such as *Pasteurella*, *Mannheimia*, *Actinobacillus*, *Avibacterium*, *Gallibacterium*, *Haemophilus*, *Histophilus*, *Lonepinella*, *Phocoenobacter*, *Vespertiliibacter* and *Volucribacter*. The new genus, *Rodentibacter* is proposed recently. The genus *Pasteurella* consists of 29 species, 3 sub-species and *Pasteurella multocida* is the major pathogenic species.The genus *Mannheimia* consists of 8 species and *Mannheimia haemolytica* is the major pathogenic species.

4. *Resistance*: *P. multocida* and *M. haemolytica* are sensitive to phenol (0.5%), bichloride mercury (1:5000), cresol (3.5%), sodium hypochlorite (1%), glutaraldehyde (2%) and ethanol (70%).

5. *Natural habitat*: *P. multocida* are most prevalent commensal in upper respiratory tract and oropharynx of domestic and wild animals. The studies also identified gastrointestinal tract, urinary tract and uterus as probable habitat of *P. multocida* in cattle and buffalo. The nasopharynx and tonsils of healthy ruminants are preferred habitat of *M. haemolytica*. In stressed animals, *M. haemolytica* are isolated from lower respiratory tract also.

6. Genome: *P. multocida* genome is 1.4-2.4 Mbp in size with GC content 37-41 mol%. The complete genome sequence of *P. multocida* (Pm70 strain) was published in 2001. Five genes and two insertion sequences of *P. multocida* type A are associated with the virulence.The plasmids (ColE1) play a major role in transmission of antibiotic resistance in *Pasteurellaceae*. Other than plasmids, multiple antibiotic resistance determinants are also chromosomally encoded within integrative and conjugative elements (ICEs) present in the genome of *Pasteurellaceae*. The ICEs contain regulatory genes associated with excision, integration and transfer between different members of *Pasteurellaceae* in the core region.

M. haemolytica possesses homologous and compatible plasmids such as pAB2 and pYFC1 which carry antibiotic resistance genes.

Isolation, growth and colony characteristics

P. multocida can be isolated in dextrose-starch agar, casein-sucrose-yeast (CSY) medium with 5% blood (bovine or ovine), chocolate agar, Mueller-Hinton agar, and brain heart infusion (BHI) agar. No growth in MacConkey's agar is observed. The optimum growth temperature is 35-37°C for 18-24 hours. In enriched media at 37°C, the colonies with 1-3 mm in diameter are produced after 18-24 hours of incubation. Two types of non-haemolytic colonies are produced by *P. multocida* in blood agar i.e. smooth/mucoid and dry/rough. The smooth colonies are like 'dew drop' and may produce changing colours when observed from different angles ('iridescent') (Figure 3, Figure 4). Greenish discolouration of blood agar is also detected. Mucoid colonies are mostly produced by pathogenic strains associated with hyaluronic acid production. Sometimes, the colonies appeared with a specific sweet odour.

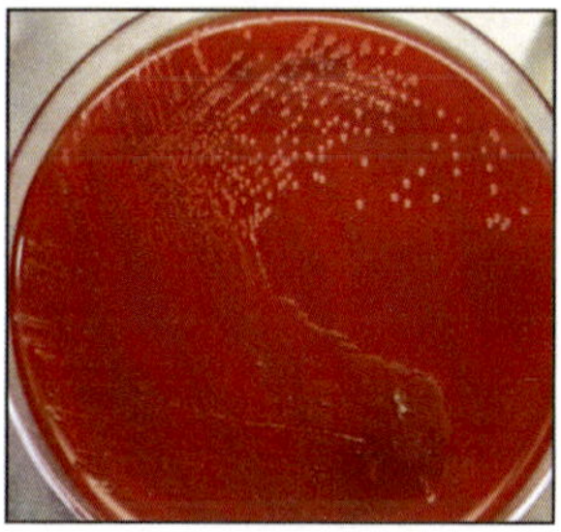

A

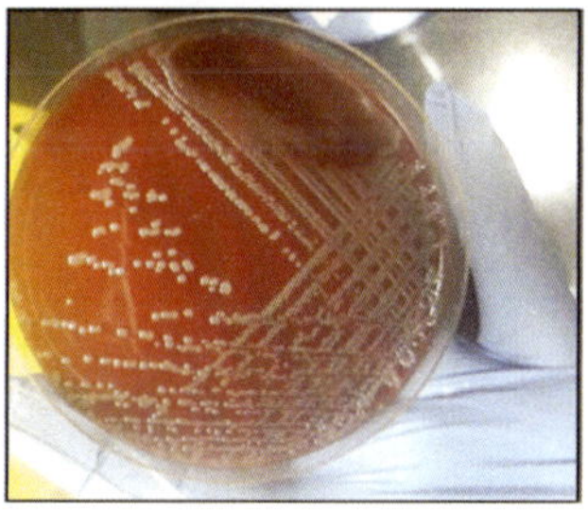

B

Fig. 3: *Pasteurella multocida* 'dew drop' colonies on blood agar **A.** Growth after 24-hours of incubation (Courtesy: Swati Sahay and Rajeswari Shome, Bacteriology Laboratory, ICAR-National Institute of Veterinary Epidemiology and Disease Informatics, Bangalore, India) **B.** Growth after 48-hours of incubation

(*Courtesy*: Joycee Jogi, Department of Veterinary Microbiology, College of Veterinary Sciences and Animal Husbandry, Jabalpur, M.P., India)

Mannheimia haemolytica produces odour less, smooth, greyish, 1-2 mm diameter colonies with narrow zone of beta-haemolysis on ovine or bovine blood agar (Figure 5). The bacteria can produce pink coloured colonies on McConkey agar.

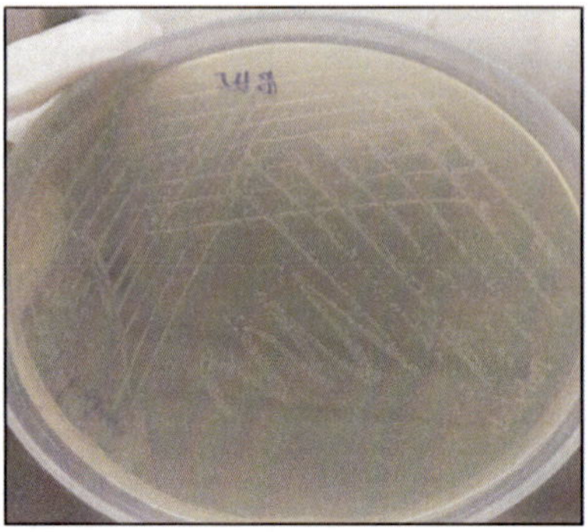

Fig. 4: *Pasteurella multocida* 'dew drop' colonies on brain-heart-infusion (BHI) agar (*Courtesy*: K. Karthik, Central University Laboratory, TANUVAS, Chennai, India)

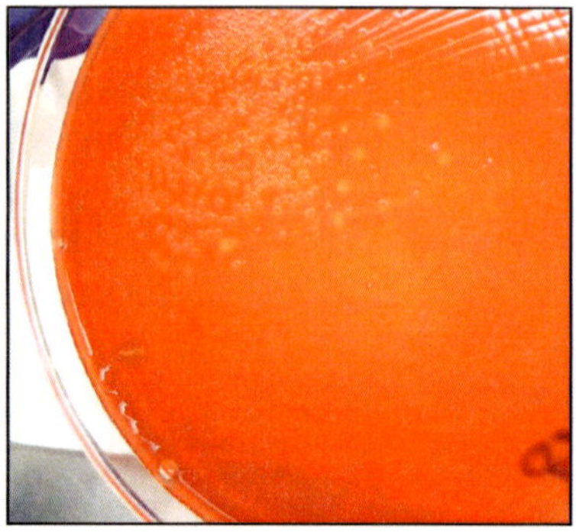

Fig. 5: *Mannheimia haemolytica* colonies on blood agar showing β-hemolysis beneath the colony (*Courtesy*: Swati Sahay and Rajeswari Shome, Bacteriology Laboratory, ICAR-National Institute of Veterinary Epidemiology and Disease Informatics, Bangalore, India)

Biochemical characteristics

Pasteurella and *Mannheimia* produce following biochemical reactions

Properties	*P. multocida*	*M. haemolytica*
Indole	+	-
Catalase	+	+
Urease activity	-	-
Ornithin decarboxilase	+	-
Carbohydrate fermentation		
Lactose	-	+
Sucrose	+	+
D-trehalose	Variable	-
L-arabinose	Variable	-
Maltose	-	+
D-xylose	Variable	+

Antigenic characteristics

Roberts (1947) developed a system of serological classification based on passive protection tests in mice. On the basis of mouse protection, he classified *P. multocida* into four types designated as types I, II, III and IV. Carter (1955) used a precipitation test and subsequently an indirect haemagglutination test and identified four serological types. He designated those four capsular types A, B, C and D. The strains that caused haemorrhagic septicaemia were grouped into Carter type B. Subsequently, he found that the strains that caused

HS in Africa did not fall strictly into any of these groups, though they were related to type B, and they were included in a separate group designated as type 'E'. The type C was not a consistent type and it was deleted. Rimler and Rhoades (1989) isolated a consistent type from turkeys which did not fit into any existing serogroups and was designated as serogroup 'F'.

Namioka and Murata (1961) identified 11 somatic types of *P. multocida* using somatic typing test. Heddleston and colleagues (1972) developed an agar gel precipitation test also for somatic typing. Using this method, 16 different somatic types were recognised. Currently, the most acceptable and widely used serotyping method is a combination of Carter capsular typing and Heddleston somatic typing. Using this method, the Asian and African HS serotypes are designated as B: 2 and E: 2, respectively. In the Carter-Heddleston system, the capsular type is expressed first, followed by the somatic type. In the Namioka-Carter system, the expression is made in the reverse order.

P. multocida shares common antigens with other closely related gram-negative bacteria. Antigenic relationships with *Yersinia paratuberculosis*, *Mannheimia haemolytica*, *Haemophilus canis*, *H. influenzae*, *Actinobacillus lignieresii, Escherichia coli* and *Neisseria catarrhalis* have been reported.

M. haemolytica is currently comprised of more than 20 serotypes and two biotypes (A and T). The serotype A1 and A2 are associated with infections in cattle and sheep, respectively, throughout the world. During viral infection or other stress conditions *M. haemolytica* serotype A2 commonly carried by healthy cattle is replaced with A1. The serotype switching (A2 to A1) occurred due to capsular switching or horizontal transfer of A1 from the infected cattle.

Toxins and virulence factors produced

Toxins

Toxigenic capsular types A and D of *P. multocida* produce an AB protein toxin known as *Pasteurella multocida* toxin (PMT, 146 kDa, encoded by *toxA*). The PMT causes host cellular cytoskeletal rearrangement through deamidation of heterotrimeric G proteins ($G_{\alpha q}$, $G_{\infty 11}$, $G_{\infty 12/13}$, $G_{\infty 13}$ and $G_{\alpha i}$) and suppression of T-cell (including T-helper cells). The PMT plays a major role in pathogenesis of atrophic rhinitis in pigs caused by *P. multocida* type-D. The PMT-mediated bone atrophy occurs through disruption of cell signaling processes in osteoblasts and osteoclasts.

M. haemolytica produces leukotoxin (105 KDa, repeat-in-toxin family, RTX) which causes activation of neutrophils and increased release of inflammatory cytokines (at low concentration) and apoptosis of pulmonary cells through formation of transmembrane pores (at high concentration).The four-gene polycistrionic operon (*lktCABD*) encodes the leukotoxin. The *lktA* acts as inactive proLKT protein, *lktB* and *lktD* helps in secreation of the toxin and *lktC* activates the inactive form by acylation. The lysis of cells by the leukotoxin is dependent on specific interaction with the lymphocyte-function associated antigen 1 (LFA-1) or beta 2-integrin present on the target cell membrane. The LktA protein contains domains with hydrophobic helices which causes spanning of host cell membrane to generate pores. The carboxy-terminal of the leukotoxin consists of glycine and aspartate-rich repeats like other RTX toxins which binds calcium and potentiates the toxin activity. *In vivo* pathogenesis studies in bovine model with leukotoxin mutant *M. haemolytica* isolates although showed reduced mortality and pulmonary lesions, other factors were also found critical for the pathogenesis.

Certain strains of *M. haemolytica* produce a zinc metalloglycoprotease (encoded by *gcp*) which can lyse *O*-sialoglycoproteins. The enzyme can enhance bacterial adhesion with the host cellular membrane. Neuraminidase (150-200 kDa) produced by *M. haemolytica* helps in colonization of the bacteria in the upper respiratory tract. The enzyme is active against N-acetyl neuraminlactose, fetuin, alpha-1-acid glycoprotein, and colominic acid.

Virulence factors

Major virulence factors produced by *P. multocida* and *M. haemolytica* are described below

Virulence factors	Function
Hyaluronidase, chondroitinase, neuraminidase	Hyaluronidase is produced by haemorrhagic septicaemia causing strains (B:2 serotype) of *P. multocida.* The enzymes help in nutrient acquisition, colonization and dissemination. Neuraminidase helps to evade host defences by blocking mucin action
LPS	Resistance to serum complement
Capsule	Capsule expressed by *P. multocida* is antiphgocytic due to hyaluronic acid components (serotype A) which helps in colonization of the bacteria in human lower respiratory tract. The serotype B capsule consists of arabinose, mannose, and galactose. Serotype D and F capsules are composed of heparin or heparin sulfate, and chondroitin, respectively. 'Fis'- protein (transcriptional regulator) regulates capsule production in *P. multocida.*
Fimbriae	Attachment to the mucosal surface
Outer membrane proteins, lipoprotein B	Act as adhesin by binding with host cellular fibronectin and helps in iron acquisition (iron-regulated OMPs) by the bacteria

Siderophore-independent iron acquisition systems, transferrin-binding receptor	Siderophore-independent iron acquisition systems (homologous to *Actinobacillus* AfeABCD system) of *P. multocida* and transferrin-binding receptors of *M. haemolytica* are associated with iron acquisition
Filamentous hemagglutinin [FhaB1 and FhaB2 (PfhB1, PfhB2)]	They act as adhesin. Precise role in virulence of *P. multocida* is unknown, although reduced expression was detected in non-mucoid strains of *P. multocida*
DNA uptake	Uptake signal sequences identified in *P. multocida* and *M. haemolytica* are associated with acquisition of new virulence genes
Type IV fimbriae (PtfA)	Possessed by *P. multocida* serotype A, B:2, D and associated with adhesion
DNA adenine methylase (*Dam*)	Regulate expression of *P. multocida* virulence genes

Pathogenesis

Transmission

P. multocida are commensal in the upper respiratory tract of different animals such as cats (70-90%), dogs (50-60%), and pigs (50%) and act as opportunistic pathogen. During immunosuppression or physiological stress condition, the bacteria penetrate the tissues and multiply. Haemorrhagic septicaemia causing *P. multocida* serotypes also occurs in the nasopharynx or tonsil of the apparently healthy animals. The nasopharynx carriage is characterized by intermittent shedding of the bacteria (active carrier), whereas the tonsillar carriage is prolonged and is without shedding (latent carriage). Introduction of an active carrier animal into the area without prior exposure to the bacteria may cause massive outbreak in susceptible animals. In endemic zone, where the animals are often exposed to the infection the prevalence will be low due to generation of active immunity in the animals. When the immunity is suppressed due to physiological stress or concurrent infection, the haemorrhagic septicaemia outbreak may occur in an endemic zone.

Exogenous transmission is possible either by direct contact or through contaminated aerosols. In poultry farm, *P. multocida* infected birds for prolonged period (carrier) are the major source of infection. The excreations coming from the mouth, nose, and conjunctiva of the carrier birds can contaminate the surroundings. Other sources of *P. multocida* infection in poultry include free flying birds, eggs, farm animals and flies (rare).

In human, most of the *P. multocida* infection occurs through bite, scratch, licks on skin abrasions by the carrier animals predominantly dogs and cats but also pigs, rabbits, guinea pigs, rats, horses, as well as wild animals such as lions, tigers, cougars and opossums. Other than bite or scratches, direct contact of injured skin and upper respiratory mucosa with contaminated animal secretions was also detected as a route of transmission specially in children, pregnant women and aged persons. Human to human horizontal and vertical transmission of *P. multocida* was also reported.

M. haemolytica reside as commensal in nasopharynx and tonsils of healthy cattle and causes endogenous infection during stress conditions associated with weaning, adverse weather, changes in feed, transportation for long distances, and concurrent viral and mycoplasmal infections.

Pathogenesis

P. multocida infection is endogenous in origin. In most of the cases, the bacteria are normally present as commensal in the upper respiratory tract or deposited through the contaminated aerosol. In the healthy and unstressed animals the cellular defense mechanisms of the lungs and the cilia help to clear the bacteria. During suppressed immunological conditions (under stress), the bacteria penetrate the tissues and multiply. Initial multiplication occurs in the nasopharynx and the lungs are filled with large number of bacteria. The virulence factors lead to release of lysosomal enzymes and inflammatory mediators by the damaged cells which contribute to severe tissue damage (Figure 6). The spindle-shaped macrophages ('oat-cells') form coils between adjacent alveoli which is considered as pathognomonic in cattle and sheep. In septicaemic pasteurellosis, severe endotoxaemia and disseminated intravascular coagulation causes fatal outcome.

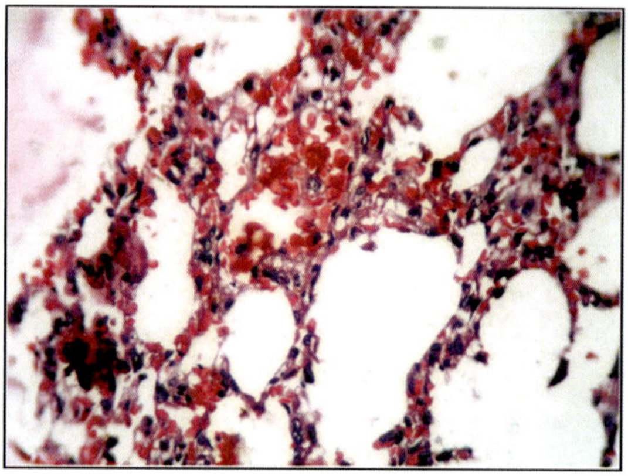

Fig. 6: Lung section showing severe congestion of alveolar capillaries of pig in natural outbreak of swine pasteurellosis (H & E, X 400) (Joycee Jogi, Department of Veterinary Microbiology, College of Veterinary Sciences and Animal Husbandry, Jabalpur, M.P., India)

M. haemolytica also causes endogenous respiratory infection in cattle co-infected with virus or *Mycoplasma*. The viral or mycoplasmal co-infection causes immunosuppression and the synergy exists between *Mannheimia* and respiratory virus or *Mycoplasma*. The primary multiplication of *M. haemolytica* occurs in nasopharynx and the bacteria reach the lungs and lower respiratory tract. The alveoli and bronchioles of the lungs are infiltrated with inflammatory cells, fibrin, blood and seroproteinaceous fluid. Pulmonary damage results acute fibrinous pleuropneumonia due to injury mediated by bacterial toxins and inflammatory cells.

Disease produced

Bacteria	Host	Disease
P. multocdia Type A	Cattle	Bovine pneumonic pasteurellosis or shipping fever Enzootic pneumonia complex Mastitis
	Sheep	Pneumonia, Mastitis
	Pigs	**Atrophic rhinitis**: Atrophic rhinitis is an infectious disease of swine characterised by serous to mucopurulent nasal discharge, shortening or twisting of the snout, atrophy of the turbinate (conchal) bones and reduced productivity. It may occur enzootically or more sporadically, depending on a variety of factors including herd immunity. The most severe progressive form is caused by infection with toxigenic strains of *P. multocida* (capsular group D and A) alone or in combination with *Bordetella bronchiseptica*. Capsular type D is most prevalent in many areas of the world, but in some regions type A predominates. Infections with *B. bronchiseptica* alone can cause a mild to moderate form with non-progressive turbinate bone atrophy. Turbinate atrophy may only be obvious at slaughter or may be detected in the live animal by use of radiography or tomography. Environmental and management factors also contribute to the severity and incidence of this disease. A large proportion of apparently normal pig herds may be infected with *B. bronchiseptica* or non-toxigenic *P. multocida* and show a mild degree or low prevalence of turbinate atrophy.
	Poultry	**Fowl cholera:** It is prevalent worldwide and affects most of the avian species. Domestic fowls including poultry, turkey and ducks are common. Turkeys are more susceptible than poultry. In poultry, death is more common in layers due to age susceptibility. Chicken less than 16 weeks of age are resistant. Change of diet acts as predisposing cause. The site of infection is generally the respiratory tract, but inoculation through oculo-nasal-oral route may also generate a typical lung lesion and bacteraemia. Following an upper respiratory tract infection, *P. multocida* may subsequently spread to the lungs and multiply before entering the bloodstream. Once in the bloodstream, *P. multocida* either multiply rapidly or localise in the liver and spleen, where initial multiplication occurs before a massive bacteraemia. Death is presumed to be due to the effects of endotoxin, as signs of acute fowl cholera have been reproduced by injection of endotoxin from *P. multocida*. In natural infection mortality rate is 0-20%. Persistence carrier state with reduced egg production is often detected. Post-mortem lesions include haemorrhages on serous surfaces and accumulation of fluid in body cavities. In sporadic chronic cases, the signs and lesions are often related to localized infections. The wattles, sterna bursae and joints are usually swollen due to the accumulation of fibrinopurulent exudates
	Rabbits	Snuffles

Bacteria	Host	Disease
P. multocdia Type B	Cattle and Buffaloes (Asia)	**Haemorrhagic septicaemia** (HS, syn: barbone): It is a major disease of cattle and buffaloes occurring as catastrophic epizootics in many Asian and African countries, resulting in high mortality and morbidity. The disease has been recorded in wild mammals in several Asian and European countries. In many Asian countries disease outbreaks mostly occur during the climatic conditions typical of monsoon (high humidity and high temperatures). The disease is caused by *P. multocida* serotype B: 2 in Asia and serotype E: 2 in Africa (Carter and Heddleston system), corresponding to 6:B and 6:E (Namioka-carter system). In wild animals, serotype B: 2, 5 is predominantly present. The association of other serotypes, *viz.*, A: 1, A: 3 with a HS-like condition in cattle and buffaloes in India has been recorded. The clinical manifestations of the typical disease caused by B: 2 or E: 2 strains include a rise in temperature, respiratory distress with nasal discharge, and frothing from the mouth, and leads to recumbancy and death. Infection with serotypes A: 1 and A: 3 predominantly involve pneumonia resulting in mortality. Septicaemia is the characteristic feature in all the disease conditions. The incubation period varies from 3 to 5 days. In per-acute cases, sudden death with observable clinical signs may be observed. Buffaloes are generally more susceptible to HS than cattle and show more severe forms of disease with profound clinical signs. Subcutaneous oedema from the mandible to the brisket is one distinctive feature of the disease in endemic areas most deaths are confined to older calves and young adults. Massive epizootics may occur in endemic as well as non-endemic areas. In the recent past, HS has been identified as a secondary complication in cattle and buffalos following outbreaks of foot and mouth disease (FMD). Case fatality approaches 100% if treatment is not followed at the initial stage of infection
P. multocdia Type D	Pigs	Atrophic rhinitis, pneumonia
P. multocdia Type E	Cattle and Buffaloes (Africa)	Haemorrhagic septicaemia (HS)
P. multocdia Type F	Pigs	Pneumonia
M. haemolytica	Cattle Sheep	Bovine pneumonic pasteurellosis or shipping fever Septicaemia (up to 3 months of age) Pneumonia Gangrenous mastitis
P. trehalosi	Sheep	Septicaemia (5-12 months of age)

Immunity: Due to non-fatal exposure to *P. multocida* the protective antibodies develop which can provide protective immunity for one year to the animals.

Diagnosis: The diagnosis of pasteurellosis is based on the clinical signs, gross pathological lesions, morbidity and mortality patterns, and confirmation by isolation of the pathogens and their conventional and molecular characterisation.

Clinical Samples: Nasal swab, swab collected from tonsil, whole blood or serum from animals and faecal sample from birds can be collected as ante-mortem samples. A blood sample or swab collected from the heart is satisfactory if it is taken within a few hours of death. If the animal died long time ago, the long bone (free of tissues) can be taken. If there is no facility for post-mortem examination, blood can be collected from the jugular vein by incision or aspiration. Blood samples in any standard transport medium should be dispatched on ice.

Laboratory examinations

Direct examination: A smear can be prepared from collected blood sample or the swabs and stained by Leishman or methylene blue or Gram's stain. *Pasteurella* and *M. haemolytica* appear as gram-negative non-sporing coccobacilli with typical bipolar staining characteristics (Figure 1, Figure 2).

Isolation of bacteria from clinical samples: Direct culture of blood sample is usually satisfactory only if the material is fresh and free from contaminants or post-mortem invaders that would otherwise overgrow any *Pasteurella*. Media, incubation condition and colony characteristics are described earlier.

Animal inoculation test: The small volume (0.2 ml) of eluted blood swabs or a portion of bone marrow in saline is inoculated subcutaneously or intramuscularly into mice. The mouse usually serves as a biological 'screen' for extraneous organisms. If viable *P. multocida* is present, the mice will die within 24-36 hours following inoculation, and a pure growth of *P. multocida* can be seen in blood smears. Pure cultures of *P. multocida* can usually be obtained from blood cultures of the mice, even when the original samples come from relatively old carcasses. The bacteria can be identified by its morphological and cultural characteristics, biochemical reactions and serological tests.

Serological tests: Following serological tests are performed in the laboratory for serotyping of *P. multocida* isolates. It is a cumbersome and time consuming procedure.

a) Rapid slide agglutination test (for capsular typing)

b) Indirect hemagglutination test (for capsular typing)

c) Agar gel immunodiffusion tests (for capsular as well as somatic typing)

d) Counter immunoelectrophoresis (for capsular typing)

e) Agglutination tests (for somatic antigen)

High titres detected by the IHA test (1/160-1/1280) are indicative of recent exposure to haemorrhagic septicaemia (HS).

Molecular biology: Diagnosis of animal pasteurellosis using nucleic acid based technique (PCR) are commonly used because for its ease in use, less cumbersome, time saving as well as economically cost effective nature. Few of the important techniques are given below.

a) *Pasteurella multocida*-specific PCR assay identify all subspecies of *P. multocida*

b) *Pasteurella multocida* multiplex capsular PCR typing system identifies all the five polysaccharide capsules (A, B, D, E and F) selectively

c) HS-causing type-B-specific PCR assay confirms presence of *P. multocida* serotype B: 2

d) *Pasteurella multocida* type A specific PCR is useful for typing of serogroup A strains.

e) Genotypic differentiation of isolates can be done by several nucleic acid based techniques.

Prevention and control

Following measures can be taken in a poultry farm to prevent fowl cholera

a) The reservoirs of *P. multocida* (carrier birds) in a poultry farm should be identified and eliminated

b) Good farm practices such as strict biosecurity, sanitation and hygiene should be maintained

c) Always young birds should be introduced in the farm and should be reared in a clean environment devoid of aged birds

d) Different species of birds and animals (pigs) should not be reared together. The farm premises should also be free of dogs and cats

e) During outbreak of fowl cholera the affected birds should be disposed and the housing, utensils and equipments should be disinfected

f) In endemic area, vaccination of birds with bacterin (killed) or live vaccines should be done. The live vaccine may cause mortality and reduced egg production but the use of aluminum hydroxide bacterins was found to be safe. The live vaccines are prepared with the low virulent strains of *P. multocida* such as CU, M-9, PM-1. In India, inactivated fowl cholera vaccines (local isolates of serovars 1, 3 and 4) are available recommended for layer and broiler breeder birds with minimal risk.

Following measures can be taken in a cattle farm to prevent haemorrhagic septicaemia (HS)

Reduction of stress is the key preventive measure for the control of HS as the shedding of *P. multocida* from the carrier animals increases with the environmental or management-associated stress such as crowding, shipment, viral infection and food and water deprivation. In large herds (> 50 animals) the incidence of HS is higher than the small herds. The occurrence of HS is more in rainy season than the others. Vaccination of cattle is performed during pre-monsoon season with alum-precipitated bacterins, aluminium hydroxide gel bacterins, broth bacterins, and oil adjuvant bacterin containing the local isolates. The oil adjuvant vaccine shows the highest efficacy which can provide immunity for one year after booster. The major disadvantage with oil adjuvant vaccine is high viscosity, short storage life and adverse local reactions. The experimental efforts to reduce viscosity often result reduction of immunity. Non-oil adjuvant vaccines such as alum-precipitated and aluminium hydroxide gel bacterins produce immunity for 5-6 months. Experimental live vaccine against HS produces variable results.

[The original chapter for the first edition of the book was contributed by Tapan Kumar Dutta, Professor and Head, Department of Veterinary Microbiology, College of Veterinary Sciences and Animal Husbandry, Central Agricultural University, Selesih, Aizawl, Mizoram, India]

21

Actinobacillus, Haemophilus Avibacterium and *Gallibacterium*

Lignieres and Spitz first isolated *Actinobacillus* from the cattle with actinomycosis like condition in Argentina in 1902. The findings were also confirmed by Nocard in 1902. Later the isolated bacterium from the cattle was named as *Actinobacillus lignieresii* in memory of Lignieres.

Pfeiffer (1892) first isolated *Haemophilus influenzae* as a cause of human influenza and it is also known as 'Pfeiffer's bacillus'. Other workers isolated and described different species of the genus *Haemophilus* from animals and birds. In 1903, Friedberger, a research assistant of Pfeiffer, isolated similar kind of bacteria from prepuce of dogs which was described later as *Haemophilus canis.* In 1925, Mitchell isolated *Haemophilus ovis* from the respiratory tract of sheep. Lewis and Shope (1931) isolated and illustrated *Haemophilus suis* from the infected pigs.Glasser found the association between fibrinous serositis, polyarthritis in pigs (Glasser's disease) and a small gram-negative rod as early as 1910, later became known as *Haemophilus parasuis.* The bacteria was first isolated by Hjarre and Wramby in 1943. De Blieck (1931) isolated a hemophilic bacterium from the birds suffering with 'infectious coryza' and named the bacteria as *Bacillus haemoglobinophilus coryzae gallinarum.* Later it became known as *Haemophilus paragallinarum* (*Avibacterium paragallinarum*).

Kjos-Hansen (1950) first described *Gallibactreium anatis* as commensal flora of healthy chicken cloaca ('haemolytic cloaca bacterium').

Properties of genus

1. *Morphology: Actinobacillus* are gram-negative small rods, measuring 1.5 μm in length and 0.4 μm in width, occurring singly, in pairs or more rarely in chains. After isolation in the laboratory the bacteria may show pleomorphism varying from coccobacilli to filamentous forms. In gram stained smear the bacteria may show both bacillus and coccus form together, known as 'morse code' appearances ('dots and dashes' appearance, Figure 1). *Actinobacillus* is non-motile (both at room temperature and 37°C), non-sporing and non-acid

fast. The pili are found in *A. pleuropneumoniae.* The capsule is detected in some strains of *A. pleuropneumoniae*. The slime layer is found on the surface of other species like *A. lignieresii, A. suis,* and *A. equuli*. The slime layer is related with stickiness of the colonies in the solid media, enhanced resistance of the colonies to the chemical disinfectants, antibiotics and desiccation.

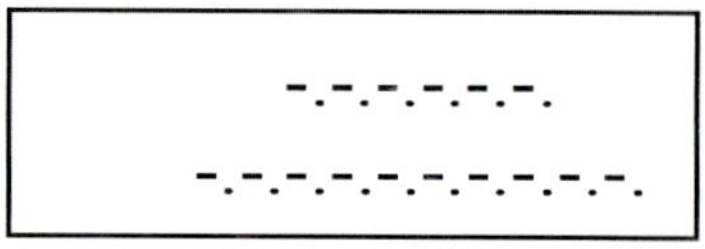

Fig. 1: 'Dot and dash' appearance

Haemophilus are gram-negative, small rods or coccobacilli, measuring about 0.5-1.5 µm in length and 0.3 µm in width (Figure 2).The bacteria may show bipolar staining characteristics like other members of *Pasteurellaceae* family. The bacteria can appear singly or in pair. Sometimes filamentous forms are found. The capsules are developed in some species like *Haemophilus paragallinarum* (*A. paragallinarum*), *Haemophilus parasuis,* and *Haemophilus influenzae*. The bacteria are non-sporing and non-motile. The pili are observed in *Haemophilus influenzae.*

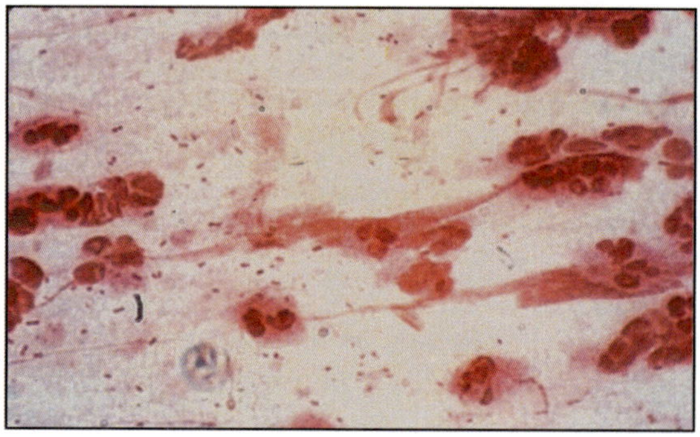

Fig. 2: Small, pleomorphic gram-negative coccobacilli of *Haemophilus influenzae* isolated from a human patient with pneumonia (*Courtesy*: Rebecca Buxton, American Society for Microbiology)

Gallibacterium are gram-negative, pleomorphic, non-sporing and non-motile bacteria.

2. *Actinobacillus* are aerobic, microaerophilic or facultative anaerobic in nature. The bacteria are chemoorganothrophic having both respiratory and fermentative types of metabolism. *Haemophilus* are facultative anaerobe and capnophilic (require CO_2 for growth). *Gallibacterium* are also facultative anaerobes.

3. *Classification*: The family *Pasteurellaceae* contains several genera like *Actinobacillus sensu stricto, Mannheimia, Pasteurella sensu stricto, Lonepinella, Phocoenobacter, Haemophilus sensu stricto, Gallibacterium, Histophilus* and *Volucribacter.* There are total 20 species or species like taxa and 2 sub-species of *Actinobacillus* reported so far. Based upon 16S rRNA phylogenetic analysis and DNA-DNA hybridizations studies, *A. sensu stricto* ('true' *Actinobacillus*) is restricted to include *A. lignieresii, A.*

pleuropneumoniae, *A. equuli* subsp. *equuli*, *A. equuli* subsp. *haemolyticus* (taxon 11 of Bisgaard), *A. hominis*, *A. suis*, *A. ureae*, *A. arthritidis* (sorbitol-positive taxon 9 of Bisgaard), *Actinobacillus* genomospecies 1 (*A. lignieresii*-phenotype isolated from horses) and 2 (sorbitol-negative *A. arthritidis*), taxa 8 (guinea pig isolate) and taxa 26 (avian haemolytic *Actinobacillus*-like) of Bisgaard. Remaining 11 species are not included within the 'true' *Actinobacillus*. Among the members of *A. sensu stricto*, only *A. pleuropneumoniae* is considered as primary pathogen.

Haemophilus has 26 species currently. The species with pathogenic significance in human, animals and birds are *H. influenzae, H. paragallinarum, H. parasuis, H. felis, H. haemoglobinophilus* (previously *H. canis*), *H. paracuniculus, H. influenzaemurium, H. somnus* (previously *H. agni*).Based on 16S rRNA gene sequences and phenotypic characteristics, *Haemophilus paragallinarum* is renamed as *Avibacterium paragallinarum* under the newly created genus *Avibacterium*. The genus *Avibacterium* comprises other species like *A. gallinarum* (previously *Pasteurella gallinarum*), *A. avium* (*Pasteurella avium*), *A. volantium* (*Pasteurella volantium*) and *A. endocarditidis* sp. nov. Recent classification also describes *Haemophilus somnus* as *Histophilus somni* under the same family *Pasteurellaceae*.

As the name of the genus *Haemophilus* suggests, the bacteria require haemin (factor 'X') and nicotinamide adenine di-nucleotide (NAD, factor 'V') in blood for their growth. However, the species with 'para' prefix require only 'V'-factor for their growth.

The genus *Gallibacterium* was created in 2003 and currently the genus consists of seven species, including 4 named species (*Gallibacterium anatis, G. melopsittaci, G. salpingitidis, G. trehalosifermentans*), 3 genomospecies (1, 2, and 3), and unnamed group V.

4. *Resistance:* 60°C temperature for 15 minute exposure and autoclaving (120°C for 15 minute) is lethal to *Actinobacillus*. The bacteria are susceptible to common disinfectants like phenol, cresol etc. *A. pleuropneumoniae* contains resistance plasmid (R-plasmid) encoding the resistance factors to sulfonamides, tetracycline and penicillin.

55°C temperature for 30 minute exposure and autoclaving (120°C for 15 minute) is lethal to *Haemophilus*. Artificial cultures die easily due to desiccation at room temperature. Experimentally the bacteria remain viable at 23.5°C in nasal mucus or blood for at least 70 days and in vaginal mucus for up to five days. The bacteria do not survive in the environment for prolonged period. The bacteria are often preserved at -70°C or by freeze drying in the laboratory.

5. *Natural habitat:* Most of the *Actinobacillus* is commensal on the mucous membrane of animal reservoirs specially in the upper respiratory tract. For example, *A. lignieresii* and *A. suis* are commonly found in the oropharynx of the cattle and tonsil or upper respiratory tract of swine, respectively. The bacteria are considered as opportunistic pathogen, causing endogenous infection in susceptible animals. The bacteria do not survive in the environment for a long time.

Haemophilus can reside in the respiratory tract of human, animals and birds. *H. somni* (*H. somnus*), *H. haemoglobinophilus* are the part of normal bacterial flora in the male and female genital tract of the cattle and dogs, respectively. *H. somnus* is also recovered from the bovine respiratory tract. *Haemophilus* are considered as opportunistic pathogen causing endogenous infection in susceptible animals (with exception of some species like *A. paragallinarum* that may act as a primary pathogen). *Avibacterium avium*, *Avibacterium volantium* are normally regarded as part of the commensal flora of the upper respiratory tract of chicken and other birds.

Gallibacterium can act as a part of commensal flora in chicken respiratory tract (nasal and tracheal passage) and digestive tract (cloaca and vagina).

6. Genome: The genome of *A. pleuropneumoniae* (KL 16 strain) is 2,357,806 bp in size with a GC content of 41 mol%. The genome consists of 2,199 putative protein-coding sequences (CDS), 62 tRNAs, and 19 rRNA-related genes. The plasmid is 7699 bp in size with the GC content of 60 mol%.

The genome of *Avibacterium* is 2.4 Mbp in size with the GC content of 41 mol%. The genome consists of several virulence factors (> 100), insertion sequences, and transposon associated with tetracycline resistance (Tn10). Earlier it was thought that *A. paragallinarum* is devoid of native plasmids. Later haemocin encoding plasmid (p250) was detected in *A. paragallinarum* strains. The haemocin is a kind of bacteriocin and can lyse a range of other gram-negative bacteria. The NAD independence for growth detected in *A. paragallinarum* is also a plasmid associated trait. The first multi-drug resistance plasmid detected in *A. paragallinarum* is designated as pYMH5.

The genome of *Gallibacterium anatis* consists of clustered regularly interspaced short palindromic repeats (CRISPR) and integrative conjugative elements (ICEs). The CRISPR acts as innate defense of the bacteria and it can degrade foreign nucleic acids. The ICEs are associated with antimicrobial resistance. The plasmids (1-4 in numbers) are also detected in *G. anatis*.

Isolation, growth and colony characteristics

Primary isolation media of *Actinobacillus* is sheep blood agar. The plates are incubated at 37°C for 24 hour with 5-10% CO_2 tension. Some species like *A. pleuropneumoniae* requires 48 hours incubation for optimal growth. The candle jar method for supplying CO_2 is satisfactory. Chocolate agar is suitable for isolation of *A. pleuropneumoniae,* as it requires factor 'V' (NAD) for its optimum growth (like *Haemophilus*). Streaking of *Staphylococcus* in blood agar can also supply the factor 'V' for optimum growth of *A. pleuropneumoniae*. The colonies of *A. lignieresii* after primary culture and 24 hours of growth are non-haemolytic, translucent or grayish, 1-2 mm in diameter, and very sticky or waxy. The stickiness is lost during subculture. Haemolysis is observed for *A. pleuropneumoniae*, *A. equuli* subsp. *haemolyticus*, *A. suis* and taxon 26 of Bisgaard (avian haemolytic *Actinobacillus*-like). All of them can produce sticky colonies like *A. lignieresii.* However, *A. pleuropneumoniae* produces two types of colonies i.e. sticky (waxy) and soft glistening. Poor growth is found in MacConkey's agar with the production of late arising, tiny, lactose fermenting colonies. *A. pleuropneumoniae* cannot grow in MacConkey's agar.

The media commonly used for isolation of *Haemophilus* are blood agar, chocolate agar, Levinthal's medium, Fildes' medium, and NAD supplemented PPLO media. The bacteria do not grow in MacConkey's agar. Chocolate agar is the most satisfactory medium for *Haemophilus* isolation from animals. *Haemophilus* are slow-growing and fastidious, and often the bacteria are overgrown by fast growing commensals.Use of dilution plating technique and antibiotics (lincomycin and bacitracin) in culture media can improve the recovery of *Haemophilus* from the contaminated clinical samples. Most species require 'X' (haemin, required for synthesis of catalase enzyme; heat stable) and 'V'-factor (nicotinamide adenine di-nucleotide, NAD or its reduced form NADH; heat labile) for their growth [except *H. somni* (*H. somnus*)]. Whereas, some of them only require 'V'-factor for their growth (designated with 'para' prefix, e.g. *A. paragallinarum*). NADH requirements for *A. paragallinarum* vary from 1.5-25 µg/ml. The 'V'-factor-independent (NAD-independent) strains have also isolated. Other growth requirements include presence of serum and 1-1.5% sodium chloride (for *A. paragallinarum*).The chocolate agar is prepared by the addition of blood in warm agar media (at 70-80°C). It contains both the 'X' and 'V' factors, liberated from lysed red blood cells in increased temperature. In the high temperature, the enzyme which can lyse the factor-V (NADase) is destroyed and the factor 'X' is heat stable. So, both of the factors are found in the media. Similarly, in Levinthal's and Fildes' media, red blood cells are lysed by heat and pepsin, respectively to liberate the growth factors. In solid media, *Haemophilus* grows better near the colonies of *Staphylococcus aureus.* It is known as 'satellitism' and cultures of

Staphylococcus are called 'nurse' or 'feeder' bacteria. *Staphylococcus* helps in their growth by synthesizing 'V'-factor. The plates and liquid media are incubated at 37°C for 48-72 hours. *A. paragallinarum, H. paracuniculus,* and *H. felis* require 5-10% CO_2 for their growth. Moist incubation may replace the CO_2 requirement. The colonies in blood agar are smooth, translucent and non-haemolytic. *H. parasuis* produces small brown to grey colonies in chocolate agar plates. *H. somni* (*H. somnus*) produces yellowish colonies in solid media. In Columbia blood agar, the colonies are surrounded by clear zone of haemolysis.

Gallibacterium can be isolated in blood agar. *G. anatis* produces β-hemolytic, smooth, greyish, non-transparent, and shiny colonies on bovine blood agar after 24-48 hours of incubation at 37°C.

Biochemical characteristics

Actinobacillus sensu stricto, *Haemophilus* and *Gallibacterium* produce following biochemical reactions

Biochemical tests	*Actinobacillus sensu stricto*	*Histophilus somni (H. somnus)*	*Avibacterium paragallinarum*	*Haemophilus parasuis*	*Haemophilus haemoglobinophilus*	*Gallibacterium anatis*
Catalase	Variable	(-ve)	(-ve)	(+ve)	(+ve)	(+ve)
Oxidase	(+ve)	(+ve)	(-ve)	(-ve)	(+ve)	(+ve)
Indole	(-ve)	Variable	(-ve)	(-ve)	(+ve)	-
Voges Proskauer	(-ve)	-	(-ve)	-	-	-
Urease	(+ve)	(-ve)	(+ve)	(-ve)	(-ve)	-
Nitrate reduction	(+ve)	(+ve)	(+ve)	(+ve)	(+ve)	(+ve)
Carbohydrate						
fermentation	(-ve)	(+ve)	(+ve)	(+ve)		
Glucose (acid	(+ve) without gas	(-ve)	(+ve)	(+ve)		
production)	(+ve) (late	(-ve)	(-ve)	Variable	(+ve)	-
Sucrose	fermentation)	(+ve)	(-ve)	(-ve)	(+ve)	-
Lactose	-	(+ve)	(+ve)	(-ve)	(-ve)	-
Xylose	(+ve) without gas				(+ve)	-
Mannitol					(+ve)	(-ve)
Ornithine Decarboxylase		(+ve)	(-ve)	(-ve)	(-ve)	-

Antigenic characteristics

A. lignieresii contains two major types of antigens i.e. somatic (heat stable) and heat labile antigens. On the basis of somatic antigens, *A. lignieresii* has six serotypes, designated as type 1-6. Among these serotypes, type 1 is restricted in cattle, whereas, types 2, 3, 4 are found in sheep. In addition to the host, the serotype distribution is also influenced by geographical locations. There is an antigenic relationship between *A. lignieresii*, *Burkholderia mallei* and *Burkholderia pseudomallei.* However, *A. pleuropneumoniae* has surface soluble antigen composed of capsular polysaccharide and lipopolysaccharide (LPS). On the basis of the soluble antigen the bacterium has 15 serotypes. Two of the serotypes (1 and 5) are sub-divided into four subtypes (1a, 1b, 5a, and 5b).The cross reactivity between the serotypes are found (e.g. between serotype 3, 6, 8) due to common LPS structure. *A. pleuropneumoniae* is also classified into two biotypes known as biotype 1 and 2, based on their nicotinamide adenine-di-nucleotide (NAD) requirements. The biotype 1 is NAD dependent, whereas, biotype 2 is NAD independent.

Page (1962) first determined three serovars (A, B, C) of *Haemophilus paragallinarum* (*A. paragallinarum*) on the basis of plate agglutination test. Other independent studies by different workers revealed three serovars (Kato and Tsubahara serotype I, II, IIII) or two serovars (Sawata serotype 1 and 2) of *A. paragallinarum*. The antigenic analysis revealed three types of antigens on the surface of *A. paragallinarum.* The three types are heat labile and trypsin sensitive (L) antigen, heat labile and trypsin resistant (HL) and heat stable and trypsin resistant (HS) antigens. The ‘L’ antigen exists in three serologically distinct forms (L1, L2 and L3) and is responsible for serospecificity. Sawata’s serotype 1 strains possess L1, while Sawata’s serotype 2 strains possess L2. The remaining antigens i.e. L3, HL, and HS are common for all the serotypes. The common antigens are responsible for the cross-reaction between the serotypes of *A. paragallinarum.* Later Kume serotyping scheme was established based on haemagglutination inhibition test. This scheme detected seven serovars arranged in three serogroups.

Haemophilus parasuis is heterogeneous and consists of 15 serotypes, designated as serotype 1-15.It is based on heat stable antigens i.e. capsular polysaccharide and lipopolysaccharide. Multiple serotypes can be detected in a herd or even the same animal. The serotypes 1, 5, 10, 12, 13, and 14 are highly virulent. The serotypes 2, 4, and 15 can cause polyserositis (moderately virulent).The remaining serovars (3, 6, 7, 8, 9, and 11) produce no clinical signs and are considered as non-virulent.

The greater antigenic variation is detected among the *Gallibacterium anatis* strains.

Toxins and virulence factors produced

Toxins

Cytotoxin: The cytotoxin belongs to 'RTX' (repeats-in-toxin structure) family, a kind of pore-forming, cytolytic protein found in gram-negative bacteria. The RTX genes are present in *A. pleuropneumoniae*, *A. suis*, *A. lignieresii* and *A. equuli* subsp. *haemolyticus.* In *A. pleuropneumoniae,* the cytotoxin has four types namely ApxI, ApxII, ApxIII and ApxIVa. The ApxI is strongly haemolytic and cytotoxic and is produced by serotypes 1, 5, 9, 10, and 11 which are associated with severe outbreaks. The ApxIII is only cytotoxic and is produced by serotypes 2, 3, 4, and 8 of *A. pleuropneumoniae*. At high concentration, the toxins can lyse red blood cells, epithelial cells, T-lymphocytes and macrophages by forming pore in their cell membrane. At sublytic concentration, they can affect oxidative metabolism of phagocytic cells.

In *A. suis*, proteins similar to ApxI and Apx II are detected.

In *A. lignieresii,* although RTX gene is detected but the expression of the toxin is not confirmed.

In *A. equuli* subsp. *haemolyticus* the RTX toxin is known as 'Aqx'. Equine granulocytes are susceptible to the toxin. The 'Aqx' toxin is not detected in *A. equuli* subsp. *equuli.*

Endotoxin (LPS): Like other gram-negative bacteria *Haemophilus* also possesses endotoxin which is responsible for pro-inflammatory cytokine (IL-1, TNF) release from the macrophages during infection. In *H. parasuis* infection, the endotoxin causes thrombosis and disseminated intravascular coagulation in liver, lung and kidney. The purified LPS of *A. paragallinarum* is toxic to chickens producing hydropericardium.

Gallibacterium toxin A (GtxA): It is secreated by few biovars of *Gallibacterium anatis* which can produce β-haemolysis in blood agar ('haemolytica' biovar). The toxin causes lysis of red blood cells and leukocytes. The C-terminus of the toxin has structural similarity with RTX toxin family. The N-terminus is associated with lysis of red blood cells or leukocytes. The GtxA has significant role in pathogenesis. The binding of the toxin with actin protein in the host immune cells may modify the cell structure and cellular signal transduction and can evade the immunity.

Outer membrane vesicles (OMVs): *Gallibacterium anatis* can release outer membrane vesicles by budding of outer membrane in the cell wall. It consists of proteins, LPS, periplasmic components and DNA. The OMV is associated with colonization, biofilm formation, and removal of antibacterial substances. *G. anatis* OMVs also contain haemagglutinin causing lysis of broiler chickens, layer birds, quails, rabbits, and pigs red blood cells.

Virulence factors

Following virulence factors are produced by *Actinobacillus*, *Haemophilus / Avibacterium* and *Gallibacterium anatis*

Virulence factors	Function
Capsule	Capsule is produced by *A. pleuropneumoniae, Haemophilus* and *G. anatis*. It is anti-phagocytic and helps in adherence of the bacteria with the host cells. The capsule of *G. anatis* is thin and disappears during sub-culture
Pili	Pili are observed in A. pleuropneumoniae and *G. anatis*. It helps in adherence of the bacteria with the alveolar epithelium and cilia of the terminal bronchioles. The fimbriae/pili in *G. anatis* belongs to F-17 family and the fimbrial protein has significant role in pathogenesis
Lipopolysaccharide (LPS)	LPS is considered as a putative virulence factor of *A. pleuropneumoniae* since LPS can induce lesions in mice similar to whole cells, but less severe and without haemolysis. The LPS can mediate adhesion of *A. pleuropneumoniae* with tracheal epithelium
Transferrin binding protein (TBP) and 'Afu-A' (Actinobacillus ferric uptake) protein	a) TBP is an outer membrane protein, detected in *A. pleuropneumoniae*. It helps in acquisition of iron by binding porcine transferrin only. It suggests that the bacterium is highly host specific. Iron is required for metabolic electron transport chain of the bacteria. b) 'Afu-A' protein is a periplasmic protein, which is involved in iron transport
Neuraminidase	It is produced by *H. parasuis*. It can remove sialic acid from the host cell surface and thus exposes the bacterial attachment site. It also interferes with the host defence system by decreasing the viscosity of mucin.
Outer membrane protein (OMP)	Virulent strains of *H. parasuis, H. somnus* possess 37KDa and 40Kda OMP, respectively. Exact role in pathogenesis is not established.
Immunoglobulin binding protein	*H. somni* possesses surface immunoglobulin binding protein that can bind Fc portion of bovine IgG. The antibody become unavailable in the serum for the complement mediated bacterial killing and the bacteria become serum resistant
Zinc-containing metalloprotease	It helps in colony establishment, nutrition, protection from the host immune system, bacterial distribution through blood circulation of *Gallibacterium anatis*. The enzyme can lyse avian IgG which helps in immune evasion

Virulence factors	Function
Biofilm	*Gallibacterium anatis* can produce biofilm which helps in persistence and antimicrobial resistance
Elongation factor-Tu (EF-Tu)	It is produced by *Gallibacterium anatis* and it has amyloid properties
Small colony variant (SCV)	The SCV is observed in *Gallibacterium anatis* associated with persistence of infection and antimicrobial resistance
Glycosyltransferase (cps16A), HyaE/ hyaluronidase (cps16B), UDP-glucose 6-dehydrogenase (cps16F)	The enzymes are associated with virulence of *Gallibacterium anatis*

Pathogenesis

Transmission

Actinobacillus

Actinobacillus lignieresii causes endogenous infection in cattle. It resides in the cattle oropharynx, tonsil, tongue and rumen. Injury or trauma of buccal cavity or stomach helps in penetration of the bacteria into the underlying soft tissues. Continuous feeding with thorny vegetations, stemmy haylages may produce such kind of buccal injuries.

A. pleuropneumoniae and *A. suis* are transmitted into susceptible pigs either by direct contact or inhalation of the contaminated dust particles. In a pig farm, high population density and poor ventilation are predisposing factors for transmission. Maternal antibodies from infected sow can pass through the colostrum and protect the piglet up to 3 weeks of age.

A. equuli ssp. equuli is responsible for major neonatal mortality in horses. It is transmitted to the neonates through ingestion and inhalation or umbilical cord. The transmission occurs either within uterus, during parturition, or after birth. Stress, colostrum deprivation and parasitism may predispose the infection. The migrating larvae of *Strongylus vulgaris* can bring the bacteria from the intestinal lumen to blood circulation. It may cross the placental barrier to infect the foetus (verminous aneurysms).

Haemophilus and Avibacterium

Haemophilus parasuis inhabits the nasal mucosa, tonsil, trachea and lungs of the healthy pigs. The vertical transmission to piglets occurs before 10 days of age. Young weaned pigs are most susceptible due to low amount of maternal antibody at the time of weaning. Stress factors like transport, pregnancy etc. contribute to the development of the clinical syndrome.

H. somni (*H. somnus*) resides in the bovine reproductive and urinary tracts. Infected cattle can shed the bacteria through the urine and other discharges. It can contaminate the pastures. In intensive system of rearing pen-mates become infected by inhalation of contaminated aerosols. Rarely the bacteria can enter the central nervous system thorough the Batson's vein directly from the reproductive tract.

Avibacterium paragallinarum colonizes the upper respiratory tract and sinuses of the poultry birds. Chronically infected and healthy birds are major reservoir of the infection. The transmission of the bacteria occurs into the susceptible birds by aerosol route or ingestion of contaminated feed and drinking water.

Gallibacterium anatis

G. anatis is commonly transmitted through inhalation route. Experimentally it was also transmitted through trans-ovarian or oviduct or trans-eggshell route but in natural infection the routes are not confirmed yet.

Pathogenesis

A. lignieresii

A. lignieresii results endogenous infection in cattle. Coarse feedstuffs produce injuries in the buccal cavity. The wound may turn into non healing deep ulcers specially in the tongue, pharynx and soft palate. The bacteria enter into the underlying soft tissues through the wound. Leukocytosis at the infection site produces characteristic lesion after a few days. In the center of the lesion, club shaped bacterial microcolonies are found. It may enlarge into granulomatous masses surrounded by connective tissues. The bacteria may disseminate into other organs (lungs) through lymphatics. The lesions produced in other organs are often confused with neoplasms.

A. pleuropneumoniae

The bacteria enter the host (pigs) through inhalation of the contaminated dust particles. The bacteria colonize in the lower respiratory tract after adhesion with the alveolar mucosa and cilia. The multiplication of bacteria and release of the toxins occurs. Bacterial LPS and the released toxins generate an inflammatory response after enhancing the recruitment of neutrophils or other inflammatory cells (macrophages) at the site of the infection. Some of the recruited neutrophils die due to the cytolytic nature of the bacterial toxins. Death of the neutrophils releases its granular contents causing further tissue damage. The inflammatory response causes focal necrotizing vasculitis, localized thrombosis, edema, and fibrinous pleuritis. Capsule of the bacteria helps in evasion of the phagocytosis by macrophages. In chronic infection, the bacteria are sequestered in fibrinous lesion or tonsillar crypts through the pili.

Histophilus somni (H. somnus)

The bacteria can survive within bovine neutrophils and alveolar macrophages. Attachment with vascular endothelial cells is crucial for pathogenesis. After the attachment it causes endothelial cells of small blood vessels to separate and thus it exposes the underlying basement membrane. The condition results in the formation of a 'thrombus' with the help of bacterial endotoxin. The lipooligosaccharide (LOS) of *H. somni* causes endothelial cell apoptosis and through antigenic phase variation it helps in bacterial evasion of immune response. Other virulence attributes like serum resistance property of the bacteria helps in survival and dissemination of the infection into the different organs like brain, heart, skeletal muscle, joints, larynx, liver and kidneys through the blood. The bacteria help in liberation of histamine, which in conjunction with anti-*H. somni* IgE may account for the early respiratory lesions. The bacteria can also produce biofilm within the host and fork head associated (FHA) proteins may be involved in the process. The formation of biofilm protects the bacteria from host defence and antibiotics.

A. paragallinarum

The capsule made of hyaluronic acid helps in attachment of the bacteria with the cilia of the nasal mucosa. Antiphagocytic capsule, bacterial endotoxin may play significant role in pathogenesis, but exact mechanism is unexplored. Major lesion is catarrhal inflammation of the upper respiratory tract with mast cell infiltration into the lamina propria of the nasal cavity mucous membrane. The mast cell infiltration is responsible for the development of the clinical signs.

H. parasuis

H. parasuis may preferentially colonize the nasal mucosa of the pigs, but the bacteria can also reside in the tonsil and trachea. The neuraminidase enzyme helps in exposing bacterial attachment sites into the nasal mucosa. The enzyme can remove sialic acid from the host cell surface and thus exposes the attachment site. The permease and aldolase enzymes help in the neuraminidase action. Some strains produce capsule and fimbriae which helps in bacterial attachment. After attachment, they can penetrate the mucosa and enter the blood stream by an unknown way. Replication of the bacteria occurs at the serosal site to produce systemic infection. Destruction of alveolar macrophages by concurrent viral infection (like porcine respiratory and reproductive syndrome virus, PRRS) helps in bacterial multiplication. Bacterial endotoxin plays significant role in lesion development.

Gallibacterium anatis

G. anatis can colonize the upper respiratory tract of healthy chicken without showing any clinical signs. The adherence and colonization takes place with the help of adhesins present on the bacterial surface. After colonization the bacteria multiply and secreate virulence factors. The secreated factors cause up-regulation of pro-inflammatory cytokines (IL6, IFNγ, TNFα) and produce tissue injuries. During stress and immunosuppression associated with co-infection (infectious bronchitis virus, *E. coli*, *A. paragallinarum*, *Mycoplasma gallisepticum*), change in environmental factors like seasonal variations, cold stress, lack of biosecurity, deficient nutrition, poor ventilation, and overcrowding may enhance *G. anatis* multiplication. The opportunistic bacteria enter different organs through the blood circulation and cause pericarditis, perihepatitis, oophoritis, follicular hemorrhage and degeneration, salpingitis, peritonitis, and enteritis.

Disease produced

Bacteria	Host	Disease produced
Actinobacillus lignieresii	Ruminants	Wooden tongue: It is pyogranulomatous lesions of the soft tissues of head and neck with odourless pus; specially in the gums, cheeks and the tongue; lungs, testes, mammary glands and draining lymph nodes of ruminants. Hard tumourous masses are produced in the tongue causing dysphagia and weight loss.
Actinobacillus pleuropneumoniae	Pig	Porcine pleuropneumonia: The disease is characterized by haemorrhagic necrotizing pneumonia affecting the caudal lung lobe and fibrinous pleuritis with high morbidity (30%) and mortality (50%). Coughing, dyspnoea (thumping), abortion, blood tinged discharge from the nose or mouth before death is common signs.
Actinobacillus suis	Pig	It is associated with septicemia, pneumonia and enteritis of pigs with the highest susceptibility for infection in suckling and newly weaned piglets
	Horse	Septicaemia, polyarthritis
	cattle	abortion

Bacteria	Host	Disease produced
Actinobacillus equuli ssp. equuli	Horse (neonatal foal)	a) Sleepy foal disease: It is a septicaemic infection of neonatal foals found worldwide. Infection of the foals occurs through ingestion, inhalation or umbilicus. Mares are carrier of the bacteria in their mouth, upper respiratory tract and alimentary tract. b) Purulent arthritis ('joint ill') c) Nephritis
Actinobacillus equuli ssp. haemolyticus	Horse	a) Endocarditis, meningitis, metritis, abortion, respiratory and wound infections
A. hominis and A. ureae	Human	b) Sporadic respiratory tract infection
A. arthritidis and Actinobacillus genomospecies 2	Horse and other animals	c) Septicaemia and arthritis
Actinobacillus genomospecies 1	Horse	Stomatitis
Bisgaard taxon 8	Guinea pig	Not reported
Bisgaard taxon 26	Duck	Sinusitis, septicaemia
Avibacterium paragallinarum	Chicken	Infectious coryza: An acute respiratory infection of growing chicken and layers characterized by nasal discharge, facial swelling, lacrimation, anorexia, and diarrhoea. Decreased feed and water consumption may reduce the growth rate and drop the egg production in layer.
Avibacterium endocarditidis sp. *nov*	Chicken	Endocarditis
Histophilus somni (Haemophilus somnus)	Cattle	Haemophilus somnus disease complex: a) Reproductive or urogenital form: Vaginitis, endometritis, infertility and abortion occurs in this form. Abortion occurs in all stages of gestation. b) Respiratory form: In this form, laryngitis, tracheitis, suppurative bronchopneumonia develop. It may be a part of 'classical shipping fever' complex. c) Septicaemic form: It can localize brain, heart, skeletal muscle, joints, larynx, liver, and kidneys. The clinical signs vary depending on the affected area and resistance of the animal. d) The nervous form is thrombotic meningo-encephalomyelitis (TME). Other signs like myocarditis, otitis, chronic and gangrenous mastitis are observed.

Bacteria	Host	Disease produced
Haemophilus parasuis	Pig Actinobacillus suis, Haemophilus parasuis, and Streptococcus suis have emerged as important pathogens of swine associated with serious clinical conditions. It has given rise to the nickname "suiside diseases")	**Glasser's disease:** It is characterized by fibrinous polyserositis, polyarthritis and meningitis, acute pneumonia without polyserositis, acute septicaemia.
Haemophilus haemoglobinophilus	Dog	Commensal of lower genital tract, rarely causes vaginitis, cystitis, balanoposthitis
Haemophilus felis	Cat	Rhinitis, conjunctivitis
Haemophilus paracuniculus	Rabbit	enteritis
Haemophilus influenzae	Human	Respiratory tract infection and meningitis
Haemophilus influenzaemurium	Rodents	Respiratory tract and ocular infection
Gallibacterium anatis	Chicken	Non-specific clinical signs such as rales, coughing, dyspnea, shaking heads, mild swelling of head, nasal discharge, diarrhea, anorexia, emaciation, and 3-18% decrease in egg production are detected. The lesions such as inflammation of ovaries and fallopian tubes, follicle degeneration, ovary regression, hemorrhagic oviducts, nonfunctional oviducts, deformed follicles and broken follicles and peritonitis are observed. In breeder birds, 0.06-4.9% mortality rate is detected

Immunity

The humoral immune response (Ig-G production) offers protection against *Actinobacillus pleuropneumoniae.* Secreatory IgA (sIgA) is also produced after infection. Probably it prevents the bacterial colonization with the mucosal surface. Transfer of serum or anti-RTX toxin-antibodies from infected animals can produce immunity in uninfected animals. Role of cell mediated immunity in protection is not established. Whereas, cell mediated hypersensitivity develops during *A. lignieresii* infection (wooden tongue) in cattle. The neutralizing antibodies are not related with the recovery of the infection.

Diagnosis

Clinical samples: Pus, exudates from the lesion can be collected as ante-mortem samples for diagnosis of bovine actinobacillosis. After post mortem, tissue biopsies and pneumonic lesions are collected in 10% formalin for histopathology.

Vaginal swab, nasal swab, blood, faecal sample, synovial fluid from the suspected animals and / or birds according to the lesion can be collected as ante-mortem samples for *Haemophilus/ Avibacterium* infection. After post mortem, tissue biopsies and pneumonic lesions are collected for histopathology. Ante-mortem samples should be disposed within 24 hours of collection to the laboratory to protect from drying.

Laboratory examinations

Direct examination: For direct examination of *Actinobacillus lignieresii* in clinical samples, the following method is followed.

Grayish-white granules are observed in the pus

↓

Granules are washed with distilled water in a sterile petri dish

↓

Granules are placed in one drop of 10% KOH in a glass slide

↓

Granules are gently crushed with cover slip and observed under low power of light microscope

↓

'Club shaped' bacterial colonies (like actinomycosis) are observed. If gram stained, at the center of the colony, gram-negative rods are found. In actinomycosis, they are gram positive rods with branching filaments.

For demonstration of *Haemophilus / Avibacterium / Gallibacterium*, the smear can be prepared from collected fluid samples or tissues and stained by Gram's stain. *Haemophilus / Avibacterium* appears as gram-negative small non-sporing rods or coccobacilli with 'bipolar staining' characteristics. *Gallibacterium* appears as gram-negative small non-sporing rods.

Isolation of bacteria from clinical samples: Media, incubation condition and colony characteristics are described earlier.

Haemolysis and cytotoxicity assay: The assays are conducted for detection of GtxA toxin activity produced by *Gallibacterium anatis*. In tris-sodium chloride buffer (10mM Tris-HCl, 0.9% NaCl, pH 7.5), the bovine blood is washed repeatedly until the fluid layer become colourless. The washed red blood cells are incubated with the test bacterial suspension (1:1) at 37°C for 1 hour. The quantification of released haemoglobin after haemolysis can be done at 540 nm by ELISA reader. For cytotoxicity assay, HD11 cell line is used in tissue culture plate (96-well). The bacterial culture is added into the wells and is incubated overnight at 37°C with 5% CO_2.

Serological tests

Actinobacillus

CFT and ELISA can be used for detection of antibodies against *Actinobacillus pleuropneumoniae*. ELISA offers better sensitivity than CFT. In ELISA, antibodies against LPS, capsular polysaccharide, 'Apx' toxins are detected. However, serotyping by detection of anti-LPS- antibodies are often confusing. Most of the serotypes possess identical O-chain of LPS and cross react. For e.g. there is cross-reactivity between LPS of serotypes 4 and 7, and serotypes 3, 6 and 8 of *A. pleuropneumoniae*. Capsular polysaccharide is better antigen than LPS. It lacks cross reaction between serotypes. The preparation and standardization of capsular antigen is a difficult procedure although. The Apx toxin of *A. pleuropneumoniae* as an antigen is also cross reactive with *A. suis* ($ApxI_{var.\ suis}$ and $ApxII_{var.\ suis}$) or haemolytic *Escherichia coli* (HlyA).

Haemophilus / Avibacterium

Haemagglutination inhibition test (HI): Three types of HI tests are commonly employed for detection of *Avibacterium* (infectious coryza) in poultry. They are i) simple HI ii) extracted HI and iii) treated HI. i) The simple HI test uses the antigen prepared from the whole bacterial cells of *A. paragallinarum* (Page serovar A). Although simple to perform, this HI test can detect antibodies only to serovar 'A'. ii) The extracted HI test is based on antigen derived from potassium thiocyanate (KSCN) extracted and sonicated cells of *A. paragallinarum.* iii) The treated HI test is based on hyaluronidase-treated whole bacterial cells of *A. paragallinarum.* Vaccinated chicken with 1:5 or more titers in simple or extracted HI is considered as 'protected' against infectious coryza. The simple HI test is suitable for detection of both the infected and vaccinated birds associated with serovar 'A'. The extracted or treated HI tests are suitable for detection of vaccinated birds associated with serovar 'C'.

Slide and tube agglutination test, agar gel precipitation test (AGPT), latex agglutination test can be used for detection of antibodies against *A.*

paragallinarum in carrier birds. The antibodies are detected 1-2 week after infection in the birds and they are present up to one year after the onset of the infection.

Indirect Haemagglutination assay (IHA) is used for diagnosis of *Haemophilus parasuis* infection in pigs. It uses supernatant of sonicated *H. parasuis* cells or boiled cells as coating antigens for sheep red blood cells. However, the test result is often unreliable.

Complement fixation test (CFT) is used for diagnosis of *H. parasuis* infection in pigs. Circulating complement fixing antibodies are demonstrated within 1 week of the onset of infection.

Enzyme linked immunossorbant assay (ELISA): Monoclonal antibody based ELISA can detect Page serovar A and C of *A. paragallinarum.* However the availability of the monoclonal antibodies is limited and the test can be used as flock test only.

Immunohistochemistry: *H. parasuis* antigen has been detected in formalin-fixed, paraffin-embedded tissues by immunohistochemistry (IHC). Major advantage is direct demonstration of the bacterial antigen in the affected tissues and its correlation with the histopathological changes. It can also detect non-viable bacteria in the tissues. The availability of the monoclonal antibodies against *H. parasuis* which act in formalin fixed paraffin embedded tissues is limited. Polyclonal antibodies against *H. parasuis* shows cross-reactivity with other bacteria like *Actinobacillus pleuropneumoniae.*

Gallibacterium anatis

ELISA based test is developed for detection of acute phase protein (ovotransferrin) in chickens experimentally infected with *G. anatis*. Fluorescent in situ hybridization (FISH) with a cyanine dye-labelled in situ hybridization probe (GAN850) targeting 16S-rRNA can be used for detection of *G. anatis*. MALDI-TOF MS (matrix-assisted laser desorption/ionization time-of-flight mass spectrometry) is used to identify the biomarkers of *G. anatis* based on size of protein molecules by producing fingerprint spectra.

Molecular biology

Actinobacillus

PCR based detection of *A. pleuropneumoniae* is described which detects *omlA* or *apxIVA* gene. Among them, *apxIVa* gene detection permits direct identification of the bacteria from infected lung tissues and nasal fluids. The PCR based serotyping of the *A. pleuropneumoniae* isolates are also carried out depending on the differences in *apx* toxin gene sequences. The typing method is known as 'RTX-PCR-serotyping'. Other genotyping methods like multilocus enzyme electrophoresis (MLEE), ribotyping are used to investigate the spread of particular genotype of *A. pleuropneumoniae.*

Haemophilus / Avibacterium

For rapid confirmatory diagnosis of infectious coryza the PCR was developed in Australia, known as HP-2 PCR. The PCR can directly detect *H. paragallinarum* (*A. paragallinarum*), including the NAD-independent isolates, in sinus swabs collected from the chicken. It can also detect the bacteria in the samples preserved for six months at 4°C. Recently, the PCR-RFLP is developed targeting the hyper-variable region of *HMTp210* gene. The technique can detect all the three serovars (A, B, C) of *A. paragallinarum*.

PCR based on 16S rRNA gene can be used for detection of *Haemophilus parasuis* in clinical samples. Detection limit is 10^2cfu/ml. However use of this PCR directly in nasal swab is inconclusive. *H. parasuis* is a commensal of upper respiratory tract in pigs and the PCR can also detect *Actinobacillus indolicus*, another commensal of upper respiratory tract. Recently for improved sensitivity, nested-PCR is developed to detect *H. parasuis* infection in pigs which can identify the bacteria even in formalin fixed paraffin embedded tissues.

In situ hybridization (ISH): This method can detect the genomic sequences of *H. parasuis* in tissues using a PCR amplified product as probe. It does not need monoclonal antibody as used in immunohistochemistry.

Molecular typing: It can be performed by digestion of the whole genomic DNA with restriction enzyme followed by the analysis of the fragments. In *H. parasuis* infection, different band patterns are observed between the isolates from diseased and healthy animals. Other modern techniques like ERIC-PCR (enterobacterial repetitive intergenic consensus), PCR-RFLP (restriction fragment length polymorphism), single locus sequence typing are used for epidemiological studies of *H. parasuis* infection in pigs. In ERIC-PCR the band pattern differs between the isolates due to deletion and insertion of different mobile elements in the genome. PCR-RFLP amplifies a single gene of the bacteria by PCR followed by restriction enzyme digestion of that PCR product to obtain a band pattern. So there is no need to isolate the bacteria. It can be applied directly in the clinical samples which is time saving and less tedious. The selected genes of *H. parasuis* for PCR-RFLP were the transferrin binding protein A (tbpA), the fragment of the 16s rRNA gene and the 5-enolpyruvylshikimate- 3-phosphate synthase (aroA).

Gallibacterium anatis

PCR (conventional/real-time) based detection and quantification of *G. anatis* can be performed efficiently targeting 16S-23S rRNA internal transcribed spacer sequence (ITS), beta-subunit of DNA-dependent RNA-polymerase (*rpoB*), DNA gyrase subunit B gene (*gyrB*), GtxA-toxin encoding gene (*gtxA*) and the fimbrial gene (*flfA*).The Loop-mediated isothermal amplification (LAMP) PCR assay is also developed for rapid detection of *G. anatis* targeting the *sodA* gene (conserved gene in *G. anatis*).

Prevention and control

Control of bovine actinobacillosis is possible with segregation and effective treatment of clinical cases. No vaccine is still available for prevention of the infection.

For prevention and control of *Avibacterium* in poultry farm following measures can be followed

a) The day old chicks should always be preferred as new stock, not aged birds. Recovered birds from infectious coryza may act as lifelong carrier without showing any syndrome

b) Infected or recovered birds should be completely eliminated from the farm with disposal of beddings and disinfection of utensils. The premises should be vacant for 2-3 weeks before introduction of new stock.

c) Vaccination of the birds with bacterin / live vaccines is the best prevention strategy. The bacterin prepared with formalin or thimerosal used as inactivating agent is found protective than other adjuvants. The bacterins generally provide protection against Page serovars (A/B/C) and the serovar should be present in the geographical location for effective vaccination. Primary vaccination in layer is done during 5-10 weeks of age which is followed by a booster at least 4 weeks later. The bacterin can provide immunity for 9-12 months. In India commercial bacterins are available consists of Page serovar 'A' (083 / Modesto/ 221 strain), 'B' (Spross strain) and 'C' (H-18 strain).

For prevention and control of *G. anatis* in poultry farm following measures can be followed

a) Immunosuppression due to concurrent infection with other bacteria /virus should be minimized by proper and timely vaccination, use of effective antimicrobials and implementation of strict biosecurity measures

b) An experimental killed vaccine consisting of *G. anatis* and *A. paragallinarum* strains produced immunity against challenge with field strains in birds. Another experimental vaccine prepared with outer membrane vesicle (OMV) of *G. anatis* produced anti-OMV antibodies in the serum. The commercial vaccine against *G. anatis* is still not available.

Differences of Bovine actinobacillosis and actinomycosis

Characteristics	*Actinobacillus lignieresii*	*Actinomyces bovis*
Specific disease	Wooden tongue	Lumpy Jaw
Abscess formation	At tongue, head, neck (soft tissue)	Jaw (hard tissue)
Granules in pus	Grayish-white, 1 mm	Yellow coloured 'sulfur granule', 1-3 mm
Osteomyelitis	(-)	(+)
Gram stain properties	Gram negative rods	Gram positive rods with branching filaments
Oxygen requirement for growth	Facultative anaerobe	Anaerobe

22

Brucella

Clinical conditions similar to brucellosis have been described since the time of Hippocrates (450 BC). J. A. Marston (1861) first described brucellosis as gastric remittent fever in Malta, the Southern European island country. Sir David Bruce (1886) first isolated small coccobacilli from an infected soldier's spleen and purified the culture in 1887, and named *Micrococcus melitensis*. Later the genus was renamed as *Brucella* in his honour. Similarly, Bang and Stribolg (1897) first isolated *Brucella abortus* from abortion material of a cow. Traum in 1914 isolated *Bacillus abortus suis*, currently known as *Brucella suis*. In 1953, *Brucella ovis* was firs isolated in New Zealand by Budlle and Boyes from the aborted material of sheep. Carmichael and Bruner (1968) first isolated *B. canis* from the aborted placenta of a dog.

In India first report of 'contagious abortion' associated with *Brucella* was found in annual report (1918) of imperial veterinary research institute (presently Indian veterinary research institute), Mukteswar, Uttarakhand and later in 1942 by Polding.

Properties of genus

1. *Morphology*: *Brucella* is gram-negative, partially acid fast, small bacilli or coccobacilli, 0.6-2 μm in length and 0.3-0.5 μm in width (Figure 1). In tissues, the bacteria are found in groups or single. In artificial culture short chains are observed. Older cultures are pleomorphic. The bacteria are non-motile and non-sporulating. Capsule like envelope is found surrounding the bacterial cell (*B. abortus*, *B. melitensis*, and *B. suis*) but true capsule is absent.

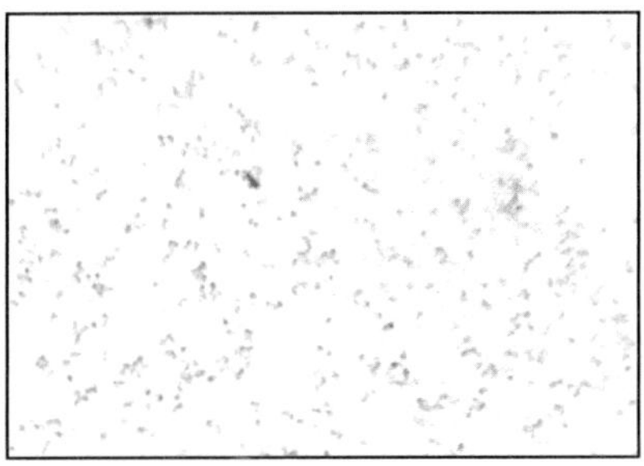

Fig. 1: Gram-negative coccobacilli appearance of *Brucella abortus* (100X) (*Courtesy*: S. Ghodasara, B.B. Bhanderi and Ashish Roy, Department of Veterinary Microbiology, College of Veterinary Science and Animal Husbandry, Anand Agricultural University, Anand, Gujrat)

Brucella can also be stained by modified Ziehl-Neelsen or Macchiavello stains and the bacteria appear red in colour in microscopic field.

2. *Brucella* is aerobic in nature. Some strains prefer increased CO_2 concentration for growth. The bacteria are facultative intracellular and can grow within macrophages of liver, spleen and bone marrow, dendritic cells and placental trophoblasts.

3. *Classification*: *Brucella* is classified within α-2 subdivision of Proteobacterium, which includes *Agrobacterium, Rickettsia, Rhodobacterium*, and *Rhizobium.* Previously it was thought that *Brucella* is a genus with single species i.e. *Brucella melitensis*. All other species were described as biovars. Currently 30 species and numbers of biovars under the genus *Brucella* are described in the list of prokaryotic names with standing in nomenclature (LPSN, https://www.bacterio.net/). The major pathogenic species, numbers of biovars and host range of *Brucella* are

   a) *Brucella abortus* (number of biovars-7)-cattle
   b) *Brucella melitensis* (number of biovars-3)-goat
   c) *Brucella ovis* (number of biovars-1)-sheep
   d) *Brucella suis* (number of biovars-5)-pig
   e) *Brucella canis* (number of biovars-1)-dog
   f) *Brucella neotomae* (number of biovars-1)-desert wood rat

Other new species are

   a) *Brucella pinnipedialis* - isolated from marine mammals (seal)
   b) *Brucella ceti*- isolated from cetaceans
   c) *Brucella microti* – isolated from common voles (*Microtus arvalis*), soil and foxes
   d) *Brucella inopinata*- isolated from a breast implant in human
   e) *Brucella gallinifaecis*-isolated from chicken faeces
   f) *Brucella lupini*
   g) *Brucella anthropi* etc.

4. *Resistance*: *Brucella* is killed by exposure to 60°C for 10 minutes and common disinfectants. Pasteurization of milk can also lyse the bacteria. The bacteria can survive up to 4 months in milk, urine and water. Most strains are sensitive to chloramphenicol, gentamicin, tetracycline and ansamycins.

5. *Natural habitat*: As intracellular bacteria *Brucella* requires host for survival and multiplication. Different species of *Brucella* has different preferred host range. In the environment survival of the bacteria depends on the low temperature and high moisture level.

6. *Genome*: The genome of *Brucella abortus* (A13334 strain) is 3.3 Mbp in size. The genome consists of two chromosomes (ChrI and ChrII) with 56-58 mol% G+C content of each chromosome. The genome has 3,338 predicted coding sequences, 55 tRNA genes (41 in ChrI and 14 in ChrII) and 9 rRNA genes (6 in ChrI and 3 in ChrII).

Isolation, growth and colony characteristics

Brucella is fastidious bacterium with the specific requirements. The growth may be improved by the addition of blood or serum, amino acid, nicotinamide, thiamine, and magnesium ion. Trypticase soya agar with 5% serum, Farrell medium containing antibiotics, Castaneda medium (for liquid clinical sample), serum agar, liver infusion serum agar, potato agar, serum dextrose agar, *Brucella* agar (albimi) are commonly used for isolation of *Brucella*. To prevent contamination, antibiotics like actidione (30mg/lit), bacitracin (7500U / lit), polymyxin B (1800U/lit) are added in the medium. *B. abortus* (biovars 1-4) needs 8-10% CO_2 for growth, while others like *B. abortus* (biovars 5, 6, 9), *B. abortus* cotton strain19 vaccine strain, *B. melitensis*, and *B. suis*, do not require CO_2. Optimum required pH is 6.6-7.4. The cultures are incubated at 37°C for 3 days to 3 weeks.

The colonies appear bluish under light. Smooth and rough types of colonies are found depending on the presence or absence of polysaccharide side chain of lipopolysaccharide (LPS). Initially the smooth colonies are small, round with entire margins, translucent, pale or honey coloured, and non-haemolytic which later become large and brown coloured (Figure 2). Rough colonies are large, flat, pale yellow with a granular appearance. *B. ovis* and *B. canis* produce rough colonies.

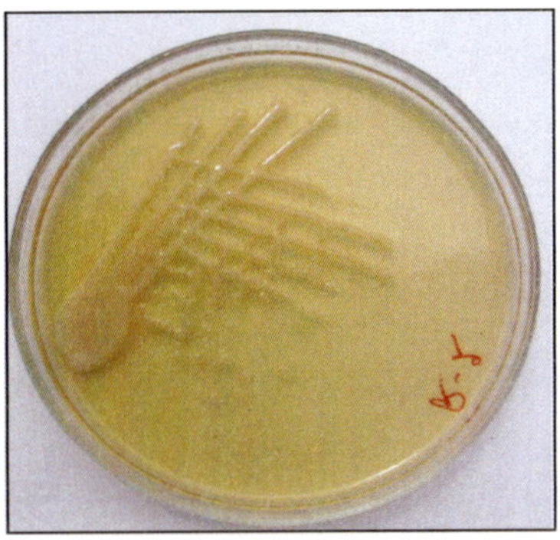

Fig. 2. Colonies of *Brucella abortus* in *Brucella* agar after 5 days incubation (*Courtesy*: S. Ghodasara, B.B. Bhanderi and Ashish Roy, Department of Veterinary Microbiology, College of Veterinary Science and Animal Husbandry, Anand Agricultural University, Anand, Gujrat)

Biochemical characteristics

Brucella produces following biochemical reactions

Biochemical test	Expected result
Catalase	(+ve) [except *B. ovis, B. neotomae*]
Oxidase	(+ve) [except *B. ovis, B. neotomae*]
Indole	(-ve)
Methyl red	(-ve)
Voges- Proskauer	(-ve)
H_2S production	(+ve) for *B. abortus, B. suis* (-ve) for *B. melitensis, B. ovis*
Nitrate reduction	(+ve)[except *B. ovis*]
Carbohydrate fermentation	
Arabinose	(+ve)
Galactose	(+ve)
Ribose	(+ve)

Antigenic characteristics

Lipopolysaccharide (LPS) is the major immunodominant antigen of *Brucella* (smooth strains). The cross-reactivity of *Brucella* with other bacteria like *Yersinia, Vibrio cholerae, Salmonella, E. coli* and *Pseudomonas* is due to structural similarity in the O-polysaccharide region of LPS. The O-polysaccharide (OPS) can be subdivided into two types i.e. A and M. These two types are present in different proportion in different species of *Brucella*. For example, in *B. abortus,* A: M is 20:1, in *B. melitensis* A: M is 1:20 and in *B. suis* A: M is 11:9.

Major outer membrane proteins (OMPs) of *Brucella* are detected as potential immunogenic and protective antigens. The proteins are classified according to their apparent molecular mass as group 2 porin proteins (36-38 kDa) and group 3 proteins (25-27 and 1-34 kDa OMPs). Group 2 porin proteins are encoded by *omp2a* and *omp2b* genes; whereas, the group 3 proteins are encoded by *omp25* and *omp31*genes. Among them, the *omp25* has been shown to be involved in virulence of *B. melitensis, B. abortus* and *B. ovis*. The omp31 is considered as major immunodominant antigen of rough strains (*B. ovis*). Other antigens like L7/L12 ribosomal protein, Cu/Zn superoxide dismutase, P39 (periplasmic protein) are observed to induce T cell proliferation and partial protection against *Brucella* in the experimental mice model.

Toxins and virulence factors produced

Toxins

No true exotoxin is produced by *Brucella*.

Endotoxin (Lipopolysaccharide, LPS): *Brucella* with smooth type of colony is more virulent than rough colony producers (*B. ovis, B. canis*). LPS is present in outer membrane of smooth type only and considered as major toxic factor. It is a non-classical LPS as compared to the classical LPS of *Enterobacteriaceae*. The LPS helps in intracellular survival of the bacteria in the following way.

i) Lipid A portion contains more numbers of fatty acids (C_{28}) in comparison to enterobacterial lipid A ($C_{12\text{-}16}$). Host immune system recognizes pathogen through different pattern recognition receptors (PRR) including toll like receptor (TLR). The TLRs can recognize pathogens by their cellular components like LPS, flagella etc. and activate the system for its lysis. In case of *Brucella*, due to altered lipid-A structure of LPS, the TLR poorly recognizes it. As well as *B. abortus* Btp1 protein (and its *B. melitensis* homologue, designated as TcpB) can also inhibit TLR signaling pathway. The TLR-inhibitory activity reduces both maturation of dendritic cells and their ability to produce pro-inflammatory cytokines such as TNF-α and IL-12. Thus *Brucella* conceals its presence from the host immune system that helps in intracellular survival.

ii) *Brucella* O-polysaccharide chain consists of a linear homopolymer of 1, 2-linked 4,6-dideoxy-4-formamido-alpha-D-mannopyranosyl residues. It provides very less numbers of the free hydroxyl groups in comparison to enterobacterial LPS for binding with C3 complement component. Thus by preventing C3 binding to its O-antigen, *Brucella* also prevents generation of pro-inflammatory complement products (C3a and C5a) which helps in immune evasion and intracellular survival.

Virulence factors

Virulence factors	Function
Type IV secretion system (Vir B)	VirB T4SS apparatus is encoded by the *virB1–virB12* genes on chromosome II of *Brucella*. It helps in adherence of the bacterium to the host cell and cell entry. Once the bacteria bind to the macrophages the vesicles (*Brucella* containing vacuole) engulf it. The acidification of the vesicle is thought to induce Vir B expression. The acidified vacuole acquires the markers of endoplasmic reticulum (calreticulin) with the help of Vir B T4SS. The strategy may activate enzymes helping in accumulation of nutrients required for the bacterial growth. These secreation systems are also involved in a variety of processes ranging from the delivery of virulence factors into the host cells, transfer of genetic material and uptake or release of DNA
Heat shock protein 60 (Hsp60)	It is a member of the GroEl family of chaperonins. It is expressed on the cell surface of *Brucella*, correlated with VirB expression. Hsp60 helps in bacterial adherence by binding to a host cellular prion molecule (PrPr).

Pathogenesis

Transmission

Brucella is transmitted by ingestion, inhalation, and coitus. The transmission can also take place through conjunctiva and skin. Aborted foetus, placenta, genital discharges from infected cows are the major source of infection in the environment. Infected milk or colostrums also helps in transmission of the infection.

Pathogenesis

Pathogenesis of *Brucella* has three sequences a) adherence b) invasion and c) establishment and dissemination within the host. LPS is the most relevant toxic factor during the infection and vaccination.

a) Adherence: Adherence to the oral mucosa is the first step of pathogenesis. Oral mucosa covering the peyer's patches is the preferred site of entry. Smooth colony forming *Brucella* are more efficient in adherence than rough strains. Specific cellular receptors for *Brucella* help in adherence. *Brucella* toxins / virulence factors like O-polysaccharide side chain of LPS, type IV secretion system (Vir B), BvrR / BvrS gene sensing system play role in adhesion.

b) Invasion: After adherence, the bacteria enter into the regional lymph nodes either in cell-free state or carried by the phagocytes. Opsonized *Brucella* is ingested via complement and Fc receptors in macrophages and monocytes, whereas non-opsonized *Brucella* remains cell-free and penetrates via lectin or fibronectin receptors. Professional phagocytes kill the majority of the bacteria through formation of phagolysosomes. Only a few numbers of bacteria can bypass the phagolysosome or other killing mechanisms and reach the replication site. Intracellular survival of the bacteria depends on adenine 5' guanosine monophosphate production that can inhibit the phagolysosome formation. Other factors like catalase, superoxide dismutase can prevent oxidative killing; stress proteins of the bacteria protect it from hydrolytic enzymes, oxygen radicals etc. LPS also helps in intracellular survival.

c) Establishment and dissemination: *Brucella* (survived from phagolysosome) enters the blood stream from regional lymph node causing bacteremia which is followed by localization into the cells of reticulo-endothelial systems in spleen, liver, supramammary lymph nodes, bone marrow, mammary glands and reproductive organs. The gravid uterus (specially placenta) and testis of cattle, sheep, goat, pig contains unidentified stimulants for *Brucella*, known as 'allantoic fluid factors'. Erythritol is one of the important elements of the fluid factors. Erythritol stimulates the growth of majority of *Brucella* (except *B. ovis*) but can inhibit *B. abortus* cotton strain 19 (vaccine strain).

In pregnant animals, *Brucella* prefers to multiply in the cisternae of the endoplasmic reticulum of the placental trophoblasts during the middle and late stage of gestation causing placentitis. The infection is transmitted into the foetus and the abortion occurs. The probable causes of abortion are described below.

a) Placentitis may interfere with the blood circulation of foetus and abortion takes place

b) Endotoxin mediated foetal stress

c) Infected trophoblasts produce cortisol, a steroidal hormone not normally generated by the placenta, which can also produce foetal stress. *Brucella* induces the synthesis of steroids and modifies the metabolism of prostaglandin precursors, such as arachidonic acid, because the hormones are used as growth factors by the bacteria.

Disease produced

Bacteria	Host	Disease produced
Brucella abortus	Cattle (biovar 1-6, 9), sheep, goat, pig	Abortion (late pregnancy period / 5 months onwards) and orchitis
	Horse	Poll evil, fistulous withers (bursitis)
	Human	Undulant fever
Brucella melitensis	Goat, sheep (major host, biovar 1-3); Camel, alpaca, llama	Abortion
	Human	Malta fever
Brucella suis	Pig (biovar 1,3) Wild boar (biovar 2) Reindeer (biovar 4) Rodent (biovar 5)	Abortion, orchitis
	Human (all biovars except biovar 5)	Undulant fever
Brucella ovis	Sheep	Contagious epididymitis in ram; sporadic abortion
	Human	Non-pathogenic
Brucella canis	dog	Abortion
	Human	Undulant fever (moderate pathogenic)
Brucella neotomae	Desert wood rat (salt lake desert at Utah)	Non-pathogenic
	Human	Moderate pathogenic

Immunity

Immunity against *Brucella* involves antigen-specific T-cell activation and humoral responses. The protection is primarily due to cell mediated immunity (Th1 mediated).*Brucella* stimulates host antigen-presenting cells to release interleukin 12 (IL12) that causes Th0 cells to differentiate into Th1 cells. The Th1 cells can secreate gamma interferon (IFN-γ) that activates macrophages to kill the intracellular bacteria. Cytotoxic T cells (CD8+) secreting IFN-γ are also able to kill *Brucella* infected macrophages and this T-cell subpopulation level is critical for protection against *Brucella.*

Diagnosis

Clinical specimens: Aborted foetus (stomach contents, spleen and lung), foetal membrane, vaginal secreations (swabs), milk, semen, and synovial fluids can be collected as clinical specimens. PM samples include the tissues of the reticulo-endothelial system (mammary and genital lymph nodes and spleen), late pregnant or early post-parturient uterus and udder. The vaginal swab taken after abortion or parturition is one of the best clinical samples for *Brucella* isolation. It avoids risk to handlers also. All the samples should be sent to the laboratory maintaining cold chain.

As *Brucella* is OIE risk group 3 organisms (organisms that can cause severe human or animal disease and may spread in the community and/or animal population but for which there is usually effective prophylaxis and treatment is available), the laboratory should have suitable facilities to handle such containment group 3 organisms.

Laboratory examination

Direct examination: A smear can be prepared from collected samples and stained by modified ZN method (Stamp method). *Brucella* appears as red bacteria against blue background. Confusion may arise with other abortion causing bacteria like *Coxiella burnetii*, *Chlamydophila abortus*, which can also be stained by modified ZN method. Milk or dairy products containing few numbers of bacteria may give false negative result in direct examination method.

Isolation of bacteria from clinical samples: Media and incubation conditions are described earlier. This is considered as gold standard method for detection of *Brucella*.

Dye-inhibition test: Albimi or trypticase soya agar is used to which at least three concentrations of basic fuchsin, thionin and safranin dyes are added (1: 50000, 1:100000 and 1: 200000).The calculated amounts of dyes are added into the melted medium from stock solutions (1% or 0.1% solution). The test bacteria and the controls are inoculated on each plate and the growth or inhibition of growth in presence of dye is observed after incubation (Figure 3, 4).

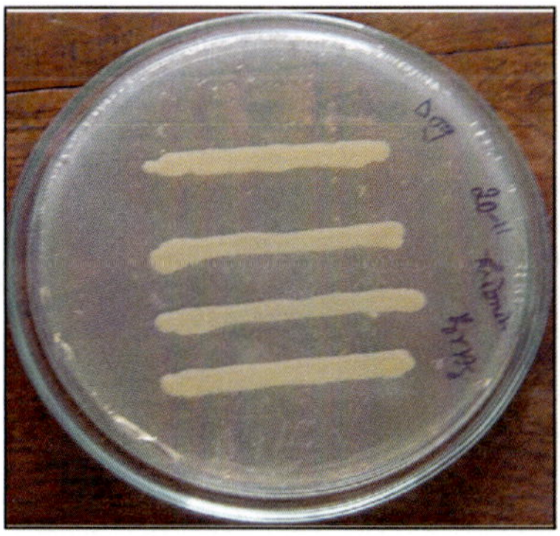

Fig. 3: Growth of *Brucella melitensis* in presence of thionin (1:50,000) (*Courtesy*: S. Ghodasara, B.B. Bhanderi and Ashish Roy, Department of Veterinary Microbiology, College of Veterinary Science and Animal Husbandry, Anand Agricultural University, Anand, Gujrat)

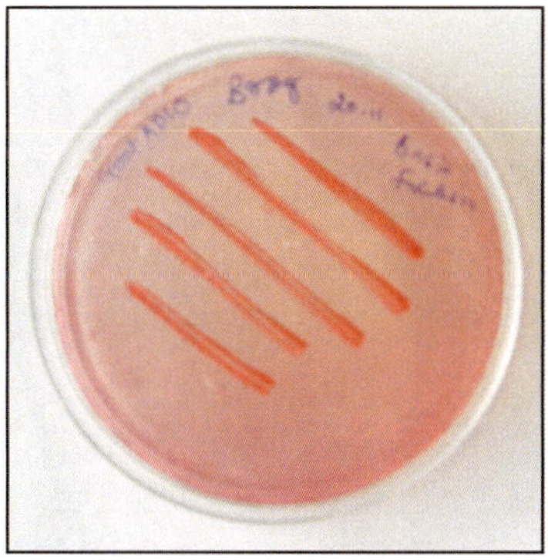

Fig. 4: Growth of *Brucella abortus* in presence of basic fuchsin (1:50,000) (*Courtesy*: S. Ghodasara, B.B. Bhanderi and Ashish Roy, Department of Veterinary Microbiology, College of Veterinary Science and Animal Husbandry, Anand Agricultural University, Anand, Gujrat)

Serological tests

Serum/ blood based tests

a) *Rose Bengal test*: It is a simple agglutination test for detection of *Brucella* immunoglobulin in serum using killed *Brucella* antigen mixed with Rose Bengal dye. The buffer of the antigen has low pH (3.65 ± 0.05) to avoid non specific agglutination. Antigen is prepared from *B. abortus* S99 or S1119-3 strain, killed with 0.5% phenol saline. Antigen should be calibrated against OIE international standard serum. In a white tile or clean plastic plate 20-30 μl test serum and equal amount of antigen is mixed with a clean glass rod. Result is read after 4 minutes. Any visible clumping is considered as positive. The test is commonly used for screening of *Brucella* infected animals in a herd. Positive result should be confirmed by other tests. Sometimes it may produce false-negative result due to prozone phenomenon, early phase of the infection and immediately after abortion.

b) *Complement fixation test (CFT)*: It is confirmatory and OIE prescribed test for *Brucella* detection. Antigen is prepared from *B. abortus* S99 or S1119-3 and should be calibrated against OIE International standard serum. Sera giving a titer equivalent to 20 international complement fixation test unit (ICFTU)/ml or more are considered to be positive.

c) *Enzyme linked immunossorbant assay (ELISA)*: Both indirect and competitive-ELISA are used for diagnosis of *Brucella*. It is another OIE prescribed test. LPS or O-polysaccharide (OPS) prepared from smooth strains are used as antigen.

d) *Fluorescence polarization assay (FPA):* The small fragment of OPS of *B. abortus* strain 1119-3s LPS is labeled with fluorescein isothiocyanate (FITC) and used as the antigen. The antigen is added to diluted test serum or whole blood and a measure of the antibody content is obtained in about 2 minutes (for serum) or 15 seconds (for blood) using a fluorescence polarization analyzer.

e) *Serum agglutination test (SAT):* Previously it was widely used for screening and control of *Brucella*. It can be done in plate or tube. Antigen contains a bacterial suspension in phenol saline. A serum containing 30 or more IU per ml is considered to be positive. SAT can detect total antibody produced against *Brucella* (IgG and IgM). Specifically IgG can be detected by the addition of 2, mercaptoethanol as IgG is better indicator of active infection. Mercaptoethanol can specifically lyse Ig-M. So use of mercaptoethanol can differentiate vaccinated and infected animals also.

Coombs developed an antiglobulin test to detect anti *Brucella*-IgG only, that helps in identification of chronic infection when anti *Brucella* IgM disappears from the circulation.

f) *Interferon gamma (IFNγ) test*: The lymphocytes are stimulated by suitable antigen of *Brucella* to secreate interferon gamma which is detected by capture-ELISA. The test can overcome the limitations of other serological tests.

g) *Brucellin intradermal test:* It is a tuberculin like skin test commonly used in unvaccinated animals. Specificity is high, but positive result should be supported by other tests. 'Brucellin' is a bacterial extract that should not contain smooth LPS to avoid non-specific inflammation. 0.1 ml brucellin is injected intradermally at the side of the neck or skin of the flank region of the suspected animal. In positive case swelling of the injection site (1.5-2 mm increased thickness) in 48-72 hours is detected.

Serological tests have following limitations

a) Vaccination against *Brucella* is practiced with smooth strain (*B. abortus* cotton strain 19). It will produce false positive reaction in serological tests as it is difficult to differentiate the test result between the infection and vaccination.

b) Due to the similarity of the O-antigenic side chain of LPS of *Brucella* and other bacteria such as *Yersinia enterocolitica* O: 9, *Vibrio cholerae, Esherichia coli* O157 and *Francisella tularensis* the serological cross reaction is produced.

Milk based tests

Screening of herd for *Brucella* can be performed easily by testing the milk from bulk tank in a dairy. In positive cases the cattle are re-tested with the blood samples.

Milk ring test (MRT): MRT is performed with bulk milk sample freshly collected from suspected lactating cows. The amount of the test sample depends on the herd size. For less than 150 cows 1 ml milk sample, 150-450 cows 2 ml milk sample, 451-700 cows 3 ml milk samples are collected. The milk samples are not frozen, heated, violently shaken and stored for more than 72 hours before the test. False positive reaction may occur in vaccinated cows, with colostrums containing milk samples and during mastitic condition. MRT antigen contains killed *B. abortus* S99 or S1119-3 cell suspension in haematoxylin stain. The test procedure includes addition of 30-50 μl of MRT antigen into the collected milk sample. The height of the milk column in the tube must be at least 25 mm. The mixture is incubated at 4°C overnight. Positive reaction is indicated by the formation of blue ring above the white milk column. In positive cases, anti-*Brucella* antibody in milk can agglutinate the antigen. The agglutinated mass comes near the surface layer along with the fat globules of the milk and makes the top layer bluish (color of the haematoxylin stain).

Milk Indirect-ELISA is a sensitive and specific test followed by milk ring test. The *competitive ELISA* should be used with whey samples only.

Animal inoculation test (Strauss reaction): Guinea pig is highly susceptible to *Brucella*. In male guinea pigs, culture is inoculated intraperitoneally. In positive cases, orchitis and peritonitis is developed. 'Strauss reaction' is not specific for *Brucella*. It should be followed by isolation and identification of the bacteria.

Molecular biology: Polymerase chain reaction (PCR) and different molecular typing methods such as PCR-restriction fragment length polymorphism (PCR-RFLP), pulsed field gel electrophoresis (PFGE) are developed to detect *Brucella* species and the serovars. First genus specific PCR was developed targeting 16S-23S genes. The first species-specific multiplex PCR assay for the differentiation of *Brucella* was based on the species-specific localization of the insertion sequence IS711 in the chromosome. It is known as AMOS-PCR or 'abortus, melitensis, ovis, suis'-PCR. The modified technique like 'Bruce ladder PCR' is developed targeting genes for glycosyltransferase (*wboA*),outer membrane protein (*omp31*),erythritol catabolism (*eryC),*ribosomal protein S12 (*rpsL)* etc. 'Bruce ladder PCR' can detect all species and vaccine strain in a single test.

Prevention and control

Following control and prevention measures are followed in different countries to control animal brucellosis

a) Detection of *Brucella* in breeding animals and removal of positive reactors from the herd before parturition (test and slaughter policy is followed in few countries)

b) The negative reactors of the same herd should be quarantined for 120 days-1 year or until completion of one gestation period. The animals should be checked for brucellosis periodically and the positive reactors should be removed.

c) Mass awareness campaign about the risk of animal brucellosis causing economic losses and public health hazard should be carried out periodically among the farmers and animal handlers by the local veterinarians or livestock regulatory authority

d) Vaccination of cattle can be done with live vaccine (*B. abortus* cotton strain 19) which reduces the rate of abortion effectively for next 5-6 lactations. The cotton strain 19 has low virulence and cannot cause abortion in cattle except in the advanced stage of pregnancy. The vaccine can cause undulant fever in human if inoculated accidentally. The optimum vaccination age is 4-8 months ('calfhood vaccination'). The calves may develop synovitis and lameness after vaccination. Vaccination at below 75 days of age in calves is not fruitful due to immature immune system. The upper age limit for vaccination is permitted up to 12 months of age. The antibody generated with cotton strain vaccination can hinder the serological differentiation of vaccinated and infected animals as the antibodies are persistent in nature. The persistence of these antibodies depends on age, dose, and route of vaccination. The persistence of antibodies increases if the calves are vaccinated at more than 12 months of age. The bulls are discouraged for strain 19 vaccination because it may develop orchitis and presence of *B. abortus* (strain 19) in the semen. The pregnant cattle are also not preferred for vaccination due to possibility of abortion. In non-pregnant but sexually matured heifers having the probability of exposure, the 'adulthood vaccination' may be done with 1/400 of the standard calf dose of the vaccine. The adultohood vaccination reduces the rate of active infection but it generates persistent carriers. It should not be done in pregnant animals and in unexposed animals present in non-endemic zone with minimal possibility of exposure. In adult cattle after vaccination the reactions like development of local swelling, high fever for 2-3 days, anorexia, listlessness and temporary drop in milk production are observed.

B. abortus RB51 is a rough strain which lacks O-side chain of LPS. It is preferred for preparation of live vaccine used in heifer calves at 3, 5 and 7 months of age. Due to lack of O-side chain the antibodies produced by the vaccine does not interfere the diagnostic serological tests. Even application of RB51 vaccine in strain 19 vaccinated cattle does not hamper sero-surveillance. The vaccine does not generate any local or systematic adverse reactions. The smooth variant of the vaccine (SRB51) with standard dose is found safe in pregnant cows and matured bulls. The bacterial strain (SRB51) does not cause abortion or persistence.

B. abortus strain 45/20 is used to produce killed vaccine. It is also a rough strain and lacks the O-side chain in the LPS structure. So, vaccination with 45/20 strain does not interfere the diagnostic serological tests. It is used in adult cattle also. Boostering is required to generate optimum antibody titer.

The live *Brucella melitensis* Rev 1 strain is used to produce the vaccine against brucellosis in small ruminants.

Government of India has launched 'National animal disease control programme for foot and mouth disease (FMD) and brucellosis' for five years (2019-20 to 2023-24) by vaccinating cattle, buffalo, sheep, goat and pig for FMD and bovine female calves of 4-8 months of age for brucellosis. It is one of the largest animal disease control program in the world and it aims to control FMD and brucellosis with vaccination.

23

Vibrio and *Campylobacter*

Since the periods of Hippocrates and Lord Buddha cholera like symptoms was described in human. The first outbreak of cholera was described in India in 1817. Filippo Pacini (1854), an Italian anatomist, observed a gram-negative bacterium associated with human cholera. Robert Koch (1884) first isolated and confirmed the association of 'comma-shaped bacteria', later designated as *Vibrio cholerae* with the disease in Calcutta (India). In 1959, Sambhu Nath De, Professor of Pathology at Nilratan Sircar Medical College in Calcutta discovered the exotoxin produced by *V. cholerae* and a simple method (rabbit ligated ileal loop assay) to study the *in vitro* effect of exotoxins. The Ganges delta of India and Bangladesh is considered as the worst affected place with cholera although the infection is widespread throughout the world. The spread of cholera in different continents occurred through six 'waves' ('pandemics') since 1817. The current seventh pandemic (7P) was originated in Indonesia (Sulawesi) in 1961 and spread throughout Asia, Africa and Latin America. In 1963, the seventh pandemic reached South Asia and circulated for more than 50 years with intermittent transmission to other continents. The recent major 7th pandemic outbreak was detected in Haiti causing more than 9400 deaths in 2010 which was originated through patients from endemic countries.

In 1886, Escherich observed *Campylobacter* like organisms in stool samples of children with diarrhoea. In 1913, McFaydean and Stockman first confirmed the bacteria as *Campylobacter* in foetal tissues of aborted sheep. Confirmatory tests were also carried out by Smith in 1918 when similar bacteria were isolated from aborted bovine foetuses. The bacteria were then known as *Vibrio foetus*. In 1963, due to certain differentiating characteristics, the organisms were separated from *Vibrionaceae* family and the new genus *Campylobacter* (means 'curved rod') under *Campylobacteraceae* family was proposed.

Properties of genus

1. *Morphology: Vibrio cholerae* is a gram-negative, curved bacillus, measuring 2-3 μm by 0.5 μm with a single polar flagellum and it shows a typical darting motility under dark-field or phase contrast microscopy.

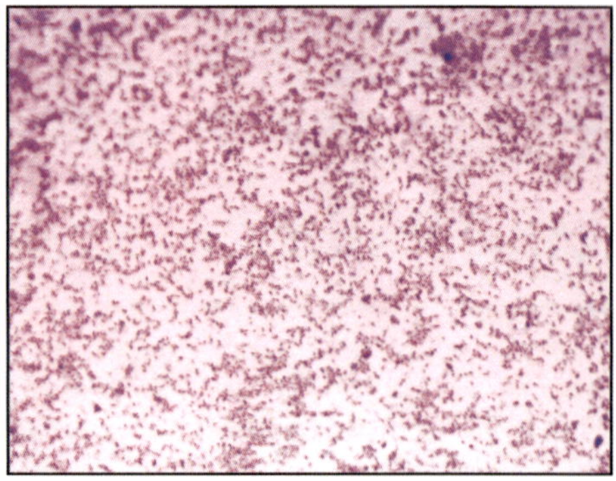

Fig. 1: Gram stained appearance of *Campylobacter jejuni* (*Courtesy*: Suman Kumar, Division of Veterinary Public Health, ICAR-Indian Veterinary Research Institute, Bareilly, U.P., India)

Campylobacter is gram negative, comma shaped rod specially in infected tissues and young cultures (Figure 1). The size is 1.5-4 µm by 0.5 µm. When two bacterial cells are found together in a microscopic field, it looks like 'S' or 'wing of gull' ('flying seagull'). In older cultures, the chains of bacteria appear as long spirals. The bacteria are motile by single unipolar/ bipolar unsheathed flagella. Motility is darting or corkscrew type, best observed by dark field microscopy. The bacteria are non-sporing. Some species contains S-layer (surface layer), a paracrystalline protein structure composed of S-layer proteins (SLPs). It is external to the outer membrane. It helps in immune evasion of the bacteria.

2. *Vibrio cholerae* is aerobic or facultative anaerobic. *Campylobacter* is microaerophilic in nature and it requires 3-5% CO_2 with 3-15% O_2 for growth.

3. *Classification:* The genus *Vibrio* belongs to the order Vibrionales and family *Vibrionaceae*. There are more than 150 species under the genus *Vibrio* and *V. cholerae* is considered as a potent human pathogen.

Previously *Campylobacter* was included under the same family *Vibrionaceae*. Due to the following differentiating characteristics the bacteria are separated from *Vibrionaceae* family and included under *Campylobacteraceae* family.

i) *Campylobacter* has unsheathed flagella
ii) *Campylobacter* is microaerophilic in nature
iii) *Campylobacter* is unable to use sugars by oxidation or fermentation
iv) *Campylobacter* is indole (-ve)
v) *Campylobacter* (29-38 mol %) has lower (G+C) value than *Vibrio* (38-51 mol %)

Currently *Campylobacteraceae* family consists of single genus namely *Campylobacter*. There are 47 species and 16 sub-species under the genus *Campylobacter*.

Important species and sub species of *Campylobacter* are

i) *Campylobacter fetus* ssp. *venerealis*

ii) *Campylobacter fetus* ssp. *fetus*

iii) *Campylobacter jejuni* ssp. *jejuni*

iv) *Campylobacter jejuni* ssp. *doyeli*

v) *Campylobacter coli*

vi) *Campylobacter concisus*

vii) *Campylobacter hyointestinalis*

viii) *Campylobacter mucosalis*

ix) *Campylobacter lari*

x) *Campylobacter helveticus*

xi) *Campylobacter upsaliensis*

4. *Resistance: V. cholerae* is susceptible to common disinfectants such as 1% chlorine, 2% tincture of iodine and potassium aluminium sulphate.

60°C temperature for 5 minute and autoclaving (120°C for 15 minute) is lethal to *Campylobacter*. The bacteria are remarkably sensitive to environmental conditions, including dehydration, atmospheric oxygen, sunlight and elevated temperature. The bacteria are also susceptible to common disinfectants like phenol, cresol etc.

5. *Natural habitat: V. cholerae* is common in aquatic environment (estuaries and brackish waters) as either free-living cells or associated with plants, green algae, copepods (crustaceans) and chironomids (non-biting midges).The copepods (crustaceans) and chironomids are considered as natural reservoir of *V. cholerae* which are consumed by fishes and water birds present in the aquatic ecosystem. A strong association between chitinous surface (copepods) and *V. cholerae* is observed. The major pathogenicity island of *V. cholerae* (*Vibrio* pathogenicity island 1, VPI-1/TCP) and type VI secretion system (T6SS) are induced by chitin, required for establishment of bacterial colony on the chitinous surface. *V. cholerae* O1 are isolated from different fishes such as sardines (*Stolephorus* sp.), mullet (*Liza* sp.), zebra fish (*Danio rerio*) and *Tilapia* sp. Both healthy and diseased fishes were detected to possess *V. cholerae* in the intestines, gills, skin, kidney, liver and brain tissue. In aquatic environment, occasionally due to deprivation of nutrients *V. cholerae* is converted into 'quiescent' (dormant) cells which can revert back to the infectious form in favourable conditions. Most of the environmental strains of

V. cholerae are non-toxigenic which can acquire the toxin genes in human gut.

In the life cycle of *V. cholerae* both 'planktonic' and 'biofilm' forms are observed. Down-regulation of motility associated genes and induction of genes associated with biofilm formation can convert the planktonic cells into biofilm. The conversion is controlled by intracellular concentration of secondary messenger cyclic diguanylic acid. Moreover, termination of motility enhances the expression of toxin and virulence factors (ctxA, tcpA) of *V. cholerae* required for establishment of infection.

Campylobacter can be recovered from water, sewage, hay, manure and other environmental sources. Few strains specifically reside in the reservoir animals and birds. *C. fetus* is commonly found in genital and intestinal tract of domestic ruminants (cattle, sheep). Specifically, *C. fetus* ssp. *venerealis* resides in the prepuce of the bull and the vagina of the cow. In cows this carriage rate is generally reduced after two breeding seasons. Whereas, *C. fetus* ssp. *fetus* commonly inhabits intestinal tract of healthy small ruminants like sheep. Other campylobacters like *C. jejuni* and *C. coli* can colonize the intestinal mucosa of most warm-blooded animals including the food animals (cattle, Sheep) and companion animals (dog, cat). In commercial broiler chickens, the colonization is commensal. *C. jejuni* is found at highest levels in the mucosal crypts of the caeca and to a lesser extent in the small intestine. The prevalence in broiler poultry is age and season related. It is uncommon among less than 2-3 week old birds, probably due to the presence of maternal antibodies. The bacteria are considered as major source of poultry meat contamination and are responsible for 20-40% human infection due to consumption of the contaminated raw and undercooked meat or re-contaminated meat following cooking. During processing of the poultry carcasses, the prevalence of *Campylobacter* increases after defeathering and evisceration and the rate decreases after scalding, chilling. So, special care during defeathering and evisceration can check the *Campylobacter* contamination of poultry carcasses.

The Natural habitat of *C. upsaliensis* is intestinal tract of healthy puppies and kittens.

6. *Genome: V. cholerae* is studied as a model bacterium in the field of bacterial study with multiple chromosomes. The genome consists of two chromosomes designated as chromosome 1 (Chr1, 3Mb) and chromosome 2 (Chr2, 1Mb). Acquisition of a large plasmid during ancient times was the origin of the *V. cholerae* chromosome 2. The origin of replication present in Chr1 (*ori1*) acts like other bacterial chromosome. The *ori1* contains DnaA boxes and GATC sites which act as major replication initiator. Division of the genome into two replicons helps in faster replication of the bacteria. The Chr2 has more

plasticity and evolves faster than Chr1. The Chr1 possesses the genes for growth and viability, DNA replication and repair, transcription, translation, cell-wall biosynthesis and different metabolic pathways. The Chr2 harbours the genes encoding ribosomal proteins (L35, L20), initiation factor (IF3), D-serine dehydratase and threonyl-tRNA synthetase. Transfer of antibiotic resistance determinants in *V. cholerae* is assisted with mobile genetic elements. *V. cholerae* integrons can incorporate antibiotic resistance cassettes by site-specific recombination in a site proximal to the promoter which controls their expression. Class 1 and class 2 integrons associated with *Tn402* and *Tn21* transposons, respectively are detected in *V. cholerae*. Transfer of integrons is induced by exposure to antibiotics and related stress. One of the largest integron, known as 'superintegron' or '*Vibrio cholerae* repeats (VCR)' is observed in Chr2. It is 126 kbp in size, contains 179 cassettes and is considered as the most variable region of the genome. The integrating conjugative element (ICE) such as SXT (100 kb) is detected in *V. cholerae* which offers resistance against sulphamethoxazole-trimethoprim, streptomycin and chloramphenicol. The SXT was first detected in a *V. cholerae* O139 strain isolated from India and currently it is common in clinical and environmental isolates of *V. cholerae* in Asia and Africa. Other than integrons and ICEs, the plasmids belonged to incompatibility groups IncC and IncJ are also detected in *V. cholerae*. Besides mobile genetic elements, the transformation acts as major way of gene transfer in *V. cholerae*. The transformation not only causes horizontal gene transfer but also repair of DNA and use of DNA as food or building blocks of bacteria. Competence for DNA uptake in *V. cholerae* depends on presence of the polymer chitin. The biotic surface rich in chitin such as exoskeleton of copepods thus acts as a preferred bacterial niche for genetic exchange.

The (G+C) content of the chromosome of *C. jejuni* is 30-33 mol%. The size of the chromosome is 3.6 Mbp. *Campylobacter* enterotoxin is encoded by the chromosome. The genome of *C. jejuni* contains several hyper-variable regions containing genes for expression of flagella and capsule. The hyper-variable sequences are homopolymeric (composed of short runs of the same nucleotides). It serves as a molecular switch to 'on' or 'off' a gene expression. The region can activate a previously suppressed gene with addition or loss of single nucleotide or stop expression of a gene. It is heritable in nature. With the help of the hyper-variable region *Campylobacter* causes 'phase variation'. The phase variation helps in rapid change of gene expression of the bacteria (antigenic drift) during its colonization into the host. So, same individual animal or the herd may show the presence of multiple serotypes of the bacteria at a time.

Isolation, growth and colony characteristics

Vibrio cholerae can be isolated in special media such as thiosulfate citrate bile-salts sucrose (TCBS) or taurocholate-tellurite-gelatin agar (TTGA) agar. Characteristic yellow and shiny colonies, 2-4 mm in diameter, sometimes with an elevated centre appear after 18 to 24 hours incubation at 35°-37°C. The suspected *V. cholerae* colonies are sub-cultured into heart infusion agar (HIA) or tryptone soy agar (TSA) at 35°-37°C for up to 24 hours. Gram staining and biochemical tests conducted on sub-cultured colonies such as oxidase test, string test, growth in triple sugar iron agar, Kligler iron agar, lysine iron agar can confirm the isolates. The string test can differentiate *V. cholerae* (strongly positive) from other *Vibrio* sp. (weakly positive).

Campylobacter can be isolated from clinical samples without any enrichment. The selective or non-selective media can be used for isolation. Sometimes the samples are filtered through 0.65 or 0.45µm filters before inoculation into the media (passive filtration method). However both the media should contain nutritional supplements including whole and lysed animal blood along with ferrous sulphate, sodium metabisulphite and sodium pyruvate (FBP) supplement. The selective media for *Campylobacter* isolation is broadly categorized into two types: charcoal based and blood based. Charcoal and blood components remove toxic derivatives of oxygen from the media. Examples of charcoal based selective media are Modified charcoal, cefoperazone, deoxycholate agar (mCCDA), Karmali agar or CSM (charcoal-selective medium) etc. Whereas blood based media are Preston agar, Skirrow agar, Butzler agar and Campy-cefex agar.

Commonly used non-selective media for *Campylobacter* isolation are blood agar with or without 0.1% sodium thioglycolate (used to reduce oxygen tension of the media) and antibiotics; serum dextrose antibiotic broth. The antibiotics used in the media are cephalosporins, trimethoprim, bacitracin, actidione, amphotericin B etc. Actidione and amphotericin B are used to prevent the growth of yeasts and moulds. Thiol media is used for both isolation and maintenance of the culture. Chocolate agar is used for antigen production of *Campylobacter*. The bacteria are microaerophilic in nature and require 3-5% CO_2 with 3-15% O_2 for growth. Optimum growth requires incubation at 37°C (for *C. jejuni* and *C. coli* 42°C) temperature for 2-5 days (24-48 hours for *C. jejuni* and *C. coli*) and pH 6.8.

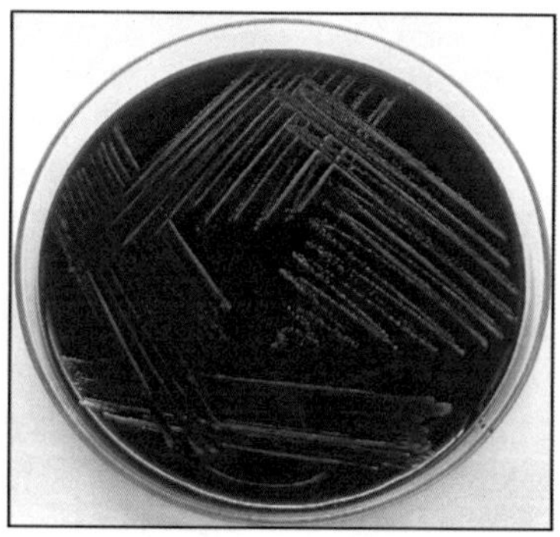

Fig. 2: Typical *Campylobacter jejuni* colonies in modified charcoal, cefoperazone, deoxycholate agar (mCCDA) (*Courtesy*: Rahul Yadav, HPVK, DI Lab, Mahendergarh, LUVAS-Hisar, Haryana, India)

C. fetus ssp. *fetus* produces non-haemolytic, smooth, 1 mm in diameter, colourless colonies (Figure 2). *C. fetus* ssp. *venerealis* produces non-haemolytic, rough, 1-2 mm in diameter, cream to tan coloured, irregular edged colonies. *C. jejuni* is also non-haemolytic and produces finely granular, irregular margin, flat, greyish colonies. On charcoal based media, the colonies may produce 'metallic sheen'.

Biochemical characteristics

Campylobacter fetus ssp. *venerealis* produces following biochemical reactions

Biochemical test	Expected result
Catalase	(+ve)
H_2S production	(-ve)
Nitrate reduction	(-ve)

Antigenic characteristics

More than 200 serovars is described in *V. cholerae* based on O-antigen. All the cholera pandemics occurred so far is attributed to O1 serogroup. It is further classified into three serotypes (Ogawa, Inaba, and Hikojima) based on O-antigen and two biotypes i.e. 'classical' and 'El Tor' based on phenotypical characteristics. The six cholera pandemics (1899-1923) occurred by classical strains and El Tor strain is associated with current seventh pandemic. The frequent switch between Ogawa and Inaba strains occurs.

Campylobacter is antigenically heterogeneous group of bacteria. *C. fetus* has three major groups of antigens i.e. S-layer protein antigen (SLPs), somatic (O) and flagellar (H) antigen. The bacteria have at least 50-heat stable serotypes based on somatic and more than 36 heat-labile serotypes based on flagellar antigens. It has antigenic relationship with *Brucella abortus*. The *C. fetus* S-layer is composed of a regular monomolecular array of subunit S-layer proteins (SLPs) of various sizes, which are the immunodominant *C. fetus* antigens. S-layer may be hexagonal or tetragonal in appearance depending upon the presence of SLPs. S-layer is present as the outermost covering of the cell; either it binds directly to the cell membrane or to the protruding structures (like LPS). This LPS binding domain of SLP is present at the amino terminal of the protein. This layer is antiphagocytic and prevents the complement mediated lysis. It can also down regulate the production of pro-inflammatory cytokines to modulate the host immune response. These SLPs are encoded by *sapA* gene locus. Antigenic variation related to SLPs can take place due to genomic rearrangements within the *sapA* locus. Electrophoretic analysis of *Campylobacter* LPS has shown that in contrast to the smooth LPS of *Enterobacteriaceae* which contains O polysaccharides of heterogeneous chain length, the O polysaccharides of *Campylobacter* have quite homogeneous chain length. The *Campylobacter* LPS is low molecular weight, conferring large number of serotypes. This antigenic diversity results from difference in the small number of sugars found in the O- chain. The flagella of *C. jejuni* are unsheathed and composed of flagellin protein having molecular weight of 57,000-66,000 Dalton. This protein is another major surface antigen of *Campylobacter*. Its amino acid sequence variation is responsible for sero-diversity based on flagellar antigen (Lior serotyping system).

Toxins and virulence factors produced

Toxins

Cholera toxin: *V. cholerae* after colonization secrete cholera toxin, an AB_5 family ADP-ribosyl-transferase which causes profuse rice-watery diarrhoea in the patients. The genes *ctxA* and *ctxB* encode cholera toxin. The genes are carried by a filamentous phage (CTXF). After release the toxin binds to the intestinal enterocytes through the interaction of the pentameric B subunit of the toxin with the GM1 ganglioside receptor on the intestinal cell. The endocytosis of the toxin molecule occurs after binding. The AB_5 cholera toxin is cleaved and the enzymatically active 'A1'is generated. Within the enterocyte the enzymatic A1 activates the G protein through an ADP-ribosylation reaction. The G protein is locked in its GTP-bound form and it continuously stimulates adenylate cyclase to produce cAMP. The high cAMP levels activate the cystic fibrosis transmembrane conductance regulator (CFTR) causing an increased efflux of ions from the infected enterocytes into the intestinal lumen. The osmotic pressure of the lumen is increased which attracts more fluid from the enterocytes. It will lead to watery diarrhoea.

Enterotoxin: It is produced by *Campylobacter jejuni, C. coli* and *C. lari*. It has structural and functional relationship with *E. coli* heat labile enterotoxin (LT) and cholera toxin (CT). *Campylobacter* enterotoxin is also heat labile (inactivated at 56°C for 1 hour or at 96°C for 10 minutes), trypsin and pH sensitive (pH 2 or 8) and has a molecular weight of 60-70 K Da. Like CT or LT, the toxin also attaches with ganglioside receptor of the host cell. It activates adenylate cyclase enzyme to increase the level of intracellular cAMP and disrupt the normal ion transport in the enterocytes, thus causing secreatory watery diarrhoea. Toxic activity of the crude toxin is progressively lost after storage for 1 month at 4°C or for 1 week at -20 or -70°C. The toxin can induce fluid accumulation in rabbit or rat ligated ileal loop assay.

Cytotoxin: It is also produced by *C. jejuni, C. coli* and *C. lari*. It is trypsin sensitive and toxic for HeLa and vero cells *in vitro*. The toxin is destroyed at 70°C temperature for 30 minutes exposure. No correlation has been observed between cytotoxin production and serotype of the bacteria.

Cytolethal distending toxin: It is heat labile, trypsin sensitive, non-dialyzable cytotoxin with a molecular weight of 30 K Da and is produced by *C. jejuni*, *C. coli* and *C. lari*. It is cytolethal to Chinese hamster ovary (CHO), vero, HeLa, human epithelial carcinoma (Hep2) cell lines. The toxin cannot induce fluid accumulation in rabbit ligated ileal loop assay. The iron is required for expression of the toxin.

Virulence factors

Major virulence factor of *V. cholerae* is toxin-coregulated pilus (TCP), a type IV pilus required for adherence and intestinal colonization (proximal part of small intestine) in mice and humans. The gene encoding TCP is located within *V. cholerae* pathogenicity island (VPI) or TCP island. RND efflux system of *V. cholerae* helps in expression of both cholera toxin and toxin-coregulated pilus.

The sheathed polar flagellum driven by sodium motive force and alternative RNA polymerase subunits (σ54, σ28 and σ54-dependent transcriptional activators FlrA and FlrC) is another virulence factor. Clockwise motility of *V. cholerae* depends on both the appendages.

Other important virulence factors produced by *V. cholerae* and *Campylobacter* are described below.

Virulence factors	Function
V. cholerae biofilm-matrix cluster (VcBMC) which comprises *Vibrio* polysaccharide (encoded by *vps-1* and *vps-2* gene clusters) and rugosity and biofilm structure modulator A (*rbm*) cluster (*RbmA, Bap1, RbmC*)	Development of biofilm structure in *V. cholerae*
galU and *gale*	UDP-glucose and UDP-galactose synthesis required for biofilm formation in *V. cholerae*
ToxR-regulated porin (OmpU), transcriptional regulators (CadC, HepA), gluthatione synthetase (GshB), DNA repair and recombination enzyme (RecO)	Development of acid tolerance in *V. cholerae* in intestinal tract
ToxR-regulated porin (OmpU)	Tolerance in *V. cholerae* to bile acids and antimicrobial peptides
Nacetyl-L-cysteine, soluble mucinase (haemagglutinin/protease , Hap)	Mucolytic agent secreted by *V. cholerae* to penetrate mucin rich barrier to colonize intestinal epithelium
TagA	A metalloprotease secreated by *V. cholerae* which specifically modify mucin glycoproteins attached to the host cell surface. It helps in colonization during the later stages of movement through the intestinal mucosa

Virulence factors	Function
Neuraminidase (NanH)	It is an extracellular enzyme in *V. cholerae* that cleaves two sialic acid groups from the GM1 ganglioside, present on the surface of epithelial cells and thus it unmasks the receptors for cholera toxin
Chitinase	Required to utilize chitin by *V. cholerae*
Surface layer (S-layer) [*Campylobacter fetus*, *C. rectus*]	a) This layer is antiphagocytic and prevents the complement mediated lysis. It can also down regulate the production of pro-inflammatory cytokines to modulate the host immune response. S-layer allows *C. fetus* to disseminate through the bloodstream b) S layer is composed of proteins known as S-layer protein (SLP), encoded by *sapA* gene. Genetic rearrangements of this locus cause expression of various SLPs resulting continuous antigenic variation of the bacteria. Consequently, the bacteria is able to avoid or delay a potentially clearing antibody response
Lipopolysaccharide (LPS)	a) It is responsible for allergic response associated with *Campylobacter* mediated abortions. b) The LPS contains N-acetylneuraminic acid (NeuAc), responsible for serum resistance. 'NeuAc' is rarely found in prokaryotes although common in eukaryotic glycolipids.
Spiral shape and presence of flagella	Shape and motility mediate colonization into the mucus filled crypts of the caeca (*C. jejuni*) and penetration of this viscous matrix.
Campylobacter Adhesins: i) CadF (*Campylobacter adh*esion to *f*ibronectin [Fn])	It helps in binding of bacteria with fibronectin protein, found in extracellular matrix or regions of cell to cell contact. So it helps in bacterial adhesion with host tissues
ii) Periplasmic/membrane-associated protein (PEB1, PEB3)	Putative adhesin of *C. jejuni*
iii) CapA (*Campylobacter a*dhesion *p*rotein *A*)	Acts as adhesin
iv) JlpA (*j*ejuni *l*ipo*p*rotein *A*)	It helps in adherence of bacteria with human epithelial cells (Hep2).
v) Cj1279c and Cj1349c protein	They act as Fibronectin and fibrinogen-binding protein
Major outer membrane protein (MOMP); encoded by *porA* gene	MOMP is known to allow passage of hydrophilic molecules across the outer membrane and provides structural stability to the outer membrane. It also helps in bacterial adhesion with host tissues.

Pathogenesis

Transmission

V. cholerae

Ingestion of contaminated water or food is the major way of *V. cholerae* transmission in human. Consumption of raw/salted/smoked or undercooked fishes such as Hilsa (*Hilsa ilisa*), whitebait was found to be associated with cholera outbreaks. High bacterial concentration (10^8 cfu) is required for initiation of infection in the small intestine as *V. cholerae* are sensitive to acidic pH. In children, aged and the persons using antacids for prolonged period, low concentration (10^4 cfu) of *V. cholerae* can produce the infection. Person to person spread is limited due to requirement of high infective dose to produce the disease. However, infected persons shed *V. cholerae* through the faeces which further contaminate aquatic environment. In the water bodies the bacteria can exist either in a planktonic state or by producing biofilm. During the persistence stage in the water bodies *V. cholerae* cells become coccoid in shape and metabolically inactive. The bacterial cells are activated and multiply when the bacteria receive signals from active bacterial cells present in the environment or host cells.

Campylobacter

C. fetus ssp. *venerealis* is transmitted to cows during coitus with infected bull or by artificial insemination with contaminated semen. Cow to cow transmission is rare. The bacteria survive in the cervix for the full gestation period and can infect the bulls during subsequent coitus. The bulls may also become asymptomatic carriers. The carrier stage depends on size and number of crypts present in the epithelium of penis, where the bacteria can persist.

C. fetus ssp. *fetus* is transmitted through ingestion of contaminated materials, drinking water etc.

C. jejuni is transmitted through faecal-oral route in poultry. After infection, caeca are the major site for bacterial multiplication followed by faecal shedding. Thus it contaminates the nearby premises. So, inadequate disinfection between chick placements and deficiency of biosecurity measures are the major risk factors. Other vectors such as litter beetles, house flies, wild birds and farm workers also help in transmission. Vertical route of transmission from breeder hen to chick is rare.

In human, major source of *Campylobacter* (*C. jejuni*) is contaminated poultry and its products. So eating undercooked poultry meat or its products and handling poultry is the major route of transmission. The poultry meat may contain high level of the bacteria at pre harvest level which is further contaminated during the time of slaughter and processing. Specially if the skin is not removed from the carcass, it contains a large population of the bacteria *in situ*. Other sources of *C. jejuni, C. coli* include undercooked contaminated pork (with intact skin), beef, mutton and raw milk. Transmission also occurs from pet animals to human, specially in children. However, person to person transmission is rare.

Pathogenesis

C. fetus ssp. *venerealis*

After introduction into the body the bacteria persist in the cervico-vaginal junction probably due to the increased blood supply during ovulatory phase of the estrus cycle. In this phase neutrophils are also abundant in the secreation, causing phagocytosis. The organisms that can escape the phagocytosis are able to multiply. *Campylobacter* S-layer and the 135 KDa proteins help in escaping phagocytosis. The protein (135 KDa) prevents binding of O-specific antibody. After multiplication, the bacteria enter the uterus during the luteal phase when the neutrophils appear less in numbers. The active invasion and multiplication in the uterus result endometritis and cessation of pregnancy. So the animal returns to estrus and this cycle continues until there is effective elimination of the bacteria by the host immune system or proper treatment. Abortions may also occur as an allergic response to *Campylobacter* endotoxin (LPS).

C. jejuni ssp. *jejuni*

The bacteria adhere with the intestinal mucosa and penetrate enterocytes. The adherence prevents the clearing mechanism of the intestine. Adherence is mediated by adhesin proteins like CadF, PEB 1, PEB 3, CapA, JlpA and LPS. Invasion occurs after adhesion with the enterocytes. It is mediated by endocytosis. Initially after invasion, the bacterial number is decreased followed by multiplication within 72 hours. The bacteria enter into the deeper tissues like parenchymal cells, granulocytes, mononuclear cells in the lamina propria and submucosa by transcytosis. Phagocytic cells appear in the lamina propria to engulf the bacteria. Severity and duration of infection depends on intracellular survival of the bacteria. Superoxide mutase and catalase produced by *C. jejuni* help in its intracellular survival within the phagocytes.

Disease produced

Bacteria	Host	Disease produced
Vibrio cholerae	Human	**Cholera:** Cholera is an acute diarrhoeal infection caused by ingestion of food or water contaminated with *Vibrio cholerae*. Cholera remains a global threat to public health and an indicator of insufficient social development. Cholera affects both children and adults and can kill within hours if untreated. Majority of infected people have mild or moderate symptoms, while a minority develop acute watery diarrhoea with severe dehydration. This can lead to death if left untreated
	Animals	Generally the animals do not develop cholera. However, cholera like outbreak was detected in dogs, cattle and bison due to exposure to high numbers of the bacteria
Campylobacter fetus ssp. *venerealis*	Cattle	**Venereal campylobacteriosis:** catarrhal vaginitis, abortion (5th or 6th month of gestation), endometritis, salpingitis, long estrus cycle (more than one month), infertility, early embryonic death
Campylobacter fetus ssp. *fetus*	Cattle	Sporadic abortion (second or third trimester of gestation)
	Sheep	Epizootic abortion (second or third trimester of gestation)
Campylobacter jejuni ssp. *jejuni*	Human	Fever, diarrhoea, abdominal cramp. **Guillain-Barré syndrome (GBS):** a demyelating disorder resulting in acute neuromuscular paralysis is serious sequelae of *Campylobacter* infection. **Reiter syndrome:** Another sequel of *Campylobacter* infection, characterized by arthropathy specially in knee joints. Both of these syndrome are auto-immune response, stimulated by the infection.
	Sheep, goat, dog	Sporadic abortion
	Cattle, pig, cat, dog	Enteritis and mastitis (cattle)
	Chicken	'Avian Vibrionic hepatitis' and enteritis
Campylobacter coli	Human, pig	enteritis
Campylobacter lari	Human	enteritis

Bacteria	Host	Disease produced
Campylobacter hyointestinalis and *Campylobacter mucosalis*	Pig	**Swine proliferative enteritis (SPE):** It is a disease complex in pigs characterized by intestinal adenomatosis, necrotic enteritis and ileitis. Thickening of the ileal wall is observed. Other organism like *Lawsonia intracellularis* may be involved.
Campylobacter upsaliensis	Human, dog	Diarrhoea

Immunity

In venereal campylobacteriosis of cattle, IgG and IgA are produced against the bacteria in the uterus and vagina, respectively. IgG is opsonising antibody and thus helps in phagocytosis. Ig-A fixes the bacteria in the cervicovaginal junction so that they cannot enter into the uterus. In carrier bulls, antibody production is low because the organisms persist at the surface of the penis that is less accessible to the host immune system. In sheep and goats, IgG and IgM are produced against *C. fetus* ssp. *venerealis* infection. The antibodies bind to the bacteria while it is in the bloodstream resulting in removal by liver and spleen. Bound antibody can also initiate complement mediated lysis of the bacteria. The sheep and goats become immune following abortion. *C. jejuni* can produce both local and systematic antibody response. IgA is the major antibody produced against flagellar antigens of *C. jejuni*.

Diagnosis

Clinical samples

V. cholerae: Fresh faeces or rectal swabs (2 swabs /patient) in transport medium are preferred clinical samples for detection of *V. cholerae*. The faecal samples should be collected within four days of onset and before beginning of antimicrobial therapy. Cary-Blair transport medium is commonly used due to high pH (8.4). Alkaline peptone water is an alternative transport medium if the culture is to be done within 6 hours. The buffered glycerol saline as transport medium is contraindicated for *V. cholerae*. Piece of sterile cotton or filter paper soaked with suspected stool sample can be collected in a sterile plastic bag (zipper) if transport medium is not available. The collected samples can be preserved at 4°C in refrigerator up to 48 hours. The samples are sent to the laboratory in insulated container or thermo flask with ice pack or dry ice.

C. fetus ssp. *venerealis*: Anestrus mucus of cows collected from a herd (10-20 animals), preputial washing of bull, foetal abomasal contents.

C. jejuni ssp. *jejuni*: The infected poultry birds shed large numbers of bacteria (>10^6 colony forming units /gm faeces). Clinical samples for isolation of *Campylobacter* are fresh faeces (without urine), caecal droppings or cloacal swabs and bile. Post mortem samples include caeca from poultry, intestinal content from cattle, sheep and pigs.

C. mucosalis and *C. hyointestinalis*: Mucosal scrapings from lesions, section of affected intestine for bacterial isolation, section of affected ileum and caecum in 10% formalin for histopathology. These campylobacters are cell associated, so faecal samples have no diagnostic value.

The samples after collection should be carried in a transport media (Cary-Blair, Stuart, Amies, alkaline peptone water) into the laboratory to prevent the drying and oxygen exposure. The samples should be protected from light, freezing (<0°C) and high temperature (>20°C).

Laboratory examinations

Direct examination: The collected faecal suspensions in normal saline can be microscopically examined for the presence of small, curved rods with 'darting motility' under phase contrast or dark field microscopy. In Gram-stained smear prepared from isolated bacterial colony, *V. cholerae* appears as Gram-negative, small and curved rods.

A smear can be prepared from clinical samples and stained by dilute carbol fuchsin (DCF) (stain is kept for 4 minutes over the smear). *Campylobacter* appears as pink coloured small curved rod arranged in a pair to produce characteristic 'S' or 'wing of gull' appearance. The bacteria can also be demonstrated by wet mounts of faeces by phase contrast or dark field microscopy. Darting motility of the corkscrew like organisms is suggestive for *Campylobacter*.

However, for demonstration of *C. mucosalis* and *C. hyointestinalis,* heat fixed smear is prepared from mucosal scrapping of lesions and stained with modified Ziehl-Neelsen (ZN) method. The organisms appear as pink coloured, curved, intracellular rods.

Isolation of bacteria from clinical samples: Media, incubation condition and colony characteristics are described earlier.

Serological tests

a) Slide agglutination test (SAT) with polyvalent O1 or O139 antiserum is available which can be conducted with fresh subculture (6 hours growth) of *V. cholerae* from a non-selective agar. The regional laboratories may send the cultures to national or international reference laboratory for confirmation of O1/ O139 serotype during outbreaks. The culture positive for SAT with polyvalent O1can be further typed with monovalent Ogawa and Inaba antiserum. If the culture shows positive reaction with both Ogawa and Inaba antisera it should be sent to reference laboratory for identification of Hikojima serotype.

b) Vaginal mucus agglutination test (VMAT): Antibodies against *C. fetus* ssp. *venerealis* can be detected in vaginal mucus 2-7 months post infection. It is a herd test used for 10-20 animals. Vaginal mucus is collected in a glass pipette and mixed with saline (1:4). This homogenised mixture is placed in a water bath (57°C) and equal amount of molten agar is added. This agar is allowed to set at room temperature. Now 0.5% phenol saline is added and the mixture is incubated at 37°C for 18 hours. It will help to extract the antibodies as clear supernatant fluid over the mixture. It is used to detect agglutinins present within it against the bacteria. The false negative reaction may occur if the mucus is collected during estrus.

c) Cervical mucus agglutination test

d) Serum agglutination test: it is not so reliable for detection of *Campylobacter* infection in cattle, sheep.

Antigen-capture-based tests: Enzyme immunoassays are commercially available for the detection of *Campylobacter* in human stool samples.

Molecular biology: Diagnostic PCR is developed for detection of *V. cholerae* DNA targeting the genes encoding cholera toxin (*ctx*), regulatory gene (*toxR*), and housekeeping genes such as *atpA*, *rpoB*, and *dnaJ*.

A *Campylobacter fetus* ssp. *venerealis*-specific 5' *Taq* nuclease PCR assay (TaqMan) is developed based on a subspecies-specific fragment of unknown identity. The assay specifically detects *C. fetus* ssp. *venerealis* strains with no detection of *C. fetus* ssp. *fetus* or other bovine venereal microflora. A multiplex PCR is also developed for detection of several *Campylobacter* species like *C. jejuni* (23S RNA gene); *C. coli*, *C. lari*, and *C. upsaliensis* (*glyA* gene); and *sapB2* gene from *C. fetus* ssp. *fetus*.

Prevention and control

Cholera

For prevention and control of cholera the strategy consists of surveillance, supply of clean drinking water, maintenance of sanitation and hygiene, social mobilisation, proper treatment, and use of oral cholera vaccine in endemic area. Providing clean water, proper sanitation and hygiene (WASH) in the countries can reduce the prevalence of cholera and other diarrhoeal diseases. The strategy (WASH) comes under the Sustainable Development Goals (SDG 6) of United Nations. The Sustainable Development Goals (SDGs / Global goals) were adopted by United Nations in 2015 as a universal call to end poverty, protect the planet and ensure that all the people in the planet enjoy peace and prosperity by 2030. Oral rehydration solution (ORS) is the choice of treatment for cholera infection. Antibiotics are contraindicated in cholera as it is not effective to reduce the infection but excessive use may promote antimicrobial resistance. Oral cholera vaccines are recommended during outbreak along with other strategies.

Campylobacteriosis

In meat processing plants proper washing, handling and freezing of carcasses can reduce bacterial contamination including *Campylobacter*. In hotel, restaurants and home meat should be handled properly and cooking at 80°C-100°C can kill *Campylobacter* contamination.

24

Bordetella and *Moraxella*

Guillame de Baillou (1673), a physician, described an outbreak of recurrent severe cough that could induce vomition and suffocation in human in Paris. The infection was described as 'Quintanætussis which was later confirmed as 'whooping cough'. The causative agent Bordetella pertussis was discovered by Jules Bordet and Octave Gengou in 1906 in Paris. The Gram-negative bacilli were isolated from sputum of Jules Bordet's son. Bordetella bronchiseptica was first isolated by Ferry (1911) and M'Gowan (1911) who considered the bacteria as the cause of distemper in dogs. Later B. bronchiseptica was known as primary cause of 'kennel cough' infection along with the Canine Adenovirus and Canine Parainfluenza virus. Moreno-Lopez named the bacteria B. bronchiseptica.

The genus *Moraxella* was named after Morax who first isolated the bacteria from human conjunctivitis in 1896.

Properties of genus

1. *Morphology*: *Bordetella* is small, Gram-negative, coccobacilli which may appear singly or in pair. The pili are detected in *B. pertussis, B. parapertussis,* and *B. bronchiseptica.*

Moraxella is Gram-negative, small rods occurring in pair (diplobacilli).The aged cultures exhibit pleomorphism, occurring in pairs or chains as short, plump rods with rounded ends. Some strains may appear as cocci (Figure 1). The capsule is present in fresh isolates of some species (except *Moraxella catarrhalis*). The bacteria are non-motile and non-sporing. *Moraxella bovis* contains numerous type IV fimbriae on its surface.

2. *Bordetella* is aerobic. *Moraxella* is aerobic, fastidious and non-fermenting in nature. Some strains prefer anaerobic condition for their growth.

3. *Classification:* The genus *Bordetella* belongs to the family *Alcaligenaceae*. The genus is comprised of 16 species such as *B. bronchiseptica*, *B. pertussis*, *B. parapertussis*, *B. hinzii*, *B. avium*, *B. holmseii*, *B. trematum*, *B. petrii* etc.

The genus *Moraxella* belongs to Moraxellaceae family. Previously it was known as *Branhamella*. Currently there are 24 species and one sub-species under the genus *Moraxella*. Most of the species are commensal except a few, which have disease producing capabilities. Important species are *M. bovis, M. ovis, M. catarrhalis, M. bovoculi, M. boevrei, M. canis, M. caprae, M. caviae, M. cuniculi,* and *M. phenylpyruvica.*

4. *Resistance:* Resistance of *Moraxella* to physical and chemical agents is not remarkable. The bacteria are susceptible to desiccation and do not survive long outside the host. The beta- lactam antibiotic resistance is observed among *M. catarrhalis* isolates from clinical cases. This resistance is associated with the production of beta-lactamase enzyme.

5. *Natural habitat: Bordetella* can localize at the epithelium of the respiratory tract in man, domestic and wild animals.

Most of the species of *Moraxella* are commensal in different warm blooded animals. *M. bovis* is commonly found in the conjunctiva, nasal cavity and upper respiratory tract of cattle (over two years of age). *M. ovis* resides in the eyes of the sheep and goat. Other species like *M. boevrei, M. canis, M. caprae, M. caviae,* and *M. cuniculi* are commonly found in the upper respiratory tract of healthy goats, dogs and cats; nasal cavity and eye of healthy goats; upper respiratory tract of guinea pigs; oral cavity of healthy rabbits and upper respiratory tract of marine mammals, respectively.

6. *Genome:* The size of *Bordetella* genome is 4.08-5.3 Mbp with 67-68 mol% GC content. There are 3800-5000 coding sequences with 18-358 pseudogenes, 3 mRNA operons, 51-55 tRNA present in the genome. The genome sequencing and analysis shows that *B. pertussis* and *B. parapertussis* are independent derivatives of *B. bronchiseptica* due to large-scale gene loss and inactivation.

The sequencing of *M. bovis* (Epp-63) genome revealed the size of the genome as 2,839,913 bp. Two plasmids (pMBO-1 and pMBO-2) are detected in the genome. The genome contains RTX (repeats in the structural toxin) toxin producing operon known as *mbx* operon. In non-haemolytic strains the *mbx* operon is absent.

Isolation, growth and colony characteristics

Bordetella can be isolated in blood agar, Bordet-Gengou agar, Smith-Baskerville culture media and MacConkey agar at 37°C. Haemolysis in blood agar is produced by both *B. bronchispetica* and *B. pertussis* strains. The pathogenic strains of *B. bronchiseptica* produce smooth, small and convex colonies. The rugged and large colonies are produced by non-pathogenic strains. *B. bronchiseptica* colonies on MacConkey agar are reddish and are surrounded by small red zone with amber discoloration of the underlying medium. No growth of *B. pertussis* is detected in MacConkey agar.

Moraxella can be isolated in blood or serum agar by incubating at 33-35°C. *M. bovis* grows best at 35°C. No growth is found in MacConkey's agar (except *M. phenylpyruvica*). After 48 hours of incubation, the colonies are 1-4 mm in diameter, smooth, translucent, friable, greyish and surrounded by a zone of beta haemolysis. Fresh colonies may corrode the agar. Characteristic growth pattern is observed at the interface of the agar and polystyrene petri dish. *M. bovis* produces two major types of colonies i.e. smooth and rough. The clinical isolates primarily produce rough colonies that are flat, dry, firm and umbonate with zone of beta haemolysis. The rough colony phenotype is associated with cell surface pili, causing auto- agglutination in distilled water, haemagglutination and pellicle formation in the surface of the liquid media. The rough colonies may transform into smooth, moist colonies that do not adhere to the growth medium.

Biochemical characteristics

Bordetella bronchiseptica and *Moraxella bovis* produce following biochemical reactions

Biochemical test	*Bordetella bronchiseptica*	*Moraxella bovis*
Catalase	(+ve)	Most strains are (+ve)
Oxidase	(+ve)	(+ve)
urease	Slow (+ve)	(-ve)
Nitrate reduction	(+ve)	Most strains are (-ve)
Gelatinase production	Apparently not done	(+ve)
Dnase production	Apparently not done	(-ve)
Phenylalanine deaminase	Apparently not done	(-ve)
Alkaline Phosphatase	Apparently not done	(-ve)
Acid Phosphatase	Apparently not done	Weakly (+ve)
Hydrolysis of Tween-80	Apparently not done	(+ve)
Litmus milk	Apparently not done	Three layer formation after 7 days incubation [upper layer is dark blue, middle layer is light blue, bottom layer is white]

Antigenic characteristics

Each *Bordetella* species (*B. bronchispetica* and *B. pertussis*) has the common 'O' and heat-labile serotype 7 antigens. One specific serotype antigen is detected in *B. bronchispetica* (antigen 12) and *B. pertussis* (antigen 1).

Major antigen of *M. bovis* is pili / fimbriae forming protein (pilin). The pili are thin, flexible appendages, often polar in location, associated with twitching motility of the bacteria. They belong to the type 4 category and are therefore structurally related to the fimbriae of *Dichelobacter nodosus, Pseudomonas aeruginosa, Neisseria gonorrhoeae* and *Neisseria meningitides*. Pili are composed of a protein, known as 'pilin'. Mature pilin has N-methyl -phenylalanine as its first amino acid and it has homologous hydrophobic N-terminal. Subculture may cause loss of pili from the bacterial surface. Loss of pili is associated with reduced virulence. Although the pili plays role in virulence, they are also required for production of protective antibody. *M. bovis* can be classified into seven serogroups (A-G) on the basis of the fimbrial antigen.

Toxins and virulence factors produced

Toxins

Endotoxin: *Bordetella* lipopolysaccharide (LPS) is highly immunogenic and an important bacterial defense against host immune responses. The LPS of *B. bronchiseptica* can efficiently mask the negative charge of bacterial outer membrane to prevent the attack of cationic antibacterial peptides (attracted towards negatively charged surface).

Adenylate cyclase toxin (ACT): The ACT is produced by pathogenic strains of *Bordetella*. It is lethal for tracheal cells and degenerating bones.

Dermonecrotic toxin (DNT): It is produced by *B. bronchiseptica* and it helps in generation of respiratory infections in dogs.

Haemolysin (cytolysin): It is a Ca^{++} dependent heat labile pore forming cytolytic toxin and is produced by *Moraxella bovis*. The toxin belongs to RTX-group of toxin (RTX= repeats in the structural toxin).It is related to the other RTX toxins like *Escherichia coli* HlyA, *Mannheimia haemolytica* LktA, *Actinobacillus pleuropneumoniae* ApxIIA and *Actinobacillus actinomycetemcomitans* LtxA. The clinical isolates of *M. bovis* produce this toxin *in vitro* (haemolytic in blood agar), although the exact role in pathogenesis is unclear. Probably it helps in establishment of infection by tissue damage and it provides iron to the fastidious *M. bovis* strains from lysed erythrocytes. Cytolytic activities are associated with ocular necrosis, pitting of the corneal epithelium, protecting the bacteria from phagocytosis by destroying neutrophils. Leakage of degradative enzymes from neutrophils into the corneal stroma results corneal liquefaction and ulceration.

Virulence factors

Virulence factors	Function
Filamentous haemagglutinin	It is 220 KDa rod shaped protein encoded by *fha*B gene and it produced by pathogenic strains of *Bordetella*
Adhesins and pertactin	Adhesion of *Bordetella* strains
Fimbriae / Pili	Out of six major fimbrial subunits *fim2* and *fim3* fimbrial subunit genes are responsible for *Bordetella* adhesion to host cells. The pili of *M. bovis* is of two types- Q-pilus and I-pilus. The Q-pilus helps in adherence of the bacteria with bovine conjunctival and corneal epithelium. I-pilus helps in maintenance of established infection
Ubiquitous surface protein A1 (UspA1), CD protein	Produced by *M. catarrhalis*, helps in adhesion of the bacteria with host tissues
Lactoferrin binding protein A (LbpA), Lactoferrin binding protein B (LbpB), Transferrin binding protein A (TbpA), Transferrin binding protein B (TbpB), CD and E porins, *Catarrhalis* outer membrane protein B (CopB).	Produced by *M. catarrhalis*, helps in acquisition of nutrients
Lipooligosaccharide (LOS), Ubiquitous surface protein A2 (UspA2).	Produced by *M. catarrhalis*, helps in establishment of infection

Pathogenesis

Transmission

Direct contact and inhalation are the major routes of *Bordetella* transmission in animals. The fluctuating temperature, high humidity, crowded housing (high stocking density) are the predisposing factors for *Bordetella* infection.

M. bovis is transmitted by direct contact, nasal and ocular discharges and by mechanical vectors like 'face fly' *(Musca autumnalis)*, 'house fly' (*Musca domestica*) and 'barn fly' *(Stomoxys calcitrans)*.The insects may carry the bacteria in the legs for up to 3 days. Predisposing factors for the outbreaks include prior ocular infection with *Mycoplasma*, infectious bovine rhinotracheitis (IBR) virus and *Thelazia*. Other factors are transportation of cattle, improper dust removal from the sheds, presence of unhygienic environment and lack of mineral or vitamin supplementation in diet. The best season for outbreak is summer. However snowfall and ultraviolet ray irradiation are also associated with the disease. Ultraviolet irradiation causes nuclear fragmentation, loosening of bovine corneal epithelial cells and epithelial degeneration. As the integrity of the corneal epithelium is disrupted, *M. bovis* may penetrate and multiply easily. Sometimes vaccination with modified live IBR vaccine may generate the infectious bovine keratoconjunctivitis (IBK) like condition. The aged cattle are less susceptible than younger ones. The breed predilection is observed. *Bos taurus*, specially with unpigmented white face is more susceptible than *Bos indicus*. No gender predilection has been definitely determined, although a higher prevalence has been reported in males.

Pathogenesis

Piliated and haemolysin producing strains of *M. bovis* are considered as pathogenic. The carrier cattle may harbour non-piliated strains in their conjunctiva and nasal cavity. Pili are required for bacterial adhesion with bovine conjunctival and corneal epithelium. The adherence helps in establishment of bacterial population by preventing the flushing of lacrimal secreation and blinking. Bovine lacrimal secreation contains secreatory Ig-A and lactoferrin. The lactoferrin prevents the bacterial iron acquisition and thus acts as bacteriostatic agent. However, *M. bovis* has its own iron acquisition system (siderophore) and outer membrane receptor for lactoferrin. After establishment, the bacteria start to multiply and secreate cytolysin. Initial necrosis and pitting of corneal epithelium occurs due to this cytolysin. The neutrophils migrate into the site to phagocytose the bacteria. The bacterial cytolysin lyses them and releases the neutrophil granules containing proteolytic enzymes. The enzymes cause further corneal damage.

Disease produced

Bacteria	Host	Disease produced
Bordetella bronchispetica	Dogs	**Kennel cough (Canine infectious tracheobronchitis)**: It is more common in dogs housed together at centers, boarding or training kennels, pet shops, shelters and veterinary clinics. It is a mixed infection primarily caused by *B. bronchiseptica*, Canine Adenovirus and Canine Parainfluenza virus. Some secondary agents like Reo virus, Canine respiratory Corona virus, Canine Herpes virus, *Mycoplasma*, *Pseudomonas*, *Pasteurella*, *Streptococcus* and coliforms are also detected. Bordetellosis comprises of two clinical forms. The most common uncomplicated form is associated with dry hacking cough, gagging and retching behaviour. The complicated form is characterized by wet cough and is common in puppies or immunocompromised dogs. The disease is associated with mucoid discharges and signs of systemic infection including pyrexia, anorexia, chorioretinitis, vomiting and diarrhoea leading to death. Incubation period ranges between 1 to 8 days showing clinical signs for 1–2 weeks.
	Young growing pigs (3-9 weeks age)	**Non-progressive atrophic rhinitis:** The infection is characterized by slight to severe rhinitis and transient turbinate bone atrophy. No clinical signs and growth retardation is observed other than nasal discharge and mild deformity of face. It is caused by *B. bronchispetica* and non-toxigenic *Pasteurella multocida* strains

Bacteria	Host	Disease produced
Bordetella pertussis	Human	Whooping cough
Moraxella bovis	Cattle	**Infectious bovine kerato-conjunctivitis (IBK) or 'pink eye'**: In UK, it is also known as 'New Forest Disease (NFD)'. It is characterized by lacrimation, blepharospasm (abnormal blinking of eyelid), photophobia, severe keratitis, corneal ulceration, ophthalmitis, blindness. No systemic involvement is observed
	Horse	Conjunctivitis
M. bovoculi	Cattle	Associated with infectious bovine kerato-conjunctivitis (IBK)
M. ovis	Sheep, goat, cattle	Infectious kerato-conjunctivitis (IK) and 'Pink eye'
M. catarrhalis	Human	Chronic bronchitis in adults with pre-existing respiratory tract infection, meningitis, endocarditis in adults, otitis media in children
M. phenylpyruvica	Cattle, sheep	Isolated from urogenital tract, brain. Pathogenicity is uncertain
	Pigs	Isolated from urogenital tract
	Goats	Isolated from intestinal tract

Immunity

Secreatory-IgA is the major antibody developed against *M. bovis* infection in cattle in comparison to anti *M. bovis* IgM or IgG. The role of antibodies in protection from the infection is not clearly established. Local cell mediated immunity is an important factor in providing protection against the infection.

Diagnosis

Clinical samples: The specimens for whooping cough are collected from suspected human by cough plate, nasopharyngeal swab and suction. The specimens for isolation of *B. bronchiseptica* include nasal swabs and deep tracheal swabs from live animals. The external naris is cleaned with 70% ethanol prior to collection to reduce the contamination. Amies transport medium is used for transport of the samples. *B. pertussis* colony numbers is decreased by 75% on transportation of specimens at refrigeration temperature (4°C).

For isolation of *M. bovis*, lacrimal swab is collected from deep in the inner canthus of the eye. The collected swab is transported to the laboratory in sterile distilled water within 2 hours. Sterile distilled water is used to prevent drying of the swab.

Laboratory examinations

Direct examination: A smear can be prepared from the collected swab and stained with Gram's stain. *Bordetella* is small, Gram-negative, coccobacilli which may appear singly or in pair. *Moraxella* appears as Gram-negative small rods, present in pair (diplobacilli). Gram stained smear from colonies reveal Gram-negative plumpy rods or cocci, present in pairs (Figure 1).

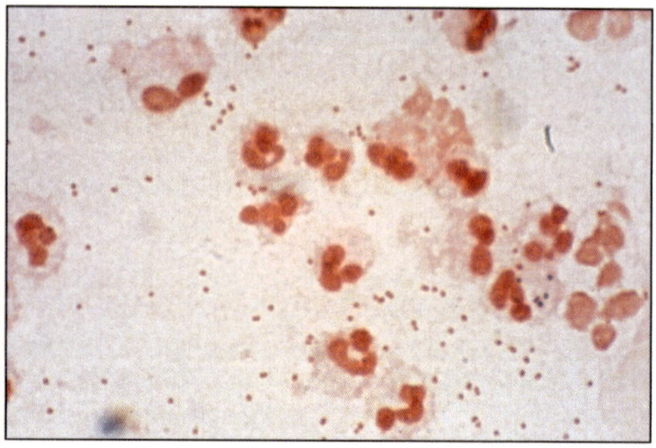

Fig. 1: *Moraxella catarrhalis* appear as gram-negative cocci, singly and in pairs. Few bacteria are visible within the cytoplasm of neutrophils (Courtesy: Rebecca Buxton, American Society for Microbiology)

Isolation of bacteria from clinical samples: Media, incubation condition and colony characteristics are described earlier.

Serological tests: Commonly employed serological tests for detection of canine bordetellosis include tube agglutination, indirect haemagglutination, micro-agglutination test and ELISA.

FAT and ELISA have developed for detection of anti *M. bovis* IgA/IgG in lacrimal secreation or serum. Several workers detected antibodies against outer membrane protein of *M. catarrhalis* in human using different serological tests.

Molecular biology: The genus (A643Bbalc and A856Bbalc) and species specific (*fim* or *fla* gene) PCRs are developed for detection of *B. bronchiseptica*.

Molecular typing methods like restriction enzyme analysis (REA) with the frequently cutting enzyme *Taq*I, pulsed field gel electrophoresis (PFGE) with rare cutting enzymes like *Sma* I, *Not* I are found highly successful in typing of *M. catarrhalis* isolates from human.

Prevention and control

Live attenuated intranasal vaccine consists of *Bordetella bronchiseptica*, canine parainfluenza virus, and canine adenovirus 2 was found effective against kennel cough. In India, the live attenuated vaccine used in kennel cough is composed of *Bordetella bronchiseptica* (B-C2 strain, 108 cfu) and canine parainfluenza virus (Cornell strain, 103 $TCID_{50}$).

The fly control is an important step in eradication of *Moraxella bovis* infection in cattle farms. Experimental use of insecticide impregnated ear tags reduced fly population and incidence of vector borne diseases. Weekly application of calves (not adult cattle) with furazolidone eye spray in the both eyes was found effective prophylaxis.

25

Gram-negative Anaerobes: *Bacteriodes Dichlobacteria* and *Fusobacterium*

Properties

1. *Bacteroides*, *Dichelobacter* and *Fusobacterium* are major gram negative anaerobes isolated from human and animals. Other gram negative anaerobes are listed below (Table-1).

2. The bacteria are tolerant to oxygen in comparison to strict anaerobes. The bacteria do not die after oxygen exposure.

3. The bacteria naturally inhabit the intestine and mucosal surfaces of human and animals. Majority of them are opportunistic pathogens. Often they cause mixed bacterial infection along with aerobes. The aerobes remove oxygen and create an anaerobic condition favourable for their growth. The aerobes may also supply other growth requirements. For e.g. *Porphyromonas asaccharolytica* requires vitamin K for its growth, supplied by another aerobic bacterium, not the host.

4. Common virulence factors are:

a) Fimbriae: It helps in adhesion of the bacteria with the host epithelial cells

b) Capsule: antiphagocytic

c) Bacterial endotoxin (LPS): LPS of gram-negative anaerobes is less chaemotactic and non-toxic in comparison to other gram-negative bacteria (*E. coli, Salmonella*).

d) Enzymes: Collagenase produced by *Porphyromonas* is a major virulence factor. However pathogenic significance of other enzymes like IgA and IgG protease, neuraminidase, DNAse, fibrinolysin is unknown.

Table 1: Common gram negative anaerobes of clinical significance

Family	Genus	Species
Bacteroidaceae	*Bacteroides*	*Bacteroides fragilis* group (True *Bacteroides*) *Bacteroides caccae* (*B. fragilis* group 3452A) *Bacteroides distasonis* *Bacteroides eggerthii* *Bacteroides fragilis* *Bacteroides merdae* (*B. fragilis* T4-1)
	Butyrivibrio	*Butyrivibrio fibrisolvens*
	Leptotrichia	*Leptotrichia buccalis*
	Anaerorhabdus	*Anaerorhabdus furcosus*
Cardiobacteriaceae	*Dichelobacter*	*Dichelobacter nodosus*
	Cardiobacterium	*Cardiobacterium hominis*
	Suttonella	
Fusobacteriaceae	*Fusobacterium*	*Fusobacterium necrophorum* *Fusobacterium equinum* *Fusobacterium nucleatum* *Fusobacterium naviforme* *Fusobacterium necrogenes*
Porphyromonadaceae	*Porphyromonas*	*Porphyromonas asaccharolytica* *Porphyromonas cangingivalis*a *Porphyromonas canoris*a *Porphyromonas cansulci*
Prevotellaceae	*Prevotella*	*Prevotella bivia* *Prevotella buccae,* *Prevotella buccalis* *Prevotella corporis*
Selenomonasceae	*Selenomonas*	*Selenomonas artemidis* *Selenomonas dianae* *Selenomonas flueggei* *Selenomonas infelix*
Campylobacteraceae	*Campylobacter*	*Campylobacter concisus* *Campylobacter curvus* *Campylobacter gracilis* *Campylobacter hominis*
Desulfovibrioaceae	*Desulfovibrio*	*Desulfovibrio desulfuricans*
Succinivibrionaceae	*Anaerobiospirillum*	*Anaerobiospirillum succiniciproducens*
Gram negative cocci Veillonellaceae Acidaminococcaceae Megasphaeraceae	*Veillonella* *Acidaminococcus* *Megasphaera*	*Veillonella parvula* *Veillonella dispar* *Acidaminococcus fermentans* *Megasphaera elsdenii*

Dichelobacter

In 1941, Beveridge first described the bacteria as *Bacteroides nodosus*, primary cause of footrot in sheep.

Properties of genus

1. *Morphology: Dichelobacter* are gram-negative straight or curved rods with distended ends. It looks like dumbbell specially those grown in the tissues (Figure 1). In the lesion, the bacteria are 3-10μm long and 0.6-0.8 μm wide. In artificial culture they are pleomorphic and may appear as long rod, filamentous or coccoid. They are capsulated but non-sporulating. The bacterial cells contain numerous type IV fimbriae arranged in a pole. The fimbriae are up to 10 μm long and 6 nm in diameter. The fimbriae help in 'twitching motility' of the bacteria. The twitching motility is the extension and retraction of fimbriae which enables the bacteria to move along the solid surfaces.

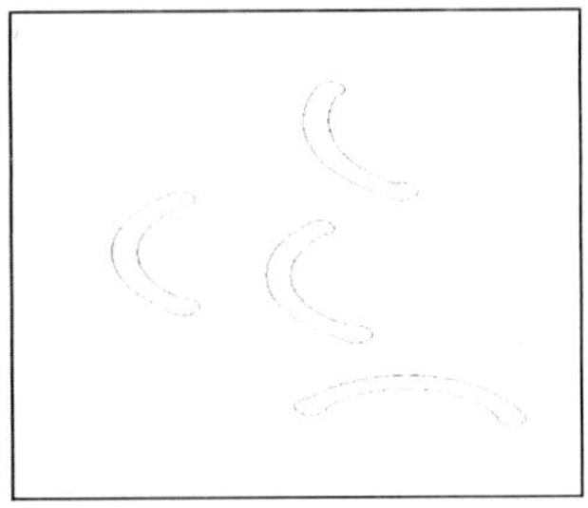

Fig. 1: Microscopic view of *Dichelobacter nodosus* (schematic)

2. *Dichelobacter* are slow growing aerotolerant anaerobe.

3. *Classification*: *Dichelobacter* belongs to the order Cardiobacteriales (γ-Proteobacteria) and family *Cardiobacteriaceae*. The only species of the genus is *Dichelobacter nodosus.* Previously it was classified under the family *Bacteroidaceae* and it was known as *Bacteroides nodosus*. Later due to genomic differences it was separated and the new family was created. The name *Dichelobacter* implies that the bacteria can colonize in cloven hoofed animals with two digits per foot. Other two genera of the family *Cardiobacteriaceae* are *Cardiobacterium* and *Suttonella*.

4. *Resistance*: The bacteria are susceptible to 50-60°C for 10 minutes exposure.

5. *Natural habitat: Dichelobacter* is an obligate parasite residing at hoof of the cattle, sheep and goats. The bacteria cannot survive in the environment for a long period. In muddy soil they are found to survive for two days. In the deeper section of the hoof they may persist without any clinical signs along with spirochaete and other aerobic bacteria. Under favourable conditions they start to multiply and the clinical signs appear.

6. *Genome: D. nodosus* genome consists of a single circular chromosome of 1,389,350 base pairs with 1,299 predicted genes. It is the smallest anaerobe sequenced till date. The (G+C) content of the genome is 44.4 mol%. Average

gene size is 973 bp with 91 coding %. The large biosynthetic array is present but the genome lacks amino acid processing pathway. Two 'pathogenicity islands' (genomic region possessing virulence associated genes and regulatory genes for pathogenicity) are detected in the genome, known as *vap* (virulence associated protein) and *vrl* (virulence related locus). The *vap* is conserved in *D. nodosus* isolates, whereas *vrl* is found in other bacteria also. The type IV fimbrial biogenesis genes (21 in numbers) and regulatory genes (10 in numbers) are scattered throughout the genome in eight locations. Two integrated elements (*intC* and *intD*) are also found in the virulence associated region of *D. nodosus* genome. However no gene is detected so far encoding type II secretion system. Little is known about the gene expression of the bacteria within the hoof of sheep. Mechanism of gene transfer in *D. nodosus* involves natural transformation, transduction or by transposon and RNAs.

Isolation, growth and colony characteristics

D. nodosus is highly fastidious and slow growing. Previously it was tried to isolate the bacteria by addition of horse serum, arginine and serine into the media. Improved and faster isolation was obtained using the simplified media of Thorley (1976) containing 4% hoof powder.

The author has personal experience of using the media for isolation of *D. nodosus* which is a nutrient agar containing 4% hoof powder, 0.15% serine and 0.5% arginine. Hoof powder is prepared from dried hoof collected from healthy sheep. The plates are incubated in anaerobic jar at 37°C. After 4 days of incubation the colonies are subcultured into the hoof agar plates containing 2% hoof powder to get pure colony. Grayish white umbonate (nipple shaped) colonies of 1-3mm diameter are found (Figure 2). Colonies are either beaded (virulent) or mucoid (less virulent).

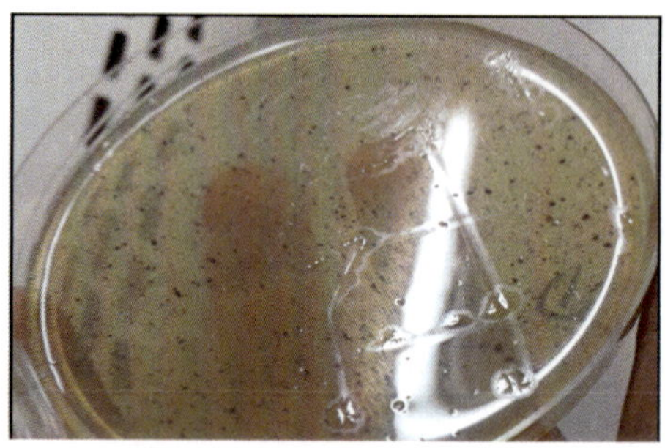

Fig. 2: Appearance of *Dichelobacter nodosus* umbonate colonies in hoof agar medium (*Courtesy*: Karthik Akshintala, Department of Veterinary Microbiology, Sri Venkateswara University, Tirupati, Andhra Pradesh, India)

Biochemical characteristics

D. nodosus is biochemically inert but following experimental results are reported in the literatures.

Biochemical Tests	Expected Results
Indole	(-ve)
Aesculin hydrolysis	(-ve)
Urease	(-ve)
Gelatin hydrolysis	(-ve)
Carbohydrate fermentation	(-ve)

Antigenic characteristics

Previously the antigenic classification of *D. nodosus* was based on capsular (K) antigen. Now this antigen is found to be identical with the fimbrial antigen. Fimbriae are composed of 'pilin' protein encoded by a chromosomal gene. On the basis of the fimbrial subunit gene (*fimA*), *D. nodosus* is classified into ten serogroups (A-I and M) and 21 serotypes (A1, A2, B1, B2, B3, B4, B5, B6, C1, C2, D, E1, E2, F1, F2, G1, G2, H1, H2, I, and M). This classification is known as 'Australian system'. An alternative system, known as 'British System' accommodates further nine serotypes (J-R), not found in the Australian system. Sequence analysis of *fimA* protein shows that there are generally more than 35 amino acid differences between two serogroups and 15 amino acid differences between two serotypes. Sometimes serogroup conversion occurs through the natural transformation or homologous recombination. In India, B, E and I serogroups of *D. nodosus* is reported to be associated with footrot.

Other antigenic components include outer membrane protein and lipopolysaccharide.

Virulence factors produced

Virulence factors	Function
Fimbriae	Type IV fimbriae is found in *D. nodosus* that helps in twitching motility. It is considered as major virulence factor. The fimbriae are composed of a protein known as 'pilin'. The pilins are mePhe pilin (type IV) as they possess N-methyl-phenylalanine at the amino terminal.
Serine proteases	Two acidic serine proteases are encoded by *aprV2* and *aprV5* gene. The enzymes can degrade substrates like casein, azocasein, elastin, hoof powder, gelatin, fibrin, collagen I, collagen III and α-keratin. The enzymes cause erosion of agar plate. Degree of erosion is correlated with the virulence.
Vap and *Vrl* pathogenicity island	The pathogenicity islands are located in the bacterial chromosome. They are one of the first pathogenicity islands identified in the bacterial genome. The *vap* region consists of *intA*, *vap* A-H and *toxA* genes. The *intA* encodes integrase enzyme

Pathogenesis

D. nodosus is considered as a primary pathogen for footrot in sheep, goat. Colonization of the bacteria requires some predisposing factors like warm and wet environment, maceration of the hoof, infection with other gram-negative anaerobic rods like *Fusobacterium necrophorum*. Infection with other bacteria produces hyperkeratosis and parakeratosis in crevices which helps in survival and multiplication of *D. nodosus*. It is invasive and it has the capacity to penetrate up to the matrix of the hoof. Probably keratinolytic protease plays a major role in destruction of the germinal layers of interdigital skin and horn matrix producing the characteristic lesion. It can separate the soft tissues of the hoof from the hard tissues of the horn. The bacteria can persist in the host for prolonged period.

Disease produced

Bacteria	Host	Disease produced
Dichelobacter nodosus	Sheep, goat, cattle, horse, pig, deer, mouflon	**Footrot:** It is an infectious syndrome of ruminant feet caused by synergistic action of certain bacterial species of which *D. nodous* is the major transmitting agent. In sheep there is exudative inflammation with foul odour followed by necrosis of the epidermis of the interdigital skin and horn matrix. It causes chronic lameness. Three clinical forms are noted i.e. virulent, intermediate and benign. The feet lesions can be scored (0-5) on the basis of its severity. In a flock more than 10% lesions with score 4 at a time is considered as 'virulent footrot'. It has major economical impact. In benign footrot infection is confined within interdigital skin. All age group of sheep is equally susceptible. The lesion in lamb feet is less severe than the adults

Immunity

Resistance to footrot is influenced by genetic factors and host susceptibility. Genetic factors are paternally inherited and involve the alleles in the ovine major histocompatibility complex class II region. British sheep breeds with coarse wool are more resistant than other breeds like Merino. Garole breed found in Sundarban delta (India) is also considered more resistant. However no systemic study is known to confirm it.

Diagnosis

Clinical samples: Exudates from the hoof lesion can be collected for the detection of the bacteria.

Laboratory examinations

Direct examination: A smear can be prepared from exudate and stained by Gram's Method. *Dichelobacter* appears as gram negative rods with knobs present at the both pole.

Isolation of bacteria from clinical samples: Isolation is tedious and time consuming process complicated by fastidious growth requirement and slow growing nature of the bacteria. The media, incubation condition and colony characteristics are described earlier.

Histopathology: Histopathological examination of the hoof lesion can be performed. However, *Dichelobacter nodosus* is found in less number than the other associated bacteria.

Serological tests: ELISA is developed using monoclonal antibodies against several protease enzymes and potassium thiocyanate extract of outer membrane protein of *D. nodosus*. In hilly area during summer, the sheep are sent to graze in alpine pastures away from the villages sometimes along with the mild footrot lesion. The lesions heal naturally before they arrive back in the villages in winter. Some of the animals still act as carrier without any visible lesion. The carriers can transmit the infection to the healthy one. A pilus anamnestic ELISA is developed to detect the carriers without lesion.

Molecular biology: The highly sensitive PCR assay for direct detection of *D. nodosus* 16SrRNA gene from footrot lesions was developed. Bacterial strain characterization and differentiation can be done by pulsed field gel electrophoresis and PCR-RFLP. The Taqman based real time PCR assay targeting 16SrRNA gene is also developed for detection of *D. nodosus*.

Bacteroides

Bacteroides are gram-negative, rod with rounded ends or spherical. The bacteria may appear singly or in pair or in short chains. They can be isolated in commonly used bacteriological media like blood agar. The colonies are 1-3 mm in diameter, smooth, entire, convex and rarely β-haemolytic. Some of the colonies become dark with age. Veterinary important species of *Bacteroides* are *B. fragilis, B. ovatus, B. asaccharolyticus* and *B. levii.*

B. fragilis is associated with neonatal diarrhoea in calves, piglets, kids and lambs; abortion and mastitis in cattle; and abscess in dogs and cats. Whereas, *B. ovatus, B. asaccharolyticus* are associated with osteomyelitis in cattle, horse, dogs and cats. *B. levii* causes mastitis in cows.

Fusobacterium

Fusobacterium are gram-negative, anaerobic fusiform rod with pointed end and has beaded appearance in stained smear. The bacteria can be isolated in blood agar. The colonies are small, smooth, α or β-haemolytic. The cultures have rancid butter odour as their metabolic end product is butyric acid. Veterinary important species are *F. necrophorum, F.* equinum and F. *nucleatum.*

F. necrophorum is associated with footrot, mastitis, metritis, 'calf diptheria' (necrotic laryngitis), equine 'thrush' (hoof lesion), 'bullnose' in pigs (associated with *Clostridium*), liver abscess in cattle (synergistic infection with *Arcanobacterium pyogenes*).

F. equinum is associated with lower respiratory tract infection including necrotizing pneumonia and pleurisy in horses.

F. nucleatum causes sporadic abortion in cattle, sheep.

Prevotella and *Porphyromonas*

They are most common gram-negative anaerobes found in the oral cavity of man and animals. The bacteria require haemin and vitamin K for their optimum growth and they can produce pigments in the isolation media. Commonly used isolation media are supplemented *Brucella* agar (with haemin and vitamin K), kanamycin-vancomycin sheep blood agar and supplemented phenylethyl alcohol agar (PEA). The colonies are circular, entire, convex, shiny, gray brown to black in colour. Pigmentation is more with prolonged incubation. Few strains are haemolytic. Both of them are either non-carbohydrate fermenting or very weak in fermentation.

Veterinary important species and disease produced

Bacteria	Host	Disease produced
Prevotella melaninogenica	Sheep, goat, cattle	Associated with footrot
	Dogs and cats	Soft tissue infections
Prevotella intermedia	Animals	abscess
Prevotella nigrescens	Animals	abscess
Porphyromonas levii	Cattle	**Summer mastitis** (synergistic infection with *Arcanobacterium pyogenes*)
Porphyromonas gingivalis	Human and animals	Dental menaces (periodonitis), **Broken mouth** (in sheep): it is characterized by exfoliation of teeth, malnutrition, weight loss, systemic health problems.
Porphyromonas intermedia	Human and animals	Dental menaces (gingivitis)

26

Leptospira and Other Spirochetes

Antony Van Leeuwenhoek (1681) first observed the spirochetes under the microscope and described them. In 1833, Ehrenberg used the name *Spirochaeta* for free living spiral shaped organisms. Obermeir (1873) first described a spirochete of pathogenic significance isolated from human patients with relapsing fever. Inada (1916) first isolated *Leptospira icterohaemorrhagiae* from human patients of Weil's disease. In 1980, Nogochi proposed the name as *Leptospira.*

In India, Taylor and Goyale (1931) first reported *Leptospira* from human patients suffering with jaundice in Andaman Islands. Ayyar (1932) first reported *Leptospira* from dogs in Chennai city.

Properties of genus

1. *Morphology: Leptospira* are gram-negative, spiral shaped organisms with hooked ends. The length varies from 6-20 μm with 0.1-0.2 μm diameter. The bacteria have a typical double membrane covering. The cytoplasmic membrane and peptidoglycan cell wall are closely associated and are surrounded by an outer membrane. Two periplasmic flagella (endoflagella) are found within the cell and are responsible for the motility. No flagella are present as extracellular appendage. One end of the flagellum is attached with the pole of the bacterial cell by insertion disc. Other end extends towards the centre of the cell and may overlap the flagellum coming from the opposite end. The endoflagella consists of a solid inner core surrounded by tubular sheaths. FlaA and FlaB proteins constitute the flagellar sheath and core, respectively.

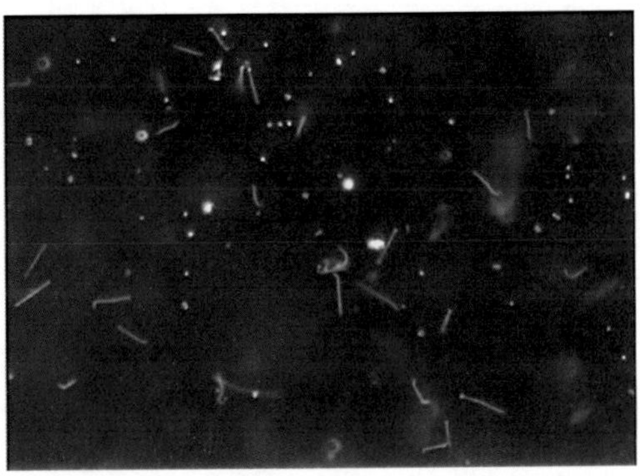

Fig. 1: Dark filed microscopic view of *Leptospira* in liquid culture medium, 20X (Courtesy: Metawee Thongdee, Mahidol University, Thailand)

The bacteria can be demonstrated by dark field or phase contrast microscopy due to their poor staining property. However using Giemsa stain, silver impregnation in the tissue section (Fontana or Levaditi's method) and fluorescent antibody technique can also make them visible (Figure 1).

2. Leptospires are obligate aerobes.

3. *Classification:* The genus *Leptospira* belongs to the family *Leptospiraceae* under the order Spirochaetales. The genus consists of 69 species out of which the major pathogenic species are *L. interrogans, L. alexanderi, L. alstonii* (genomospecies 1), *L. borgpetersenii, L. inadai, L. fainei, L. kirschneri, L. licerasiae, L. noguchi, L. santarosai, L. terpstrae* (genomospecies 3), *L. weilii, L. kmetyi* and *L. wolffii*. The recent classification considered the previously described 'genomespecies' as 'species'. The major saprophytic species are *L. biflexa, L. wolbachii, L. meyeri, L. vanthielii, L. terpstrae* and *L. yanagawae.* The pathogenic and saprophytic species can be differentiated. The growth of pathogenic strains is inhibited by the purine analogue 8-azaguanine, whereas saprophytic strains grow normally in the presence of this compound. Similarly, unlike *L interrogans*, *L. biflexa* can grow at low temperature (11-13°C). The species such as *L. inadai, L. broomii, L. fainei, L. wolffii* and *L. licerasiae* are considered as 'intermediate' with uncertain pathogenicity.

Both *L. interrogans* and *L. biflexa* contains more than 200 and 60 serovars, respectively. Most of the serovars use certain species of animals as maintenance host with same or different animals as incidental / accidental hosts (Table). The serovars with pathogenic significance are *pomona, bratislava, canicola, hardjo* and *icterohaemorrhagiae*. The serovars with similar antigenic composition are placed into 'serogroup' for easy diagnosis. The term 'serogroup' has no other taxonomic significance. At present there are 26 serogroups (e.g. Pomona, Australis, Canicola, Sejroe). The serovars are written in italics, whereas, the serogroups are written without italicization, e.g., *Leptospira* (generic name) *interrogans* (species name) serovar Icterohaemorrhagiae.

4. *Resistance*: Leptospires are killed by drying, heat (at 60°C for 1 minute), soap, bile salt, detergent, acidic pH and putrefaction. The culture can be preserved at -20°C for 3 months in the laboratory.

5. *Natural habitat*: The bacteria survive in the warm, moist environment with neutral to alkaline pH (6.6 and above). Presence of groundwater favours their survival. They can not stay alive in dry soil, sea water and sewage for a long period. The infection is common in tropical and sub-tropical countries. Leptospires commonly reside in the proximal convoluted tubule of the mammalian kidney and sometimes in the genital tract. Rodents and wild carnivores are the most frequent 'maintenance or reservoir hosts'. Although

the bacteria are isolated from a wide host range like amphibians, arthropods, birds, reptiles and marsupials. Some serovars adapt a particular species of animal for persistence. Reservoir hosts may excreate the bacteria through the urine for extended period without any clinical signs.

6. *Genome:* The chromosome of *Leptospira* is circular DNA molecule with GC content of 35-41 mol%. The genome size varies from 3.9-4.6 Mb. 'LeptoDB' (www.leptonet.org.in) is the database which contains wide range of genomic and proteomic information of *Leptospira*. Currently the database contains information of 17 complete genomes and 496 draft genomes. Previously it was thought that the pathogenic leptospires are devoid of naturally occurring plasmids. Recently the plasmids (pGui1 and pGui2 in *L. interrogans* strain Gui44; plasmid lcp1, lcp2, lcp3 in *L. interrogans* strain 56609) are detected in pathogenic strains of *Leptospira*. Mechanism of gene transfer is not established.

Isolation, growth and colony characteristics

Leptospires can be isolated in enriched liquid or semisolid media (0.1-0.2% agar) containing vitamin B1 and B12, long-chain fatty acids, and ammonium salts. Long-chain fatty acids act as the sole carbon source. Previously several broths (Fletcher, Korthoff, Noguchi and Stuart broth) containing rabbit serum were used for isolation which helps in enrichment. At present, the most widely used medium is EMJH (named after *E*llinghausen, *M*c Cullough, *J*ohnson and *H*arris who introduced it) or Tween-80/ BSA medium containing oleic acid, bovine serum albumin (BSA) and Tween 80 (polysorbate). Sometimes a combination of Tween 80, Tween 40 and BSA is used. Tween is the source of the fatty acids and BSA helps in detoxification of the fatty acids to promote the bacterial growth. A few strains require the addition of pyruvate or rabbit serum for primary isolation. The media contamination may be controlled by the addition of a variety of antimicrobials such as 5-fluorouracil, nalidixic acid, fosfomycin or a mixture of rifamycin, polymyxin, neomycin, 5-fluorouracil, bacitracin and actidione.

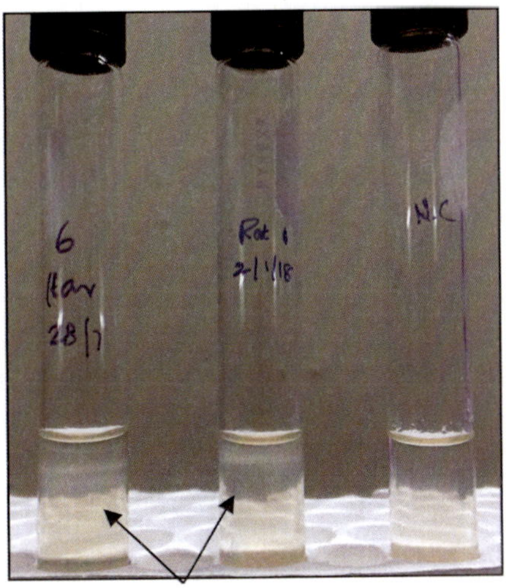

Fig. 2: 'Dinger's disc or ring' in semisolid agar media (Courtesy: Eazhisai Radhakrishnan, Department of Veterinary Microbiology, Madras Veterinary College, TANUVAS, India)

After inoculation, the media are incubated at 29-30°C for 16-26 weeks under aerobic condition. Primary cultures from animal tissues may be isolated better at 37°C. Some serovars like *pomona* show early growth within 7-10 days of incubation. Periodic observation of the culture under dark field microscopy is necessary before discarding them.

In semisolid agar (Dinger's media) the growth occurs below the surface where it gets the optimum oxygen tension. The growth becomes more turbid after prolonged incubation. This zone of growth is known as 'Dinger's disc or ring' (Figure 2).

In room temperature the culture can be maintained in semisolid (with haemoglobin) or liquid media with frequent transfer into the fresh media (every 3-12 weeks). For prolonged preservation of culture, the liquid nitrogen is preferred.

Biochemical characteristics

L. interrogans produce following biochemical reactions

Biochemical Tests	Expected Results
Catalase	(+ve)
Oxidase	(+ve)
Urease	(+ve)
Lipase	(+ve)

Antigenic characteristics

Based on the antigenic structure *Leptospira* is classified into several serovars. Lipopolysaccharide (LPS) present in the outer membrane constitutes the major antigen for *Leptospira*. It is structurally and immunologically similar with LPS of other gram-negative bacteria with relatively less toxicity and less biological activities (rabbit pyrogenicity, mouse lethality, Schwartzman reaction and B-cell mitogenicity). Leptospiral lipid- A (anchoring unit of LPS) contains some unusual compounds including a modified glucosamine disaccharide unit which is phosphorylated and methylated. The LPS is serovar specific. Other antigenic components of *Leptospira* are flagellar antigen, lipoprotein, porin (OmpL1) and the type two secreation system (T2SS)-secretin GspD.

Toxins and virulence factors produced

Toxins

Haemolysin: Some serovars (*pomona, autumnalis, icterohaemorrhagiae*) produce haemolysin (sphingomyelinase) associated with haemoglobinuria, haemolytic anaemia and tissue damages. The haemolysin provides iron and fatty acids available to the bacteria. It is encoded by *sph* gene. At least seven *sph*-like genes were detected among the pathogenic *Leptospira* (*sphA-G*). The *lai* serovar can release a postulated pore-forming haemolysin (encoded by *SphH*) not a sphingomyelinase.

Cytotoxin: The pathogenic serovars (e.g. *pomona*) can secreate cytotoxin.

Endotoxin: Leptospiral endotoxin also has the potentiality to release the pro-inflammatory cytokine (TNF-α) from the monocytes.

Virulence factors	Function
Outer membrane lipoproteins a) Lip32 b) Loa22 c) LenA, LenB, Len C, Len D, Len E and Len F d) LigA and LigB proteins (Leptospiral immunoglobulin like protein; Lig proteins are anchored to the outer membrane and have 12-13 tandem bacterial immunoglobulin-like repeated domains)	These surface proteins help in adherence of the bacteria with the different host cell types a) Lip32 binds laminin, collagen II, IV, V and plasma fibronectin of host. It is restricted to pathogenic species only. b) It also helps in binding extracellular matrix. Its absence reduces virulence. c) The proteins are associated with invasion and colonization. The proteins can bind complement regulatory factor-H and host laminin. d) Fibronectin, fibrinogen, collagen and laminin binding protein. It is restricted to pathogenic species only

Pathogenesis

Transmission

a) The leptospiral infection takes place in the susceptible animals ('incidental' or 'accidental host') by direct transmission through the contaminated urine, placenta, foetal tissues or indirectly through the contaminated environment (water, fomite, feed). The bacteria enter either through the breached mucous membrane (genital, nasal, ocular, intestinal) or broken/water soaked skin during direct transmission. The streams and ponds contaminated with the urine of rodents and carnivores are the major source of infection for domestic animals and human. Aerosols generated from the urine in cattle shed is another potential source of the infection.

b) Venereal transmission through the coitus takes place in pigs and cattle (*bratislava* and *tarassovi* serovar in pigs, *hardjo* in cattle)

c) Vertical transmission may occur from the dam to the foetus (*hardjo*). Milk from acutely infected cow is a source of infection for the calves as well as human.

d) Leptospirosis is considered as most wide spread zoonosis specially in warm and humid areas. Human gets infection through abraded skin or mucosa, drinking of contaminated water. It may be an 'occupational hazard' occurring among veterinarians, animal handlers who have close contact with the infected animals without proper precautions.

Pathogenesis

Incidental hosts

Leptospires establish a systemic infection after exposure of mucous membranes, conjunctiva or broken skin to contaminated water or soil. For tissue invasion adhesion with the host cells is the prerequisite step. Pathogenic leptospires bind to endothelial, fibroblast, kidney epithelial and monocyte/ macrophage cell lines (*in vitro*). The bacteria adhere to the extra cellular matrix (ECM) components such as collagen type I, type IV, laminin, fibronectin of host tissues through the bacterial adhesin (Lip32, Loa22, LenA-F, LigA, LigB). All the adhesins are expressed in virulent leptospires and some of them are expressed under physiologically relevant conditions of temperature, pH or osmolarity.

Adhesion is followed by a brief period of presence in blood (leptospiremia). It will generate circulating antibodies which make an effort to clear the bacteria by complement mediated lysis. The phagocytic cells also make the same effort. Leptospires can survive transiently within the phagocytic cells, although they are not intracellular in nature. The bacteria can resist the immune mechanisms and spread to different organs such as liver, spleen, meninges and specially the kidney within third day of the infection. The cell surface receptor (proteoglycan GAG motifs) is present in the proximal convoluted tubule of kidney which may help in colonization into the kidney. The infection is cleared from the other organs within 7 days (except kidney) with the help of the circulating antibodies. The incidental host suffers from different symptoms and the infection may localize and persist into the kidney. Thus leptospires are shed through the urine (leptospiruria).

The venereal route of transmission results colonization into the reproductive tract only. Invasion of placenta (third trimester of pregnancy) results either abortion or birth of weak offsprings. The offsprings infected prior to third trimester of pregnancy may be born with antibodies. Some serovars (*bratislava, hardjo*) can persist in the genital tract of cattle. In genital tract the local IgA response is produced which can protect the bacteria from the IgG mediated opsonization. The lack of opsonization and subsequent phagocytosis helps in persistence of the bacteria in the genital tract.

Maintenance hosts

In maintenance hosts, after colonization in the kidney, leptospiruria occurs for longer duration with high intensity in comparison to the incidental hosts. The molecular mechanism behind this persistence with immune evasion is poorly understood. However, the following hypothesis is given by different workers.

Mechanism of renal immune evasion

a) Anti-leptospiral antibodies (IgG) present in renal tubules is unable to kill *Leptospira* due to the absence of complement

b) Down regulation of specific leptospiral antigen expression in the renal tubule and urine may facilitate immune evasion despite the presence of *Leptospira*-specific antibody. It helps in hiding the bacteria from the specific antibodies. Sometimes antigenic variation also helps in the immune evasion.

c) There is a delay of lymphocyte infiltration into the kidney after leptospiral invasion. The invasion occurs within 7 days of the infection. Whereas, the infiltration takes place after one month. Meantime, the colonization is almost complete.

Disease produced

Leptopiral species and serovars with their maintenance, incidental hosts and disease produced is described below

Bacteria (*Leptospira interrogans* serovar)		Host and Disease produced		
Serogroup	Serovar(s)	Maintenance Host	Incidental Host	Disease produced
Pomona	*pomona*	Pig, wild animals	Pig, cattle, horse	Abortion, chronic nephritis, recurrent iridocyclitis in horses ('Moon blindness')
Australis	*bratislava*	Pig, horse	Pig, horse	Abortion, repeat breeding ('repeat breeder syndrome'), infertility
	australis	-	-	-
Canicola	*canicola*	Dogs	Dog, pig	Interstitial nephritis, abortion (pig)
Sejroe	*hardjo*	cattle	cattle	Abortion, infertility, agalactia ('milk drop syndrome'/ 'flabby udder mastitis')
	sejroe	-	Dog	-
Icterohaemorrh-agiae	*icterohaemorr-hagiae*	Brown rat (*Rattus norvegicus*)	Cattle, pig, dog	Abortion
	copenhageni	Rodents	Human, dog	-

Maintenance host is specific for a serovar, but the incidental host may vary. The well adapted serovars in the maintenance host (e.g. Bratislava in pigs) persist in the kidney or genital tract for a long time with low antibody titer. In incidental hosts the bacteria cause severe acute infection with high antibody titer and rapid elimination from the kidney.

Immunity

Anti- *Leptospira* antibodies play the protective role against the infection in human and animals like dogs, pigs, guinea pigs and hamsters. The antibodies target either serovar specific lipopolysaccharide (LPS) or the conserved protein (Lip32). The immunity can be passively transferred through the convalescent human or animal serum. The antibodies either lyse the bacteria directly in presence of complement or the antibodies enhance phagocytosis by macrophages and neutrophils. However in cattle the antibodies are not protective and Th1 response plays dominant role in the protection.

Diagnosis

Clinical samples

Mid-stream urine, whole blood, serum, milk from the animals with clinical signs, internal organs after post-mortem such as kidney, organs of aborted fetuses (liver, lung, brain, adrenal gland) may be collected. Whole blood (5 ml) is collected in 0.5 ml of 1% sodium oxalate or 0.1 ml of 1% heparin (anticoagulant). Treating the animals with diuretics prior to the urine collection produces better results. The urine should be collected and tested for consecutive three weeks.

The samples to be used for culture (kidney or other tissue, whole blood) is diluted with 1:10 bovine serum albumin (1% BSA) containing 5-fluorouracil at 100–200 μg/ml concentration and is transported to the laboratory. If BSA is not available, the sample can be inoculated directly into the media besides the collection site. The sample in transport medium can be preserved at 2-5°C to prevent other bacterial contamination and tissue autolysis. However, the kidney should not be frozen. Leptospires remain viable in the unfrozen kidney for several days after death of the animals. Isolation from the whole blood is often unsuccessful because leptospiraemia occurs for a brief period and it is not always associated with the clinical signs.

Laboratory examinations

Direct examination

Dark field microscopy

Urine: Formalin is added into the urine sample (1.5 ml of 10% formalin in 20 ml urine) to make it alkaline. In acidic urine, morphology of the leptospires is distorted. By addition of formalin the bacteria are killed but the intact morphology is retained. The bacteria can be preserved for several days to observe under dark field microscopy for the presence of leptospires. Negative finding is inconclusive as it only indicates the absence of the bacterial shedding through the urine.

Kidney tissue: A small part of the tissue is taken from inside of the organ with a sterile pasteur pipette. It is macerated with sterile distilled water and observed under dark field microscopy.

Typical spiral shaped organisms with hooked ends appear under dark field microscopy (Figure 1).

Fluorescent antibody technique (FAT)

Cryostat sections or smears from the foetal kidney can be used for FAT. Morphology of the organisms is retained better in the foetal kidney of pigs than the calves which are often autolysed.

Isolation of bacteria from clinical samples: It is the most sensitive method for detection of leptospires if the bacteria are present in sufficient number in the samples, the sample is properly transported and the tissues are not autolysed. The media, incubation condition are described earlier.

Immunohistochemistry: It helps in detection of leptospiral antigens in tissues, specially in chronic cases which are previously treated with the antibiotics. In these cases demonstration of the intact bacteria is not always possible.

Serological tests: Leptospiral antibodies appear within a few days of the onset of the infection and the antibodies persist for several months or years. Sometimes in chronic cases the antibody level becomes undetectable.

a) Microscopic agglutination test (MAT): It is most widely used serological test for diagnosis of acute leptospirosis. It uses live antigen. It can specifically detect the serovars or the serogroups. There is cross-reaction between the serovars and the test cannot differentiate the antibody resulting from infection or vaccination. MAT titer of >1:400 in the presence of clinical signs and appropriate history of animal contact is considered as positive for leptospirosis in unvaccinated individual animal. Whereas, herd titer more than >1:100 indicates endemic infection in unvaccinated animals.

b) ELISA: It is quite sensitive, but lacks the serovar specificity of the MAT. In veterinary diagnostics ELISA is commonly used for identification of recent infections and for screening herds in the regions where vaccination for leptospirosis is not practiced. The test uses a wide variety of antigen preparations, like leptospiral whole cell preparation to recombinant lipoproteins such as LipL32, LigA or porin (OmpL1). However, the reliability on ELISA alone for leptospira diagnosis is low.

Molecular biology: The genus-specific PCR is developed and evaluated in clinical samples and the PCR can amplify DNA from both pathogenic and non-pathogenic serovars of *Leptospira*. Improved sensitivity is achieved by quantitative-real time PCR either using TaqMan probes or SYBR green fluorescence. Initially pulsed-field gel electrophoresis (PFGE) and multilocus variable-number tandem-repeat analysis (MLVA) were applied for typing of *Leptospira*. Later it was found that the techniques cannot differentiate all species and clades. Currently whole genome sequencing (WGS) and core genome MLST (cgMLST) approach are considered as high-resolution typing method.

Prevention and control

a) Strict biosecurity measures should be followed in the animal farms

b) The semen used in artificial insemination should be free of leptospires. Sometimes sero-negative bulls can act as carriers for *Leptospira*. PCR should be employed for detection of *Leptospira* DNA in the semen

c) Detection and elimination of carrier animals from the farm

d) In *hardjo* endemic zone, annual vaccination of bulls, replacement heifers, and 2-3 year old females (few weeks before release of the bulls) is practiced.

Borrelia

Sakharoff (1891) first described a spirochete from acute septicaemia in geese in Caucasus, later known as *Borrelia anserina*.

Properties of genus

1. *Morphology: Borrelia* is a gram-negative, spiral bacterium with 5-6 loose coils. The bacteria are 14-15 µm long and 0.3 µm wide. The bacteria are better stained with Giemsa, crystal violet and dilute carbol fuchsin, acridine orange and silver stain. In the wet mount preparation, the bacteria are visualized by dark field microscopy like *Leptospira*. Like other spirochetes, *Borrelia* also consists an outer membrane encasing an axial fibril containing 15-20 endoflagellas.

2. *Borrelia* is slow growing microaerophiles.

3. *Classification*: The genus *Borrelia* belongs to the family *Spirochetaceae* under the order Spirochaetales. The genus consists of 58 species and 2 sub-species currently. Pathogenic species are *B. anserina, B. burgdorferi senso lato, B. theileri* and *B. coriaceae.*

B. burgdorferi senso lato consists of four subgroups i.e. *B burgdorferi senso stricto* (found in North America and Europe), *B. garinii* (Europe and Asia), *B. afzelii* (Europe and Asia) and *B. japonica* (Japan). Lyme disease in human and animals (dogs, horses) is mostly caused by *Borrelia burgdorferi sensu lato* (s.l.). *Borrelia burgdorferi* s.l. can be divided into 15 genomic groups or 'genospecies' such as *B. burgdorferi sensu stricto, B. garinii, B. afzelii, B. japonica, 'B. andersonii', B. tanukii, B. turdi, B. valaisiana, B. lusitaniae, 'B. bissettii', B. sinica, 'B. californiensis', B. spielmanii, B. americana* and *B. carolinensis*. Recently *B. miyamotoi* is detected to cause lyme disease like syndrome in human.

4. *Resistance: Borrelia* does not survive in the environment for a long period. In the blood samples containing citrate, the bacteria can survive a week in room temperature, months at 4°C, indefinite period at -20°C.

5. *Natural habitat: Borrelia* cannot live outside the host. Both hard and soft ticks (*Ixodid* sp., *Argas persicus, Ornithodoros* sp.) act as vector for pathogenic *Borrelia.* In certain stage of the life cycle the ticks acquire the infection from recently infected animals. The larvae of the ticks feed in the summer on small mammals and migratory birds. The larvae moult into the nymphs which feed on small mammals and migratory birds during the spring. The nymphs and adults also feed and breed on large mammals like dogs and human. Sometimes uninfected larvae pick up the infection from the small mammals in summer which was infected by the nymph in the last spring.

6. *Genome: Borrelia* is a unique prokaryote to possess a linear chromosome with a number of linear or circular plasmids (21 numbers in *B. burgdorferi sensu lato*). The plasmids possess essential genetic elements encoding major outer surface proteins (osp) which act as adhesin, transport or binding proteins. The genes do not encode any protein related to biosynthetic pathways (like *Mycoplasma*). The sequencing of *B. burgdorferi sensu lato* (B31) genome is completed recently.

Isolation, growth and colony characteristics

Isolation of *Borrelia* is difficult due to its slow growth and microaerophilic requirements. Modified BSK (Barbour-Stoenner-Kelly) media are generally used for isolation of *B. burgdorferi sensu lato.* It is an enriched serum broth containing antibiotics (kanamycin and 5-flurouracil). The media after inoculation is incubated at 33°C. *B. anserina* cannot be isolated in artificial bacteriological media. It is grown in embryonated hen's eggs like virus. The inoculation route is either the chorioallantoic membrane (CAM) or yolk sac. The CAM route produces better numbers of isolates.

Biochemical characteristics: *Borrelia* ferment glucose and other carbohydrates.

Antigenic characteristics

Borrelia contains muramic acid, ornithine in their cell wall and numerous outer surface proteins (osp) in their outer membrane. There are 150 numbers of 'osp' detected from *B. burgdorferi sensu lato.* No true lipopolysaccharide in the outer membrane is detected. Some strains possess its analogue. The spirochete shows remarkable antigenic variations for which vaccination is not so much successful against borreliosis. In response to host immune system, there is rapid recombination between outer surface proteins (between ospA and ospB of *B. burgdorferi sensu lato*). It can generate different antigenic structure of *Borrelia* in the host which helps in immune evasion.

Virulence factors produced

Virulence factors	Function
Outer surface protein ospA ospB	It helps in attachment of the spirochete to the tick mid gut. It helps in invasion of endothelium
Erp surface protein (ospEF)	The Erp surface proteins bind complement inhibitor factor H and help in persistence of the infection

Pathogenesis

Transmission

Borrelia is mainly transmitted between animal to animal and animal to human by ticks. The ticks can transmit the infection up to one year. Other arthropods are short term vectors. *Borrelia* is also transmitted through blood products, urine, milk and placenta (transplacental transmission).

Pathogenesis (Lyme disease)

After bite with infected tick the spirochete is transmitted into the susceptible hosts (human, dog, cattle, horses, cat). Primarily the bacteria multiply in the skin and later invade the blood circulation. In the circulation the bacteria are either phagocytosed or lysed by the antibody-complement complex.

The antibodies are primarily generated against the outer surface proteins. The antibody titre rises very slowly by unknown mechanism. Bactericidal antibodies are generated after 3-5 weeks. Survivor of the antibody mediated lysis can localize within the host cell. For localization in the host cells *Borrelia* follows different ways of immune evasion, as described below.

a) Antigenic variation of *Borrelia* helps in immune evasion
b) *B. burgdorferi sensu lato* can hide within the folds of cellular membrane, less exposed to the host immune system or antibiotics
c) *Borrelia* can transform themselves into cyst, spheroplast, L-form within the host under unfavourable conditions to remain dormant. In favourable conditions the dormant forms can revert into the motile vegetative form.

The motile and ospB expressing *Borrelia* can cross the endothelium through the breaking of tight junction or transcytosis (transport of organism from one side of the cell to the other). The microbial invasion of central nervous system, cardiac muscle, joints can take place. After synovial cell invasion the spirochetes cause inflammation through the increased level of cytokines like IL8, TNFα. The LPS analogue or 'osp' of the bacterium is responsible for it. The inflammation of the cells is the key developer of the symptoms.

Disease produced

Bacteria	Vector	Host	Disease produced
Borrelia anserina	Tick (*Argas persicus, A. miniatus, A.reflexus*)	Chicken, duck, geese, turkey, pigeons, pheasants, wild birds	**Avian spirochaetosis:** It is characterized by fever, depression, greenish diarrhoea, paralysis, anaemia, enlarged and mottled spleen. Higher mortality is found in young birds
Borrelia burgdorferi sensu lato	Tick (*Ixodes* sp.)	Human, dog	**Lyme disease:** In dogs, it is characterized by swelling of joints (carpal), pain, lameness, fever, lethargy, anorexia. Sometimes nephropathy with renal failure occurs, known as 'Lyme nephropathy' or 'Lyme Nephritis'. Rarely, myocarditis, heart block, CNS involvement is found.
Borrelia theileri	Tick (*Rhipicephalus sp., Boophilus sp., Margaropus sp.*)	Cattle, sheep, horse	**Tick spirochaetosis:** It is characterized by fever, weakness, weight loss and anaemia.
Borrelia coriaceae	Tick (*Ornithodoros coriaceus*)	Cattle, deer	Epizootic bovine abortion

Immunity

Humoral immunity plays dominant role in protection against *Borrelia burgdorferi* infection.

Diagnosis

Clinical samples: Blood, serum, synovial fluid (Lyme disease suspected cases), cerebrospinal fluid can be collected from live animals. The blood collected during fever is preferred. After post mortem, liver and spleen can be collected.

Laboratory examinations

Direct examination: Dark field Microscopy or Giemsa stain can directly demonstrate the organisms in the blood film, synovial fluid/ liver/spleen smears. Sometimes FAT is used like other spirochetes for direct examination of the smears.

Isolation of bacteria from clinical samples: The media, incubation condition are described earlier. However, it is tedious and time consuming process to isolate *Borrelia* from clinical specimens.

Serological tests: Agar gel precipitation test (AGPT), ELISA can detect the antibody against *B. anserina, B. burgdorferi sensu lato* in the collected serum samples. ELISA followed by western blot is the most sensitive way to detect *Borrelia* antibody that persists for months or years. The blot can differentiate the vaccinated and infected animals. Recently developed ELISA can detect the antigenically conserved invariable region of *B. burgdorferi sensu lato.* It does not cross react with other *Borrelia.* However, in endemic zone of Lyme disease healthy dogs are often sero-positive.

Molecular biology: The PCR is developed for detection of *B. burgdorferi sensu lato* using primers for the *ospA* gene or 23S RNA gene. Taqman-real time PCR is also developed for rapid and quantitative detection of *B. burgdorferi sensu lato*.

Treponema

Schaudinn and Hoffmann (1905) first described *Treponema pallidum* as a causative agent of human syphilis. The genus *Treponema* belongs to the family *Spirochaetaceae* under the order Spirochaetales. The pathogenic species include *T. pallidum ssp pallidum*, *T. paraluis-cuniculi*, *T. brennaborense.* Morphologically *Treponema* is slender, spiral shaped filaments with pointed ends and small coils present throughout the length. It can be stained by Giemsa or India ink. They can be observed under dark field microscopy.

No satisfactory method for isolation of *T. paraluis-cuniculi* has been developed. Although *T. brennaborense* can be isolated by enrichment in Oral Microbiologie and Immunology Zurich-Pat (OMIZ-Pat) medium for 1 h at 37 ^{O}C followed by inoculation into OMIZ-Pat agar. It is incubated at 37°C in anaerobic jar with gas pack. Diffuse colonies are observed within 5-10 days.

T. pallidum ssp *pallidum* causes human syphilis (chancre), still a dreadful disease of human civilization. *T. paraluis-cuniculi* and *T. brennaborense* are responsible for venereal disease in rabbits ('Rabbit Syphilis') and digital dermatitis in cattle ('hairy foot warts'), respectively. Digital dermatitis is an acute or chronic inflammatory disease of the bovine foot which is characterized by painful lesions, typically found along the coronary band, red in colour and has a foul odour. Other gram negative anaerobes (*Dichelobacter nodosus, Fusobacterium necrophorum*) are also involved in digital dermatitis but *Treponema* plays a central role.

Brachyspira

The genus *Brachyspira* belongs to the family *Spirochaetaceae* under the order Spirochaetales. Pathogenic species are *B. hyodysenteriae, B. pilosicoli, B. aalborgi, B. alvinipulli.* Several species of *Brachyspira* were previously included under the genus *Serpulina* which only contains non-pathogenic species (*Serpulina intermedia*) at present.

Brachyspira are loosely coiled, slender, flexible gram negative spirochetes. They can be better stained by Romanowsky type stain.

Brachyspira are aerotolerant (oxygen tolerant) anaerobe. They can be isolated in blood agar containing spectinomycin (400μgm/ml) or colistin and vancomycin. The plates are incubated at 42°C in anaerobic chamber containing 10% CO_2 for 10 days. *B. hyodysenteriae* colonies are strongly haemolytic whereas colonies of *B. pilosicoli* are weakly haemolytic. *B. hyodysenteriae* is indole positive.

B. hyodysenteriae causes 'swine dysentery' found in growing pigs. Whereas *B. pilosicoli* causes 'post weaning colonic spirochetosis' in pigs, dogs and birds. *B. aalborgi* causes colonic spirochetosis in human and other primates. *B. alvinipulli* causes colonic spirochetosis in poultry. The colonic spirochetosis (CS) is characterized by rapid onset of diarrhoea which persists for 7-10 days followed by reduced feed efficiency, fall in growth rate.

27

Mycoplasma

The word '*Mycoplasma'* is originated from the Greek word *mykes* (fungus) and *plasma* (formed). It was first used by Albert Bernhard Frank (1889), a German biologist. He thought it was a fungus. An older name for *Mycoplasma* was pleuropneumonia-like organisms (PPLO), referring to organisms similar to the causative agent of contagious bovine pleuropneumonia (CBPP).It was later found that the fungus-like growth pattern of *Mycoplasma mycoides* is unique to the species. It was first isolated in 1898 by Edmond Nocard and E. Roux from bovine lungs. *Mycoplasma pneumoniae* was considered as a virus previously. Eaton and his co-workers cultured the causative agent of human primary atypical pneumonia (PAP) or 'walking pneumonia'. It was known as 'Eaton's agent'. In the early 1960s, Leonard Hayflick, in Philadelphia, was first to isolate and cultivate the causative agent of primary atypical pneumonia and identified the agent as a *Mycoplasma pneumoniae*.

Properties of genus

1.*Morphology*: *Mycoplasma* have no cell wall and therefore are resistant to the antibiotics used to inhibit the cell wall synthesis like penicillin, cephalosporin and vancomycin. The bacteria are the smallest prokaryote (0.3-0.8μm). They are pleomorphic due to absence of the rigid cell wall. The different shapes include ring, globules, filaments and elementary bodies. Due to their plasticity in shape and size, they can be passed through the membrane filter with pore size of 0.45μm. The cell membrane is constituted of trilaminar structure enriched with phosphoprotein, lipoprotein, glycolipid, phospholipid and sterol. So *Mycoplasma* require sterol for their growth.

Despite of their close similarity with gram-positive bacteria, *Mycoplasma / Ureaplasma* can't retain the stain of crystal violet/ Gram's iodine. Gram staining is not ideal for their visual inspection due to the absence of cell wall. Contrast phase microscopy, dark phase illumination techniques can be used for their visualization.

They usually divide by binary fission. However, some of them have a reproductive cycle.

2. *Mycoplasma* is aerobe or facultative anaerobe.

3. *Classification:* Many taxonomists have classified *Mycoplasma* in the phylum/division Firmicutes because of their low (G+C) content and similarity in 16SrRNA gene sequence with other Gram-positive bacteria such as *Clostridium*, *Lactobacillus* and *Streptococcus*. However some literature assigned *Mycoplasma* in the phylum/division Tenericutes.

Mycoplasma belongs to the class Mollicutes. 'Mollicutes' is originated from two Latin words i.e. 'mollis' (means soft) and 'cutes' (means skin). All the bacteria that lack a cell wall and the genetic capability to synthesize peptidoglycan come under this class. Two major orders under this class are Mycoplasmatales and Acholeplasmatales.

There are two families under the order Mycoplasmatales i.e. Mycoplasmataceae and Metamycoplasmataceae which comprises of four genera i.e. *Mycoplasma, Ureaplasma Mesomycoplasma* and *Metamycoplasma*, 207 species and 7 sub-species.

The pathogenic *Mycoplasma* belongs to *Mycoplasma mycoides* cluster. It comprises of six closely related mycoplasmas such as *Mycoplasma mycoides* subsp. *mycoides* Small Colony biotype (MmmSC) and Large Colony biotype (MmmLC), *M. mycoides* subsp. *capri* (Mmc), *Mycoplasma capricolum* subsp. *capricolum* (Mcc), *M. capricolum* subsp. *capripneumoniae* (Mccp) and *Mycoplasma* sp. bovine group 7 of Leach (MBG7). Other veterinary important mycoplasmas are *M. bovis* (cattle), *M. agalactiae* (goat, sheep), *M. bovigenitalium* (cattle), *M. dispar* (cattle), *M. gallisepticum* (poultry) and *M. meleagridis* (turkey).

Important species of *Metamycoplasma* are *M. cloacale*, *M. equirhinis*, *M. faucium*, *M. gateae* and *M. hominis*. Major *Mesomycoplasma* species are *M. bovoculi*, *M. conjunctivae*, *M. dispar*, *M. flocculare* and *M. hyopneumoniae*. Major *Ureaplasma* species are *U. cati*, *U. diversum*, *U. felinum* and *U. urealyticum*.

4. *Resistance:* Most of the mycoplasmas are moderate to highly susceptible to tetracycline, tiamulin and erythromycin. The bacteria are resistant to penicillin, ampicillin and methicillin. They are frequent contaminants of cell culture and very difficult to remove. The bacteria are resistant to UV radiation and photodynamic action of methylene blue. Majority of mycoplasma strains are destroyed at 45-55°C for 30 minutes. The bacteria can be preserved at -70°C in liquid nitrogen· The bacteria are sensitive to various disinfectants like chlorhexidine and cetrimide and physical methods like supersonic vibrations and desiccation.

5. *Natural habitat: Mycoplasma* is ubiquitous in nature and it can be detected in all mammalian species. In human mycoplasmas are usually associated with mucous membrane and are predominantly detected in throat, lower respiratory and urogenital tracts. Asymptomatically the infected animals also carry the bacteria on mucosal surface including oral, nasal, conjunctival, intestinal and genital mucosa. Ear canal of the goat is also a major reservoir of caprine mycoplasma.

6. *Genome: Mycoplasma* genome is extremely small (0.58-1.35 Mb) with low (G+C) content (23-40 mol%) due to their evolution from Gram-positive bacteria via degenerative gene deletion.

Isolation, growth and colony characteristics

Mycoplasmas have limited metabolic option and it cannot be grown in normal bacteriological media. The bacteria require protein supplement like 20% horse serum, beef infusion, yeast extract and peptone for the growth. The fresh serum also provides some labile accessory factors. In addition, amino acid and crude DNA are required for their growth. Some of the species require specific ingredients for their growth like vaginal mucus by *M. agalactiae* and nicotinamide by *M. synoviae*. Penicillin and thallium acetate are added into the media to prevent the contaminants. *Mycoplasma* broth or agar is commercially available media used for its isolation.

The optimal temperature for growth is 36-37°C and the optimum pH requirement is 7.3 to 7.8. The plates are placed in a sealed container within the incubator. Increased humidity with CO_2 tension (5-10%) enhances the growth. It can be performed by the addition of wet blotting paper or cotton into the container along with flushing of CO_2 with nitrogen or lighting a candle within the container. Instead CO_2 incubator can be used. The broth or agar plates are incubated for 4-5 days with daily inspection for the growth.

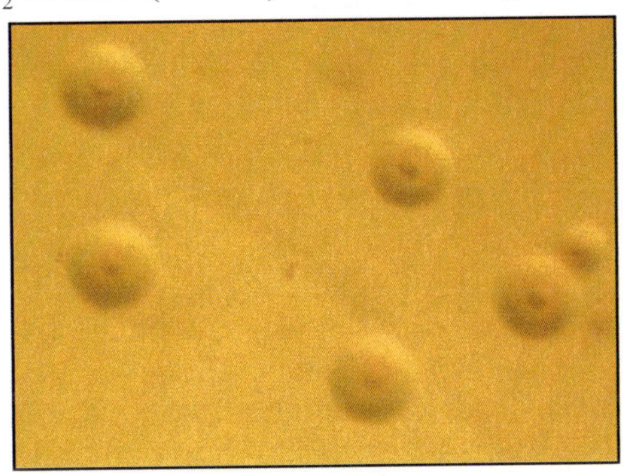

Fig. 1: Microscopic view of mycoplasmal fried egg colonies (*Courtesy*: K. Manimaran, Department of Veterinary Public Health and Epidemiology, Veterinary College and Research Institute, Orathanadu, Thanjavur, Tamil Nadu Veterinary and Animal Sciences University, India)

In *Mycoplasma* broth, the growth is indicated by change of pH which causes colour change of the indicator. Whereas the plates are checked for the colonies under 'dissecting microscope' or low power objective in a light microscope with reduced light intensity. On solid media the bacteria produce granular growth and appear as round colonies with thickened center and delicate periphery. The colonies are small, translucent or glistering with some degree of central elevation or depression which often resembles fried egg. It is known as 'fried egg' or 'nipple shaped' colony (Figure 1, Figure 2). It is very difficult to remove the colonies from the agar. Caprine *Mycoplasma* may grow on sheep blood agar and produces small colonies with alpha haemolysis.

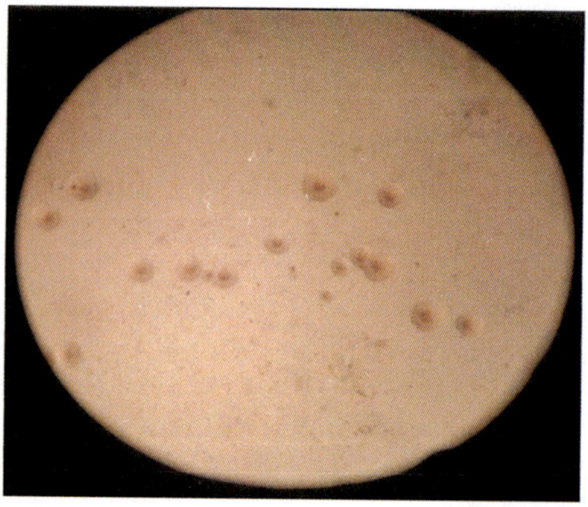

Fig. 2: Microscopic view of mycoplasmal colonies (*Courtesy*: R. S. Gandge, Department of Microbiology, Mumbai Veterinary College, Maharashtra Animal and Fishery Sciences University, India)

Mycoplasma can also be isolated in chicken embryo by inoculating through the chorioallantoic membrane (CAM) route.

Antigenic characteristics

Most of the mycoplasma possess cell membrane bound glycolipids and proteins that can act as hapten. Antibodies to the glycolipids are often exploited for several antigen-antibody reactions like complement fixation test. Glycolipid with similar antigenic structure was detected in host cells (central nervous system). Thus, the antibodies to glycolipid may cause host cell damage and this is implicated in neurological manifestation of *M. pneumoniae*. Many of the *Mycoplasma* (*M. pneumoniae* and *M. arthritidis*) act as super antigens and stimulate the signal for pro-inflammatory cytokine secreation. *M. bovis* causes apoptosis of the bovine lymphocytes. It is noteworthy that *Mycoplasma* infection is mostly chronic in nature. *Mycoplasma* uses unique immune evasion mechanism to establish persistent infection in the host. The capsular polysaccharide (galactin) prevents the phagocytosis of *M. mycoides* and *M. dispar*.

Toxins and virulence factors

During their growth and metabolic interaction with the host cells *Mycoplasma* produces several cytotoxic metabolites like glycoproteins, proteases, phospholipases, carbohydrates, haemolysin, ammonia and endonucleases which played vital role in pathogenesis. It is suggested that accumulation of such compound often triggers extensive tissue damage. The host cells often die with the leakage of essential and vital components. For example, *M.*

pneumoniae produce hydrogen peroxide which may cause oxidative injury to the host cell.

Mycoplasma neurolyticum produce a membrane associated cytotoxin which is highly neurotoxic in nature.

Mycoplasma can also synthesize molecular moieties that trigger pro-inflammatory cytokine synthesis leading to pathogenesis called 'modulin'. The modulins are often responsible for release of pro-inflammatory cytokines and chemokines responsible for inflammation and further infiltration with mononuclear phagocytic cells.

Pathogenesis

Transmission

The transmission takes place predominantly via direct contact with the infected animals, inhalation and venereal route. Mechanical transmission through milkers' hand or fomites is important in bovine and caprine mastitis. In poultry, vertical transmission by egg was noted. Contaminated milk may be the major source for calves as well as for goat kids. There is no information regarding the role of ectoparasites in transmission. However, the ear mite seems to play a role in caprine mycoplasmosis.

Pathogenesis

Mycoplasmas are metabolically and nutritionally compromised. They have to depend on the host cell or environment for essential nutritional requirements like protein, sterol and raw materials for DNA synthesis. The intimate attachment of *Mycoplasma* with the host cells is required. Mycoplasmas have definite host cell and tissue specificity. The attachment is mediated by host cell receptors usually containing sialic acid moieties. Due to highly pleomorphic plastic nature of the organism they can easily take the shape and contour of the host cell receptor. On the other hand mycoplasmas possess a high molecular weight protein called 'cytadhesin' responsible for such intimate attachment. Following adherence to the host cells, mycoplasmas may mediate the infection in various ways depending upon the nature of the toxin released by the bacteria. Most of the mycoplasmas compete with the host cells for the vital nutritional components which may often lead to loss of structural and functional integrity of the host cell. Non-fermenting mycoplasmas use arginine hydrolase pathway for ATP generation. Thus, the host cells are deprived of arginine and the protein synthesis is disrupted with exhaustion of arginine reserve.

Most of the mycoplasmas have definite site of predilection with the mesenchymal cells surrounding the serous membrane like bone joints, urogenital system and respiratory system. In respiratory tract the bacteria cause defoliation of cilia and impairment of the mucociliary defense. It may invite other pathogens to invade and as a result the pneumonia develops. Again mycoplasmas can cause infection synergistically with other pathogen to increase the disease severity. For example, *M. hyopnemoniae* can cause infection in association with porcine respiratory and reproductive syndrome virus in pigs.

Many mycoplasmas (*M. bovis, M. pulmonis, M. gallisepticum*) have their unique genetic ability to rapidly change the structure and expression of the outer surface lipoprotein to avoid identification by the host immune system.

Diseases produced

Pathogen	Host	Disease
M. gallisepticum	Chicken, Turkey	Chronic respiratory disease (CRD) is characterized by nasal discharge, coughing, sneezing, sinusitis, respiratory rales, conjunctivitis and frequently infraorbital sinusitis in turkeys. Clinical manifestations are usually slow to develop and the infection may have a long course.
M. meleagradis	Chicken, Turkey	Infectious synovitis particularly of the wing and hock joint and air sacculitis
M. synoviae	Turkey	Air sacculitis, toe and leg abnormalities and decrease egg hatchability
M. iowae	Turkey and chicken	Air sacculitis, toe and leg deformity, decreased hatchability
M. hyopneumoniae	Pigs	Enzootic porcine pneumonia characterized by coughing, chronic pneumonia, reduced growth rate, feed efficiency and prostration
M. hyosynoviae	Young and feeder pigs	Arthritis characterized by swollen hock joint and osteoarthritis
M. hyorhinis	Young Pigs	Polyserotitis and arthritis
M. mycoides sub sp. *mycoides* Small Colony type	Cattle	Contagious bovine pleuroneumonia (CBPP) is characterized by respiratory distress evident after exercise, fibrinous pneumonia with necrosis, inflammation of the lung membranes. It is prevalent in Subsaharan Africa, parts of Middle East, Central Asia including India (Assam)
M. bovis	Cattle	Mastitis, arthritis and abortion
M. bovigenitalum	Cattle	Mastits, abortion and endometritis
M. diversum	Cattle	Genital tract infection
M. mycoides sub sp. *mycoides* Large Colony type	Sheep and goat	Respiratory disorders with pneumonia in kids
M. mycoides sub sp. *capripneumonae* (F-38 and PG-3 strains)	Sheep and goat	Contagious caprine pleuroneumonia (CCPP) is characterized by coughing, fever and extensive pleurisy and pneumonia
M. capricolum sub sp. *capricolum*	Sheep and goat	Mastisis, pneumonia, septicemia and arthritis.
M. agactiae	Sheep and goat	Contagious agalactia characterized by mastitis, polyarthritis and keratoconjunctivitis
M. ovipneumoniae	Sheep and goat	Pneumonia along with *M. haemolytica*
M. conjunctivae	Sheep and goat	Keratoconjunctivitis.

Laboratory examinations

Clinical samples

The clinical samples are throat or nasopharyngeal swab, bronchoalveolar lavage, tracheal aspirate, affected tissue specimen (lung or ear canal), exudates and milk. Genital *Mycoplasma* may be isolated from urethral, vaginal and cervical swabs, semen and urine. Other important sites where the bacteria can be located are synovial fluid or aspirate, amniotic fluid, blood, cerebrospinal fluid and pericardial fluid. The biopsy specimens include endometrium, fallopian tubes, placenta and aborted foetus. Because of the fastidious nature of the bacteria, the specimens should be collected and deposited into the laboratory as soon as possible. Various commercially available media can be used for transporting swabs. Standard *Mycoplasma* broth may also be used for this purpose. In the laboratory, the samples can be preserved at 4^0C for 24hours and at -70^0C for a week. During transport the samples should be carried with dry ice or liquid nitrogen. Urogenital secretion or urine should be centrifuged to collect the precipitate for inoculation.

Laboratory examinations

Direct examination: Contrast phase microscopy, dark phase illumination techniques can be used for direct visualization of *Mycoplasma*. It is inconclusive when it is not supported with other tests.

Isolation of bacteria from clinical samples: Media, incubation condition and colony characteristics are described earlier. Direct or indirect immunofluorescence on colony impressions, colony epifluorescence or immunoperoxidase staining of the colonies may be employed.

Serological tests: In growth inhibition test (GIT) antisera impregnated disks or antisera are placed in wells for demonstration of mycoplasmal growth inhibition in and around the well. Similarly metabolic inhibition test (MIT) is based on colour change using a pH indicator. Other tests include CFT, ELISA and FAT.

Digitonin sensitivity test: For differentiation of *Mycoplasma* and *Acholeplasma*, digitonin sensitivity test is performed. Large zone of inhibition will be noticed around the paper disc impregnated with 1.5% of digitonin in case of *Mycoplasma.*

Dienes' staining: It can differentiate mycoplasmal colony with bacterial L-form. Both of them appear similar physically. The L-form colonies decolourize rapidly with the application of Dienes' stain, whereas, mycoplasmal colonies retain the stain.

Molecular biology: PCR based detection of specific DNA sequences, RAPD based method for strain differentiation, restriction enzyme analysis and sequencing of 16SrRNA are the alternative methods practiced currently.

Prevention and control

Following measures can be taken to prevent and control *M. gallisepticum* infection in poultry farms

a) Using breeding stock free of *M. gallisepticum*

b) Maintenance of strict biosecurity measures

c) Vaccination: The killed *M. gallisepticum* bacterin can be used to reduce the colonization of the infection but the bacterin cannot eliminate it. Formaldehyde, binary ethylenimine, liposome, iota-carrageenan and saponin are used as inactivating agents. The bacterins are not preferred in long term control program in poultry farms specially with multiple age groups. In pullet and layers, live vaccine containing *M. gallisepticum* Connecticut F strain is used. In broilers experimental vaccination with live F strain provided protection against airsacculitis. Later before administering F-vaccine priming with another live vaccine containing more attenuated strains (6/85 and ts-11) was suggested as Connecticut F strain was found highly virulent in few birds. Priming generated better resistance against *M. gallisepticum*. The ts-11 strain is temperature sensitive strain (reduced growth at 39°C) generated from an Australian field isolate (strain 80083). The ts-11 strain is non-pathogenic for chicken and turkey as it cannot produce cytadhesin (GapA). The 6/85 strain is also non-pathogenic for chicken but isolated from turkeys showing clinical syndrome. The recombinant fowl pox- *M. gallisepticum* vaccine was experimentally produced which was found safe in chickens. In India, live vaccine (strain MG 6/85) against *M. gallisepticum* is commercially available which can be administered in the chickens above 6 weeks of age. The commercially available killed bacterin (strain MG S6/85) can be administered at 3 weeks of age but not preferred just before laying.

Haemotrophic *Mycoplasma*

This group is constituted of the bacteria previously known as *Eperythrozoon* and *Haemobertonella*.

Properties of the genus

1. *Morphology*: Gram-negative, obligate intracellular bacteria that were not grown successfully in artificial culture. The bacteria are rod-shaped, spherical or ring-shaped and are found individually or in chains across the red blood cell surface. They do not contain cell wall and are small (0.3-3 μm in diameter) pleomorphic bacteria. However, they are enclosed by a single limiting membrane. They are found in shallow depressions and deep infoldings on the erythrocyte surface.

2. *Eperythrozoon* and *Haemobertonella* multiply by binary fission. They are dependent on host cells for amino acids, cholesterol, vitamins, and fatty acids. For such complex and specific growth requirements it is not possible to isolate the bacteria in artificial media.
3. *Classification:* *Haemobartonella* and *Eperythrozoon* were earlier classified under the family *Anaplasmataceae.* On the basis of few properties such as lack of cell wall, use of the codon UGA to encode tryptophan and 16S rRNA gene sequences *Eperythrozoon* and *Haemobartonella* are reassigned under the genus *Mycoplasma.* Although it is still under debate and the bacteria are given the '*Candidatus*' status under the genus *Mycoplasma*. They are commonly known as 'haemotropic mycoplasma' or 'haemoplasma'.
4. The bacteria are susceptible to tetracycline.
5. *Genome:* The full-length genome of *Eperythrozoon suis* is 745 Kbp. In *Mycoplasma hemofelis* (*Haemobartonella felis*) the average genome size is about 1200 Kbp. They have low (G+C) content.

Pathogenesis

Transmission

a) *Eperythrozoon* and *Haemobartonella* are transmitted mechanically by arthropods. Lice and ticks are the main ways of transmission but fleas and mosquitoes may also cause transmission.

b) *Haemobartonella felis* can also be transmitted within uterus.

c) Transmission may occur via surgical procedures through blood contamination of instruments (Mules operation in sheep, needle contamination during vaccination).

Pathogenesis

The adherence mechanism of the haemotrophic bacteria on the surface of erythrocyte is still unclear. It seems that several gene(s) encoding adhesins and bacterial fibrils play a crucial role on their adherence on the RBC surface. The interaction of the pathogens on the surface membrane of the RBCs may cause certain degree of disruption and destruction of the erythrocytes with increased cellular fragility.

Host immune response seems to play a major factor for anaemia. Haemotrophic bacteria are removed from the surface of the RBCs by spleenic and lymph node capillary endothelial cells and the macrophages. IgM cold agglutinins and other auto-antibodies were reported with haemotrophic bacteria infections.

The antibodies misdirected against the non-parasitized RBCs are responsible for massive damage and anaemia.

Diseases produced

Pathogens	Host	Vector	Diseases
Haemobartonella felis/ Mycoplasma haemofelis	Cat	Flea	Feline infectious anaemia is characterized by acute fatal haemolytic anaemia or chronic weight loss and weakness
Mycoplasma haemocanis / Haemobartonella canis	Dogs	*Rhipicephalous sanguineus*	Canine Haemobartonellosis is characterized by progressively fatal anaemia and death. Clinical manifestation is not apparent.
Epierythrozoon (Mycoplasma) ovis	Sheep	Mosquito, sand fly, sheep ked (*Melophagus ovinus*)	Caprine/ Ovine epierythrozoonosis is associated with anaemia and cranial edema and high mortality in kids
Epierythrozoon (Mycoplasma) suis	Pigs	hog louce, mosquitoes (*Aedes aegypti*) and bitting flies (*Stomoxys calcitrans*)	Porcine epierythrozoonosis with symptoms like acute haemolytic anaemia, weakness, poor growth and sudden death

Diagnosis

Diagnosis is based on demonstration of the pathogen in the blood smear. Other diagnostic tests include serological tests like indirect fluorescent test (IFT), ELISA and molecular tools like PCR and sequencing of amplified products.

[The original chapter for the first edition of the book was contributed by Samiran Bandyopadhyay, ICAR- Indian Veterinary Research Institute, Eastern Regional Station, Kolkata, India]

28

Rickettsia, *Neorickettsia*, *Ehrlichia* *Anaplasma* and *Coxiella*

History of rickettsial infections went back to 16th century and it has long been associated with famine and war. Epidemic typhus had major impact to decide over the outcome of several wars. The epidemic alone killed or caused great sufferings to over 1,00,000 people during World Wars. However, the causative agent was not determined until the early part of the 20th century. Rocky Mountain spotted fever (RMSF) was the first detected rickettsial infection in 1896 in Idaho Valley, USA. It was originally known as 'black measles' due to its clinical appearance in the form of characteristic spotted rash throughout the body. Howard Taylor Ricketts, an American pathologist for the first time described the causative agent of Rocky Mountain spotted fever and was able to isolate it in the laboratory animals during 1902-1909. He was a dedicated scientist and on several occasions injected himself with the pathogen for experiment. The causative pathogen of Rocky Mountain spotted fever, *Rickettsia rickettsii* was named after him. Later, the family *Rickettsiaceae* as well as the order Rickettsiales was named after him. Ernest William Goodpasture, an American pathologist and physician, invented the methods of isolation and culturing the rickettsial pathogens in chicken embryos and fertilized chicken eggs.

Properties of genus

1. *Morphology*: *Rickettsia* is minute, Gram-negative coccobacillus or short rod. They are usually 0.8-2.0 µm long and 0.3-0.5 µm wide. They do not possess any kind of flagella and so they are non-motile. Rickettsial cells are enclosed in loosely attached capsule. Beneath the capsule the bacteria have 7-10 nm thick typical Gram-negative cell wall consist of glucosamine, muramic acid, amino sugar, LPS, peptidoglycan, a major 135 kDa outer membrane protein (OmpB) and a 17 kDa lipoprotein. In spotted fever group *Rickettsia*, a surface exposed protein (OmpA) was also detected in the cell wall. However, the teichoic acid is absent in all the rickettsial groups. The bacteria have a 5-7 nm thick trilaminar cytoplasmic membrane. They have 70S ribosome in the cytoplasm. *Rickettsia* can be stained with Giemsa, Castaneda, Gimenez and

Macchiavello stains but poorly with Gram's stain. They appear deep red with Gimenez and Macchiavello, and purple with Giemsa.

2. *Classification:* The established genera under the family *Rickettsiaceae* are *Rickettsia*, *Neorickettsia*, *Diplorickettsia* and *Orientia.* The family *Piscirickettsiaceae* consists of a single valid genus *Piscirickettsia* and few other 'child taxa'. The genera *Ehrlichia*, *Cowdria*, *Coxiella* and *Wolbachia* are removed from the *Rickettsiaceae* family. Another family *Anaplasmataceae* was created to include *Ehrlichia*, *Anaplasma* and *Wolbachia.*

The genus *Rickettsia* is sub-divided into two groups

i) Typhus group: It contains *R. typhi* and *R. prowazekii*

ii) Spotted fever group: It encompasses *R. africae*, *R. akari*, *R. australis*, *R. conorii*, *R. japonica*, *R. honei*, *R. japonica*, *R. montana*, *R. rickettsia* and *R. ripicephali.*

According to the recent classification based on sequence analysis of conserved genes like 16s rDNA, citrate synthase, and outer membrane proteins there are 30 species under the genus *Rickettsia.* The major pathogenic species are *R. akari*, *R. conorii*, *R. felis*, *R. prowazekii*, *R. rickettsii* and *R. typhi.* Other important rickettsiae are *Neorickettsia helminthoeca*, *Diplorickettsia massiliensis*, *Piscirickettsia salmonis* and *Orientia tsutsugamushi.*

3. *Rickettsia* is obligatory intracellular bacterium and resides in cytoplasm or nucleus of host cells. The bacteria multiply by binary fission.

4. They have the ability to exchange ATP for ADP in intracellular environment and are not viable on storage because of loss of their intracellular pool of ATP and various coenzymes. They are able to synthesize ATP via glutamate metabolism. So glutamate is the key nutrient for *Rickettsia.*

5. *Resistance*: *Rickettsia* is relatively fragile and cannot survive outside the host or extracellularly under ordinary conditions. In the dried biological samples like blood or faeces of the vectors they may remain viable for several months. The cultures can be preserved at -70°C. They are easily inactivated by physical and chemical agents such as 1% lysol, 2% formaldehyde, 5% hydrogen peroxide, 70% ethanol and hypochlorite solution containing 50-500 ppm chlorine.

6. *Natural habitat*: *Rickettsia* is normally parasite of the arthropods and replicate in the gut epithelium. They are maintained in the arthropod vectors by transovarian transmission. Following multiplication in the gut the bacteria are spread into the salivary glands and the vectors become infective to the hosts.

7. *Rickettsia* has both the properties of virus and bacteria. Like virus, they require live cells for their growth and multiplication. Therefore all the rickettsiae are cultivated in the cell culture or embryonated hen's egg except *Bartonella* (*Rickettsia*) *quintana* which can grow on artificial media. Like bacteria, they also possess typical Gram-negative cell wall structure.

8. *Genome:* The single chromosome is present at the center of the rickettsial cell. The molecular weight of the chromosome is $100\text{-}150\times10^6$dalton. Rickettsial genome has close resemblance with the eukaryotic mitochondrial genome. As the rickettsial pathogens are metabolically compromised they do not contain any gene for anaerobic glycolysis or the genes involved in the biosynthesis and regulation of amino acids and nucleosides. *Rickettsia* and eukaryotic mitochondria use other resources (nuclear or host) for generation of ATP. However, rickettsial genome contains a complete set of genes encoding for the tricarboxylic acid cycle (TCA) and the respiratory chain complex. The deciphered genome of *R. prowazekii* is 1,111,523 bp long and it contains 834 protein-coding genes. Recent evidence indicates that both *Rickettsia* and viruses share some genome fragment(s). Thus, it is not uncommon to see that human patients with rickettsial infections express immune response against Retrovirus (HIV) and Flavivirus (dengue fever).

Isolation

Rickettsia cannot live or grow in cell free artificial media and are grown either in tissue or embryo cultures. Chicken embryos are commonly used for their growth and multiplication. They require various exogenous cofactors from animal cell. Growth generally takes in the cytoplasm of the cells. However, spotted fever group of rickettsial pathogens grow in the nucleus. Embryonated hen egg during 5th or 6th day of development is highly susceptible to the bacteria. Yolk sac route of inoculation is preferred. For optimum growth the egg after inoculation should be incubated at 33°C-35°C for 7-10 days.

Cell culture is not always ideal for isolation of *Rickettsia*. However, cell lines like mouse fibroblasts, MRC5, Vero, L-929, HeLa, HEp-2, and Detroit-6 are used. In cell culture, several weeks are required for optimum growth depending upon the rickettsial species.

Rickettsia may also be propagated in arthropods or by inoculation into adult male guinea pigs and mice. However, the process is cumbersome, time consuming and requires ethical approval.

Antigenic characteristics

Rickettsial pathogens possess three types of antigens

a) *Group specific soluble antigen*: The group specific antigens are the surface antigens and can be separated by centrifugation and washing of the bacteria.

b) *Species and strain specific antigen:* These antigens are associated with the cell wall of the bacteria.

c) *Alkali stable polysaccharides*: The polysaccharides are found in some rickettsial strains and few strains of *Proteus*. The common antigenic determinant present in both the bacteria is the basis of Weil-Felix reaction used for the diagnosis of rickettsial infection in human.

Toxins and virulence factors produced

Rickettsia produces two types of toxins which can have severe impact over the host. They have endotoxin like lipopolysaccharide (LPS) which is different from other Gram-negative bacteria. Rickettsial LPS can stimulate protective antibody response in the host. Therefore, the endotoxin activity can be neutralized by the antiserum.

The rickettsial pathogens produce a haemolysin which can cause haemolysis of sheep and rabbit RBCs.

Intravenous administration of UV irradiated *Rickettsia* in rats and mice was proved fatal and was reported to cause death by damage in capillary endothelial cells, loss of plasma, decrease in blood volume and shock.

Spotted fever group of rickettsial pathogens are known to liberate phospholipase A2 that degrades phospholipids in the cell membrane causing haemolysis and other degenerative changes in various tissues and internal organs. Several necrotizing toxins are also detected from rickettsial pathogens which can cause damage to the endothelial cells, thrombosis, thrombocytopaenia and disseminated intravascular coagulation.

Rickettsia has the outer membrane protein (Omp) on their surface acting as an adhesin to attach to the host cells via a protein dependent receptor (virulence factor).

Pathogenesis

Transmission

Rickettsia is transmitted by bite or faeces of an infected arthropod vector. *Rickettsia* replicates in the gut epithelium of the arthropods and later migrates into the salivary gland and the ovarian tissues. Faeces of the vectors are major source of infection. Other portals of infection like ingestion of contaminated food or inhalation of dried faeces of the vectors is also possible. The contamination of respiratory tract or conjunctiva with faeces of infected vectors rarely causes infection. The reservoirs of rickettsial infection are flying squirrels (typhus fever), rodents (murine or endemic typhus) and migratory birds (scrub typhus).

Pathogenesis

Rickettsial organisms cannot multiply outside the host cells. However, they are able to synthesize protein independently. In the vectors (ticks or other arthropods) they multiply in the epithelium and are transferred into the salivary glands or ovarian tissues. On entry into animal host, they attach themselves with a protein dependent receptor on the host cell membrane by their outer membrane protein-A functioning as adhesin.

Rickettsial pathogens are endocytosed into the blood vessels. The bacteria multiply in the cell cytoplasm escaping the phagosome by lysis of phagosomal membrane using their phospholipase. The bacteria acquire nutrients from cytosol as well as nucleus. Infected endothelial cells produce reactive oxygen species (ROS) that cause degradation of the membrane through lipid peroxidation. Haemolysis and other degenerative effects are common due to degradation of phospholipids of host cell membrane by phospholipase A_2 produced by *Rickettsia*. The pathogens can gradually disseminate into whole body via blood stream. Thrombi formation is very common because of hyperplasia of infected endothelial cells of the blood vessels.

Disease produced

Organisms	Vector	Host	Diseases
Rickettsia rickettsii	Tick (*Dermacentor* sp.)	Human, rodents, dog	Rocky Mountain spotted fever (RMSF) is characterized by anorexia, vomition, diarrhoea, lymphadenopathy, ecchymotic mucous membrane, dyspnoea, joint and muscle pain
Rickettsia prowazekii	Lice (*Xenopsylla cheopis*)	Human	Epidemic typhus, Brill-Zinsser disease (high fever, chill, headache, myalgia, macular rash, malaise, pneumonia, gangrene of extremities)
Rickettsia typhi	Fleas	Humans, squirrel fleas, flying squirrels, wild rodents	Endemic typhus (Fever, headache, myalgia and malaise); murine typhus
Rickettsia felis	Flea	Cat, human	Cat flea typhus

Organisms	Vector	Host	Diseases
Rickettsia akari	Mite	Mites, wild rodents	Rickettsial pox (fever, papulovascular rash)
Rickettsia conorii	Tick	Human	Buttonneuse fever
Rickettsia africae	Tick	Human	African tick bite fever
Rickettsia sibirica	Tick	Human	North Asian Tick typhus
Rickettsia japonica	Tick	Human	Japanese spotted fever
Rickettsia australis	Tick	Human	Queensland tick typhus
Rickettsia (Bartonella) quintana	Human body louse	Human	Trench fever
Orientia tsutsugamushi	Mites	Human, dogs	Scrub typhus
Piscirickettsia salmonis	unknown	Salmon fish	Piscirickettsiosis

Diagnosis

Clinical samples: Heparinized blood collected during acute phase of infection is useful for direct or immunocytologic detection of *Rickettsia*. Blood can be stored at 4°C if isolation and detection is done within 24 hours after collection. Punch biopsy samples (3 mm) collected from skin lesions and biopsy specimens from chronic hepatitis may serve the purpose. It is always better to collect the specimen from the patients before the treatment starts. Endolymph of ticks and different organs of the hosts after post mortem can also be collected as samples.

Laboratory examinations

Direct examination: Impression smear prepared from the blood, organs of the infected animals and endolymphs of the ticks may be stained for visualization of the bacteria or it can be processed for direct or indirect immunofluorescence tests. In tissue smear *Rickettsia* are usually seen as bipolar rods occurring near cells or free in the cytoplasm. *R. rickettsii* can be detected in the nuclei of infected cells.

Direct and indirect immunofluorescence techniques are also employed for detection of *Rickettsia* and these techniques have better sensitivity and specificity in compared to classical staining methods. In direct immunofluorescence technique, fluorescein conjugated antiserum is used for detection of antigen in the frozen and paraffin embedded formalin fixed tissue sections.

Monoclonal antibodies against lipopolysaccharide of *Rickettsia* (typhus group) are also used to detect the pathogen by immunoperoxidase staining of formalin fixed, paraffin embedded tissues specimen from the affected patients.

Isolation of Rickettsia from clinical samples: Due to their high pathogenicity, isolation of rickettsial pathogens is performed only in few laboratories equipped with appropriate safety provisions. Heparin anti-coagulated plasma and buffy coat from the suspected patients are excellent source of pathogens for isolation. The isolation techniques are described earlier.

Serological tests

a) Indirect immunofluorescence assay (IFA), enzyme immune assay (EIA) is commonly performed to detect IgG specific to rickettsial antigen. Negative results and low titer is possible in early phase of infection.

b) Latex agglutination test kits are available, containing latex beads coated with an extracted rickettsial protein-carbohydrate complex with LPS. It is used to detect anti-rickettsial IgM. This is effective only in acute phase of infection.

c) Complement fixation test is very specific but its sensitivity is low.

Although, IFA and western blot are preferred, presence of species specific OmpA, OmpB and group specific LPS antigen impedes the development of species specific serodiagnosis. Diagnostic tools involving recombinant rickettsial antigens are a promising option for this purpose. A recombinant 56-kDa surface protein from *Orientia tsutsugamushi* was demonstrated to be effective for serodiagnosis of scrub typhus.

Animal inoculation test: The test is practiced for detection of endemic (murine) typhus. When an adult male guinea pig is inoculated with blood from a patient with endemic typhus or with a culture of *R. typhi,* it develops severe fever and a characteristic scrotal inflammation. Due to formation of inflammatory adhesions between the layers of tunica vaginalis, the testes cannot be pushed back to abdomen. This is known as 'Neil-Mooser reaction' or 'tunica reaction'.

Molecular biology: Polymerase chain reaction (PCR) is widely employed to detect rickettsial pathogens in peripheral blood, buffy coat, plasma, tissue specimen, tissue aspiration from patients and arthropod vectors. The 17 kDa lipoprotein gene is known to be conserved among all the pathogenic *Rickettsia* and is used as principal target in PCR. Other genes like citrate synthase, 16S rRNA and OmpA are also amplified by PCR. The restriction fragment length polymorphism (RFLP) is used for species-specific identification.

Coxiella

The disease was first detected among abattoir workers in Brisbane (Australia) by Edward Holbrook Derrick in 1933. As the etiology was unknown during that period, it was referred as Q ('Q' stands for 'query') fever. Sir Frank Macfarlane Burnet, an Australian virologist first identified the agent as *Rickettsia* and Herald Rea Cox and Gordon Davis at the Rocky mountain laboratory (RML) in United States isolated the organism from tick. *Rickettsia burneti* was later renamed as *Coxiella burnetii*.

Properties of the genus

1. *Morphology: C. burnetii* is an obligate intracellular, pleomorphic coccobacillary bacterium with Gram-negative cell wall measuring 0.2-0.4 µm wide and 0.4-1 µm long. Gimenez method of staining is suitable for demonstration of the bacteria in clinical samples. The bacteria are obligatory intracellular in nature. The intracellular replication takes place within the vacuole present in host cellular cytoplasm. The vacuole containing *C. burnetii* is gradually converted into the phago-lysosome with the characteristics of acidic pH and secreation of acid hydrolysate and cationic peptide. *C. burnetii* liberates basic proteins which help in buffering the acidic environment of the phago-lysosome.

There are two forms of *C. burnetii*, known as 'small cell variant (SCV)' and 'large cell variant (LCV)'present in the growth cycle. The SCV is metabolically inactive, endospore like, non-replicating form, whereas, the LCV acts as the replicating form. SCVs appear as small rods with condensed chromatin, thick envelope and internal membrane. LCVs are larger in size and the cells contain disseminated chromatin. The LCV cell is covered with typical Gram-negative cell wall.

2. *Classification*: Previously it was considered under the family *Rickettsiaceae*. At present, based on gene-sequence analysis *Coxiella* is placed under the order Legionellales and family *Coxiellaceae.* The established species under the genus is *C. burnetii*.

3. *Resistance:* The SCVs of *Coxiella* are extremely stable in the environment. The SCV is resistant to heat and drying and can remain infectious in milk (> 40 months), meat (> 1 month), water, soil, dried blood and wool (7-10 months). They are able to survive in phago-lysosome at pH 5.0. Due to its survival in soil and aerosol, it can be transmitted as an airborne infection. The SCV can withstand holding method of milk pasteurization (63°C for 30 minutes) and is at borderline of inactivation in flash method (72°C for 20 minutes). They are also resistant to ultraviolet ray, desiccation and common

disinfectants like sodium hypochlorite, quaternary ammonium and phenolic compounds. However, it can be inactivated by 2% formaldehyde, 1% lysol and 5% hydrogen peroxide. The increased resistance of SCV to physical and chemical disinfection is associated with high number of cross-links in their peptidoglycan, up-regulation of genes encoding the proteins associated with oxidative stress response, cell wall remodeling, and arginine acquisition. Due to stability in the external environment and spread through inhalation route *C. burnetii* is categorized as biological threat agent and it can be used in bioterrorism.

4. *Natural habitat*: *C. burnetii* (SCV) can persist in the environment for prolonged period. The cattle, sheep and goats are natural reservoir of the bacteria from which the zoonotic transmission into human may occur. The kangaroo and wallabies in Australia and sloths were also found to be the source of *C. burnetii* infection in human. The bacteria are also isolated from hard ticks (*Dermacentor andersoni, Haemaphysalis humerosa*), soft ticks, bed bugs, flies and mites. The ticks are probably not essential for the bacterial transmission in domestic animals.

5. *Genome*: In 2003, the first genome of *C. burnetii* (RSA493 strain) was sequenced. The genome consists of a chromosome (1,995,275 bp) and a plasmid (QpI11, 37,393 bp). It contains 719 hypothetical coding sequences, 83 pseudogenes and 29 insertion sequences (IS). Later whole genome sequencing of other strains revealed that *C. burnetii* strains share strong similarity at genome level ('pangenome').

Isolation

Coxiella are routinely propagated in various cell lines such as monkey kidney cells, HeLa, Vero, DH82, L929, XTC and mouse macrophages. The cell lines inoculated with the specimens are kept in shell vials. The vials are incubated at 37°C with 5% CO_2 for 5-7 days.

Recently few laboratories developed experiential medium for cell-free cultivation of *C. burnetii* such as Vero cell extract medium (VCEM) and acidified cysteine citrate medium (ACCM2). However isolation of *C. burnetii* in solid artificial media is still not possible.

Pathogenesis

Transmission

Ruminants act as primary reservoir and shed *C. burnetii* through faeces, urine, milk, sperm, reproductive discharge and birth products. The shedding of the bacteria may also take place from other reservoirs such as birds, reptiles, ticks and marine mammals. Parturient dogs and cats are also important source of human infection. Transmission of *C. burnetii* to human occurs chiefly through the inhalation route. Consumption of raw milk from infected cow and goat may result symptomatic infection in humans. It causes occupational hazards for farmers, veterinarians and abattoir workers. Human to human transmission is rare although transmission of *C. burnetii* took place in few nosocomial cases and during transfusion of contaminated blood. In animal farms, transmission of *C. burnetii* occurs through inhalation of dust particles containing SCVs, direct contact and introduction of new animals without quarantine. Although the bacteria are commonly isolated from ticks, flies, mites and bed bugs the ticks are not found necessary for transmission of infection from the reservoirs.

Pathogenesis

Following entry through respiratory routes, the SCVs of *C. burnetii* invade monocytes and macrophages in human and animals. Alveolar macrophage and Kupffer cells are susceptible and may become infected following haematogenous dissemination. *C. burnetii* can withstand low pH of the phagolysosome. Metabolism and multiplication is enhanced in acidic environment. Replication through binary fission occurs exclusively inside the phagolysosome. The organism may localize in the female reproductive tract and mammary glands.

Disease produced

Bacterium	Host	Disease
Coxiella burnetii	Human, ruminants (cattle, sheep and goats), pets, reptiles, birds and many species of arthropods like ticks, mites, fleas, lice and flies, crayfish and amoebae	**Q-fever:** Mostly *C. burnetii* causes mild infection in animals although some severe cases have been reported. Sporadic abortion, infertility and birth of weak offspring were reported in ruminants specially in sheep. In human, the infection is self-limiting and occurs in both acute and chronic forms. Common symptoms of acute form in human may include chest pain with breathing, clay-coloured stools, cough, fever, headache, jaundice, muscle pain, and shortness of breath. Symptoms of chronic form include chill, fatigueness and prolonged fever. Q-fever is detected throughout the world except New Zealand

Diagnosis

Clinical samples: In human, blood, serum, cardiac valves, surgical tissue biopsy specimens are collected for detection of *C. burnetii.* The handling of the bacteria requires biosafety level 3 (BSL3) facilities as they are categorized as potential biological threat agent. The clinical specimens can be stored at -80°C in the laboratory intended for isolation of the bacteria.

Laboratory examination

Diagnosis is based on combination of direct cytological examination, propagation of the organism, serology and detection of the organism through molecular techniques. Giemsa, Gimenez and modified ZN stained smear from placental and vaginal discharge may reveal clumps of red coccobacilli. The organism can also be demonstrated from placental smear using immunofluorescence based techniques.

The serological techniques are considered as first line diagnostic techniques in human. Different tests like CFT, micro-agglutination, indirect immunofluorescence and ELISA are used to detect specific antibodies. The indirect immunofluorescence is considered as reference technique. Anti-*C. burnetii* phase I and phase II antibodies are associated with persistent and primary infection in human, respectively. The antibody titer (phase II IgG or IgM) should increase four fold in the sera collected 3-6 weeks (convalescent phase) after the primary collection (acute phase). Detection of *C. burnetii* – specific interferon-gamma (IFNγ) in clinical samples is the new diagnostic assay.

DNA probe and polymerase chain reaction (PCR) are much more sensitive techniques for early detection of *C. burnetii* in human and animals targeting 16S-23S RNA, plasmids, superoxide dismutase, *com1* gene, and IS*1111* repetitive elements. The real-time PCR (qPCR) targeting IS*1111* of *C. burnetii* is found most sensitive and less time consuming than conventional PCR. Immuno-PCR can detect *C. burnetii* in sera samples collected during the first two weeks of the infection with better sensitivity than ELISA or indirect immunofluorescence.

Prevention and control

C. burnetii infection in livestock farm is not significant enough to introduce any specific control program. Experimental vaccination trial with bacterin successfully prevented the infection in animals.

Following precautions should be taken by the high-risk professionals to prevent the zoonotic infection.

a) Milk and milk products should not be consumed without pasteurization

b) Vaccination of high-risk professionals in few countries such as Australia was successful.

Anaplasma

The intracellular pathogen *Anaplasma marginale* was first described by Sir Arnold Theiler in 1910. The pathogen is endemic worldwide specially in tropical and subtropical countries. Bovine anaplasmosis was formerly known as 'gall sickness'. In 1978, J.W. Harvey first reported *Anaplasma platys* in dogs suffering with the clinical syndrome known as 'canine infectious cyclic thrombocytopenia'. Madewell and Gribble (1982) first detected *Anaplasma phagocytophilum* to cause 'granulocytic anaplasmosis' in dogs in California.

Properties of the genus

1. *Morphology*: *Anaplasma* are small (0.3-0.4μm), Gram-negative, obligate intracellular, non- motile and pleomorphic (coccoid to ellipsoidal) bacteria. In the mammalian cells they are present within the membrane bound cytoplasmic vacuoles where they obtain the nutrients. They may appear in the mammalian cells as small dense core or large reticulate forms. The inclusion body (morula) formed within the cells is up to 4 μm in size. *Anaplasma phagocytophilum* are Gram-negative cocci (0.2-2μm) which can produce inclusion bodies / morulae within the monocytes. *Anaplasma platys* appears as spherical, oval or bean shaped blue inclusions (0.35-1.25 μm) in platelets. The morulae appear bluish- purple when stained with Romanowsky and Giemsa, in contrast to the deep violet coloured nuclear material of the host cells. They are poorly stained by Gimenez method. However, acridine orange can be used for easy staining of *Anaplasma*. The bacteria do not form spore or other resistant forms. Unlike other Gram-negative bacteria, *Anaplasma phagocytophilum* lacks peptidoglycan layer. There is no evidence of lipopolysaccharide or lipooligosaccharide. It lacks the genes necessary for the synthesis of lipid A and peptidoglycan.

2. *Anaplasma* multiply by binary fission.

3. *Anaplasma* is able to carry out major metabolic pathways including glycolysis, citric acid cycle and the pentose phosphate pathway. It is able to metabolize sugars such as pentose, fructose and mannose.

4. *Classification:* According to recent taxonomic classification based on 16s rRNA gene and *groESL* operon sequence analysis, *Anaplasma* with other genera like *Ehrlichia* and *Wolbachia* belong to the family *Anaplasmataceae*. Currently the genus consists of 17 species. Major pathogenic species are *A. bovis, A. ovis, A. merginale, A. centrale, A. phagocytophilum*, *A. phagocytophila, A. platys* and *A. caudatum*.

5. *Resistance:* Due to absence of peptidoglycan *Anaplasma* are fragile cells and are highly susceptible to stress and decontaminants like alcohol, sodium

hypochlorite, silver nitrate, iodine and potassium permanganate. They are susceptible to tetracycline but resistant to beta-lactam group of antibiotics, aminoglycosides, macrolides, chloramphenicol and sulfa drugs. Fluoroquinone derivatives are found effective against the bacteria.

6. *Natural habitat:* The ticks (*Dermacentor*, *Ixodes, Rhipicephalus* and *Boophilus*) are the common vectors of the bacteria. Male ticks and biting flies may be responsible for mechanical transmission. In the ticks *Anaplasma* are maintained by transstadial transmission. Domestic and wild ruminants like cervids (deer) and rodents are the natural reservoirs. Recently intermediate hosts like helminths and snails are recorded.

7. *Genome:* A. *marginale* has a circular genome of 1200 kbp size with (G + C) content of 56 mol%. *A. phagocytophilum* also has a circular genome composed of 1471282 base pairs which can encode 1264 proteins. *A. phagocytophilum* genome contains no plasmids. *Anaplasma* requires sterol to maintain physical integrity of the membrane. However, they lack genes related to the biosynthesis or modification of cholesterol or other related sterols. All sterols are therefore directly taken from exogenous sources without extensive modification before incorporation into the membrane.

Isolation

Due to obligate intracellular nature *Anaplasma* cannot be isolated in artificial bacteriological media. Isolation can be done by inoculation of fresh or frozen blood from suspected animals into the laboratory animals. Moreover, *A. marginale* and *A. phagocytophila* can be cultured by inoculation of blood in tick cell lines. *A. phagocytophilum* can also be propagated in human granulocyte cell lines.

Antigenic characteristics

Anaplasma has immunodominant major surface proteins (msp) which are important for their immunogenic characterization. The proteins range from 36 to 49 kDa in size. The proteins are generally expressed by genes containing hyper variable sequences flanked by conserved sequences both at 5' and 3' ends. In *A. phagocytophila*, there are two major antigenic membrane proteins, p44 and msp2 on the membrane surface and both of which are approximately 44 kDa in size. *A. marginale, A. centrale* and *A. ovis* also possess a restricted set of msp gene(s) necessary for their multiplication in ticks. The major surface proteins are responsible for haemagglutinating activity and also act as adhesins. Additionally, the bacterium has a type-IV secretion system by which it is able to transfer virulence factors into the host.

Pathogenesis

Transmission

Mechanical transmission of *A. marginale* is possible by biting of blood sucking insects. The red blood cells of the insects are infected. Additionally, mechanical transmission also occurs through needles, dehorners, ear taggers, castrating knives, surgical, tattoo instruments and specially during blood transfusion. Face flies, houseflies, and other non-biting insects do not transmit the infection. Mechanical transmission of infected red blood cells must occur rapidly as the blood parasite does not survive more than a few minutes outside the host.

Anaplasma can also be transmitted through the biological vector. The parasite receives nourishment and may even multiply in the biological vector. Several biological vectors were recorded for anaplasmosis. The bacteria can remain active throughout the lifecycle of the tick and can be transmitted several months later.

A. phagocytophilum is zoonotic important and can infect humans through bite of infected ticks carrying the bacteria.

Pathogenesis

Infectious bacteria reside and replicate within the salivary gland of the vector and when the vector feed on the susceptible host the bacteria are transmitted. Within the host, infected erythrocytes are disrupted and the bacteria are released. They can invade other fresh erythrocytes. *Anaplasma* can damage erythrocytes by direct interaction and damage to the erythrocytic membrane. In the infected RBCs, *Anaplasma* forms vacuoles within the cytoplasmic membranes of the red blood cells and then undergo binary fission to form dense blue-purple round/cube shaped inclusion bodies.

The host during the infection develops auto-antibodies against infected RBCs. Thus, it may lead to autoimmune disorders causing haemolytic anaemia. The uninfected red blood cells are also destroyed in the process. When the number of blood cells being destroyed exceeds the number of blood cells that the body can produce, the animal becomes anaemic. It takes 4 to 8 weeks for clinical signs to appear after the animal is infected.

During the convalescent period the immunity against the pathogen declines and in absence of proper therapeutic measures, animals may become asymptomatic lifelong carrier and source of infection. Major surface proteins (msp) play a crucial role in the interaction of *A. marginale* with host cells that undergo antigenic change and selection in cattle, thus contributing to maintenance of persistent infections.

Disease produced

Bacteria	Host	Vector	Diseases
Anaplasma ovis	Sheep, goat	Rhipicephalus, Dermacentor, Ixodes, Boophilus	Ovine and caprine anaplasmosis (Anaemia, depression, fever, anorexia and low mortality)
Anaplasma marginale *Anaplasma central*	Cattle	Rhipicephalus, Dermacentor, Ixodes, Boophilus	Bovine anaplasmosis (Fever, anorexia, anaemia, icterus, hepato-spleenomegaly, weight loss, decreased fertility). A. centrale infection is mostly asymptomatic
Anaplasma bovis	Cattle	Amblyomma, Rhipicephalus, Hyalomma	Tropical bovine anaplasmosis (anaemia, weight loss, abortion)
Anaplasma caudatum	Cattle	Ixodes	Bovine anaplasmosis (anaemia, icterus, splenomegaly, erythrophagocytosis, cholestasis)
Anaplasma phagocytophila	Human, Horse, wild and domestic ruminants	Ixodes ricinus	a)Equine granulocytic anaplasmosis (thrombocytopaenia, leukopaenia, anaemia, myocardial vasculitis) b)Human granulocytic anaplasmosis (Fever, myalgia, headache, arthralgia, lymphadenomegaly, conjunctivitis, dysuria, and peripheral edema) c)Tick borne fever in wild and domestic ruminants (fever, anorexia and drop in milk yield)
Anaplasma phagocytophilum	Dogs	Ixodes ricinus, I. persulcatus	Lethargy, anorexia, fever, pale mucous membranes, tense abdomen, vomition, diarrhoea, lameness due to immune-mediated (neutrophilic) polyarthritis, mildly enlarged lymph nodes, tachypnea, surface bleeding (petechiae, melena, epistaxis) may occur. Rare signs include collapse, mild cough, scleral injection, uveitis, limb edema, polyuria and immune-mediated thrombocytopenia/anaemia.
Anaplasma platys	Dog	Rhipicephalus sanguineus	Canine infectious cyclic thrombocytopenia (generally asymptomatic but may be with anaemia, fever, depression, anorexia, uveitis, epistaxis, lymphadenopathy and ecchymotic or petechial haemorrhages)

Diagnosis

A presumptive diagnosis is made on the basis of clinical signs, haematological observations in the animals from endemic areas.

Laboratory examinations

Direct examination: Direct examination of blood smear is a crucial step for early diagnosis. *Anaplasma* appears as dense, homogeneously staining blue-purple inclusions (0.3-1.0 μm in diameter) in Giemsa stained thin blood films. *A. marginale* inclusions are usually located at margin of the RBC. In *A. centrale* infection the inclusion bodies are located centrally. *A. caudatum* cannot be distinguished in blood films. Possibility of *A. phagocytophilum* morula detection in clinically infected canines is more (60%) than other similar bacteria.

Serological tests: The serological tests for diagnosis are indirect fluorescent antibody technique (FAT), rapid card agglutination, complement fixation test (CFT) and msp5 ELISA.

The *msp5* gene encodes a 19 KDa protein conserved in all recognized *Anaplasma* species. An indirect ELISA (msp5 ELISA) was developed for the serological diagnosis of bovine anaplasmosis with purified recombinant major surface protein 5 (MSP5) of *Anaplasma marginale* produced in *E. coli.*

Ehrlichia

Ehrlichia ruminantium was first identified as the causative agent of 'heartwater' by Edmund Cowdry (1925), an American parasitologist when he successfully demonstrated the bacteria in the tissue of infected animals and ticks and named the organism *Rickettsia ruminantium*. This was later changed to *Cowdria ruminantium* and currently known as *Ehrlichia ruminantium*. In 1935, Donatien and Lestoquard first isolated *Ehrlichia canis* from the dogs infested with ticks and were suffering with fever and anaemia in Algeria. The genus *Ehrlichia* was named after the famous German microbiologist Paul Ehrlich. During the Vietnam war the dogs of United States army showed similar symptoms, known as 'tropical canine pancytopenia', later renamed as 'canine monocytic ehrlichiosis'(CME).

Properties of genus

1. *Morphology:* The ehrlichiae are group of small, Gram-negative, pleomorphic, obligate intracellular coccoid to ellipsoid bacteria that infect different blood cells in various animals and human. *E. canis* produces 1-20 inclusion bodies in the cytoplasm of canine endothelial cells of pulmonary vessel and reticuloendothelial cells of the alveolar septal wall. The inclusions

never fuse with one another or with the lysosomes. The inclusion bodies consist of vacuoles filled with 2-40 numbers of round to ovoid elementary bodies. Each of the elementary body is 0.5-0.9 µm in diameter. Each of the elementary body is covered with a cell wall and trilaminar plasma membrane. The cytoplasm of elementary bodies is divided into dense and pale areas. Each of the elementary body can undergo binary fission to generate initial bodies. The initial bodies are enclosed in vacuole to produce 'morula'. The inclusion bodies / morulae appear as deep bluish purple in blood slides stained with Giemsa, Gimenez, Romanowsky, Wright and Diff-Quick stains (Figure 1).

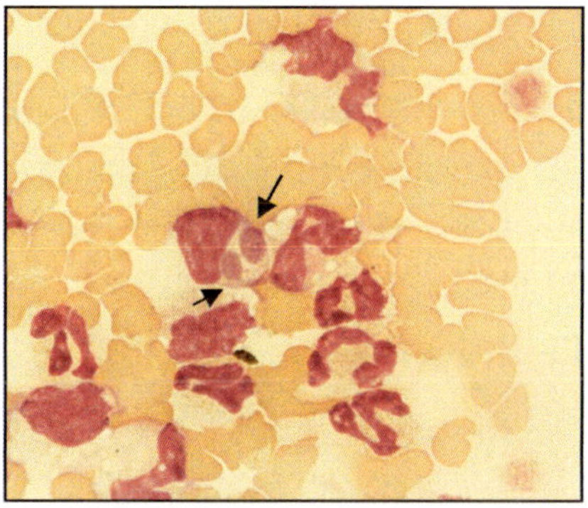

Fig. 1: Demonstration of *Ehrlichia canis* (morula) in canine monocyte (*Courtesy*: Gad Baneth, Director, Koret School of Veterinary Medicine, Hebrew University, Israel)

2. *Classification*: According to the recent 16S rRNA gene sequence analysis *Ehrlichia* belongs to the family *Anaplasmataceae.* The genus currently consists of 19 species. The pathogenic species are *E. canis*, *E. chaffeensis*, *E. ewingii*, *E. muris* and *E. ruminantium*.

3. *Natural habitat:* The tick (*Rhipicephalus sanguineus* sensu lato, brown dog tick; *Ixodes persulcatus*) usually acts as vector of *E. canis*. The temperature above 6°C and sufficient humidity are required for survival of the ticks. The ticks undergo hibernation in the cracks of kennels and houses during winter in temperate countries. The ticks show highest activity during spring to autumn season. Chronically infected animals without clinical manifestation may serve as reservoir of *Ehrlichia*. Wild white-tailed deer (*Odocoileus virginianus*) severs as reservoir for *E. chaffeensis*. Likewise, rabbits and deer serve as natural reservoir for *E. ruminantium*.

4. *Genome:* Little is known about genomic organization of *Ehrlichia*. The study with *E. ruminantium* revealed that the genome size ranges from 1,499,920 to 1,512,977 bp long. The (G+C) content is around 27-28 mol%. *E. canis* genome consists of a single circular chromosome of 1,315030 bp to encode 925 proteins, 40 stable RNA species, 17 putative pseudo genes and several noncoding regions.

Isolation

Ehrlichia can be cultivated in mammalian or tick borne cell lines. *E. ruminantium* can be grown in monocyte-macrophage cell lines from mice and dogs and also in a human leukaemia cell line (HL60). Whereas, *E. phagocytophila* is cultivated in two continuous cell lines, IDE8 and ISE6, derived from the temperate hard tick *Ixodes scapularis*. *E. chaffeensis* can be successfully cultivated in mouse embryo, Vero, Buffalo green monkey (BGM) and L929 cells. Mouse macrophage cell line (J774) and canine histiocyte cell line can be used to culture *E. canis* and *E. muris*, respectively.

Pathogenesis

Transmission

The infection occurs through salivary secreations during ingestion of a blood meal following tick bite. Mechanical transmission through contaminated inanimate inoculating objects or through blood transfusion from infected animal is also possible. If the adult tick (*Rhipicephalus sanguineus*) engorges on the dog during the acute stage, it can transmit *E. canis* to other dogs for at least 155 days following detachment. *E. canis* is maintained in tick population (*Rhipicephalus sanguineus*) by transstadial transmission i.e. the tick acquires the bacteria by feeding on an infected dog in either the larvae or nymph stage and then the tick transmits the infection to another dog as either the nymph or adult stage. All canine breeds are susceptible to *E. canis* but severe infection occurs in German Shepherd and Siberian Huskies. No age and sex predisposition to *E. canis* infection was detected in dogs. *E. canis* is not considered as zoonotic pathogen.

E. ruminantium is extremely fragile and cannot persist outside of the host for few hours and is transmitted only by ticks of the genus *Amblyomma.*

Pathogenesis

In canine ehrlichiosis the mononuclear cells are attracted to the site of tick bite and the cells also carry the engulfed pathogens into the lymph nodes. However, the pathogens are disseminated to various locations including endoreticular cells of lymph nodes, spleen, liver and the pathogens multiply in mononuclear macrophages as well as in the lymphocytes. The bacteria are released by exocytosis and cell lysis. The infection may lead to varieties of haematological and immunological disorders and coagulation dysfunction. Development of extensive vasculitis may lead to platelet consumption and sequestration leading to thrombocytopaenia. Moreover, development of anti-platelet antibodies may also have a role for this. Due to persisting thrombocytopaenia, haemorrhage may take place as exhibited in the form of bilateral epistaxis.

In bovine ehrlichiosis (heartwater disease) *E. ruminantium* is engulfed by the mononuclear phagocytic cells from the general blood circulation. Further replication takes place in lymph nodes and spleen. Damage may occur in the microvasculature of brain leading to increased intracerebral pressure with central nervous system disorders.

Diseases produced

Bacteria	Host	Vector	Diseases
E. canis	Dogs	*Rhipicephalus sanguineus, Amblyomma americanum*	Canine monocytic ehrlichiosis(CME) is characterized by fever, anorexia, lymphadenopathy, splenomegaly, hepatomegaly, occulonasal discharge, cough and dyspnoea, thrombocytopenia, leukopenia, anaemia with bilateral epistaxis, edema (in hind legs, tail, or scrotum), abortion or neonatal death, skin ulcers, lameness and/or polyarthritis, anterior uveitis, corneal opacity, hyphema, retinal vessel tortuosity, chorioretinal lesions, subretinal hemorrhage, retinal detachment and blindness. The clinical signs are more severe than canine anaplasmosis.
E. ruminantium	Ruminants	*Amblyomma*	Heart water disease characterized by fever, convulsion, nervous disorders, anorexia, prostration and sudden death.
E. ewingii	Dogs, Human, Deer	*Amblyomma, Rhipicephalus, Dermacentor*	Granulocytic Ehrlichiosis characterized by polyarthritis, fever, thrombocytopenia, ataxia and paresis.
E. chaffeensis	Human, dog, goat, lemur	*Dermacentor*	Monocytic Ehrlichiosis
E. muris	Wild mouse	*Haemaphysalis*	Fever, splenomegaly, lymphadenopathy

Diagnosis

Clinical samples: The peripheral blood collected with EDTA and splenic aspirates are the best clinical samples for PCR based confirmation of *E. canis*.

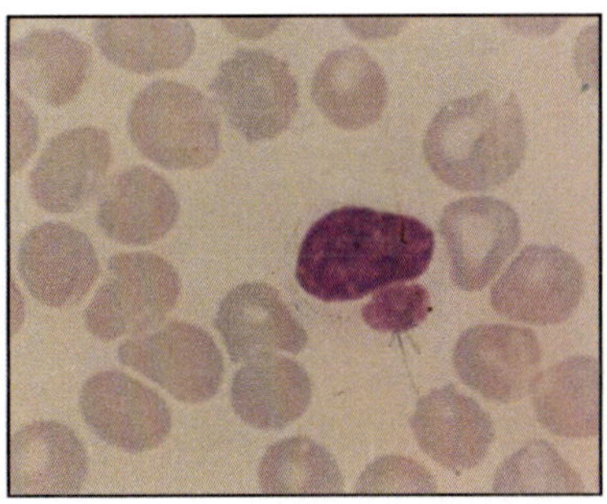

Fig. 2: Demonstration of *Ehrlichia canis* (morula) in canine monocyte (Courtesy: Bindu Lakshmanan, Department of Veterinary Parasitology, College of Veterinary and Animal Sciences, Kerala Veterinary and Animal Sciences University, Kerala, India)

Laboratory examinations

Direct examination: Canine ehrlichiosis can be diagnosed by demonstration of morula in peripheral monocytes present in smear prepared from buffy coat. The morulae are well-defined, round to oval, eosinophilic to basophilic, dark blue to purple coloured bodies found in membrane-lined vacuoles within the cytoplasm of the mononuclear cells (Figure 2). It is although difficult to detect morula in the infected canines and only 4-6% clinical cases shows morula in the blood slides. The possibility of morula demonstration is more in smears prepared from splenic aspirates. Bovine ehrlichiosis is detected by microscopic demonstration of the bacteria in brain endothelial cells in smear or tissue section.

Serological tests: Indirect immunofluorescence antibody test (IFA) and ELISA can be used to detect the antibodies against *E. canis*. Usually IgG titers of > 1:80 are considered diagnostic but the recent research indicates that titers < 1:80 should be considered as suspect and the test should be repeated within 2-3 weeks. The major disadvantage of the serological tests is that it can only predict the past exposure of the animals to the pathogen and it cannot confirm the current infection. Usually 12-14 days is required to develop anti-*E. canis* antibodies in dogs. Another drawback is that the immunodominant proteins of *E. canis* cross-react with those of *E. chaffeensis*. The studies have shown that serological testing by IFA could not distinguish between these two species. Co-infection with *E. canis* and *Anaplasma* can take place in the same animal as both of the bacteria are transmitted by same arthropod vectors. The cross-reaction between *E. canis* and *Anaplasma* is generally not detected in IFA except when titer of one of the pathogen is very high and the follow up is prolonged.

Molecular biology: PCR amplification and sequencing is the most sensitive method for the detection of ehrlichiosis in animals and human.

Prevention and control

Following measures can be adapted to control canine ehrlichiosis.

a) Outdoor exposure (garden, pasture, and kennel) of the pet dogs should be reduced to prevent the infestation of ticks ('peridomestic parasitism'). Local seasonal variation of tick infestation in outdoor should be known to the owners. However, indoor tick populations are maintained throughout the year specially in kennels and day dog care centers. The tick repellants and ectoparasiticides should be used with advice of qualified and registered veterinarians.

b) No commercial vaccines are currently available against *E. canis*, *A. phagocytophilum*, and *A. platys*.

[The original chapter for the first edition of the book was contributed by Samiran Bandyopadhyay, ICAR- Indian Veterinary Research Institute, Eastern Regional Station, Kolkata, India]

29

Chlamydia

The word 'chlamydia' comes from the Greek word 'chlamys' means 'cloak draped around the shoulder'. It describes how the intracytoplasmic inclusions produced by the bacterium appear under the microscope ('draped' around the host cell nucleus). *Chlamydia* was first discovered by a Czech zoologist and parasitologist, Stanislaus von Prowazek in 1907 in Berlin. Originally because of its structure it was thought to be a virus. In 1963 it was recognized as a bacterium rather than a virus.

Properties of genus

1. *Morphology: Chlamydia* are Gram-negative, non-motile, pleomorphic and obligate intracellular bacteria. The Gram-negative cell wall consists of cytoplasmic and outer membrane. However, they lack peptidoglycan layer. Moreover, they also encode major outer membrane protein (MOMP), the key antigenic determinant used for serological differentiation of chlamydiae.

They are poorly stained by Gram's stain. Chlamydiae are readily stained by Castaneda (blue in appearance), Giemnez and Macchiavello (red in appearance) methods. However, Giemsa staining is preferable to stain the inclusions (chlamydial micro colony) in the cell culture. Inclusion bodies of the Chlamydiae are basophilic in nature. The staining of the inclusion bodies may differ depending on the species. In *C. trachomatis*, the inclusion bodies contain glycogen matrix and can be easily stained with iodine solution.

Chlamydiae possess both RNA and DNA and some bacterial enzymes. So they can hydrolyze glucose, pyruvate and glutamate. Due to restricted metabolism they are unable to generate ATPs. Therefore, to meet the energy requirements they need to utilize host cell derived ATPs. So they are also known as 'energy parasites'.

2. The life cycle of *Chlamydia* is unique consisting of two phases. The infectious forms are known as 'elementary bodies' (EBs) and the non-infectious intracytoplasmic forms are called 'reticulate bodies' (RBs).

3. *Classification*: All the chlamydiae were earlier placed in the order Chlamydiales, family *Chlamydiaceae* and single genus *Chlamydia*. According to the recent revised classification, all chlamydiae are placed under the class Chlamydiae and two orders i.e. Chlamydiales and Parachlamydiales. There are seven families, 15 genera and 40 species currently under these two orders. Major pathogenic species are described below.

a) *Chlamydia abortus*

b) *Chlamydia trachomatis*

c) *Chlamydia psittaci*

d) *Chlamydia pecorum*

e) *Chlamydia pneumoniae*

f) *Chlamydia avium*

g) *Chlamydia suis*

h) *Chlamydia felis*

i) *Neochlamydia hartmannellae*

j) *Parachlamydia acanthamoebae*

4. *Resistance:* Chlamydiae are delicate bacteria and are easily inactivated at 56°C or at 60°C for 10 minutes exposure. It is susceptible to wide range of disinfectants like alcohol, sodium hypochlorite, silver nitrate, iodine and potassium permanganate. Because of lipid rich membrane, the bacteria are susceptible to chloroform and ether. Chlamydiae can be preserved at -70°C and liquid nitrogen for months. They are susceptible to broad range of chemotherapeutic agents like sulfonamides, tetracycline, macrolide, rifampicin, chloramphenicol and enrofloxacin.

5. *Natural habitat:* The mammals, birds and reptiles are the usual and natural hosts of the *Chlamydia*. Most of the chlamydiae have specific hosts. The mucous membranes of the genital region, throat and eyes are the usual habitats for *Chlamydia*.

6. *Genome: Chlamydia* has genome of approximately 1-1.3 Mbp in length. Chlamydial organisms contain both DNA and RNA. The RNA content is much higher in reticulate bodies. The elementary body contains a rigid cell wall and a DNA genome with a molecular weight of 6.6 X 10^8 Dalton. It has cryptic DNA plasmid of 7,498 base pairs. It also contains an open reading frame (ORF) for a gene involved in DNA replication. Additionally, the elementary body contains an RNA polymerase responsible for the transcription of the

DNA genome to start growth cycle. Ribosome and ribosomal subunits are conspicuous in these bodies. Whereas, in reticulate bodies electron dense DNA is uniformly dispersed in the cell cytoplasm. In the developing elementary body, it is concentrated into compact nucleoid and in mature elementary body it occupies most of the cell.

Earlier due to their small structural size and intracellular existence, Chlamydiae were confused with virus. However, there are some basic differences between virus and Chlamydiae.

Difference between virus and *Chlamydia*

Virus	Chlamydia
Either DNA or RNA is present in virus	Chlamydiae contain both DNA and RNA
Cytoplasmic membrane and outer membrane are absent in virus	Cytoplasmic membrane and outer membrane are present
Ribosome absent	Ribosome present
Metabolically inactive	Chlamydiae have their own metabolic system
Resistant to antibiotics	Sensitive to antibiotics

Difference between *Rickettsia* and *Chlamydia*

Rickettsia	Chlamydia
Rickettsiae can synthesize ATP	Chlamydiae are unable to synthesize ATP
Multiply by binary fission	Follow complicated biphasic life cycle for growth
It is mainly arthropod-borne infection	Transmission can occur by direct contact and ingestion of contaminated materials. It may be sexually transmitted also

Isolation

As chlamydial metabolism is restricted and they exploit host cell machinery for their energy, the bacteria require live cells for their growth. Like virus, the isolation of *Chlamydia* can be done in the yolk sacs of embryonated hen eggs, experimental animals and cell culture. Fertile chicken eggs (6-8 days old) are inoculated through the yolk sac route. The yolk sac of the embryo dying three or more days after incubation is examined for chlamydial inclusions.

Mice are ideal laboratory animals for isolation of chlamydiae. The mice usually die within 10 days of intranasal, intracerebral or intraperitoneal inoculation and the EBs can be isolated from viscera and peritoneal exudate.

The cell lines irradiated or treated with a metabolic inhibitor (cycloheximide @ 2μg/ml) can be used for isolation of chlamydiae. McCoy, HeLa, monkey kidney cells, mouse fibroblast cells, fish and lizard cells are generally used depending upon the species. Prior to inoculation into the cell culture, suspected clinical samples (faeces, placenta, urine, semen, conjunctival fluid) should be decontaminated with antibiotics like gentamicin (50 μg /ml), vancomycin (75 μg/ml) and nystatin (500 unit/ml).The inoculated cells should be incubated at 35°C to 37°C for 48-72 hours and stained for intracytoplasmic inclusion bodies. Fluorescein conjugated monoclonal antibody is in use now-a-days. It is more sophisticated and sensitive technique to detect inclusion body.

Antigenic characteristics

Chlamydia possesses genus, species and serotype specific antigens. The genus or group specific antigen is also called complement fixing antigen. It is heat stable and lipopolysaccharide in nature like other Gram-negative bacteria. The species-specific antigens are present on the cell surface of the chlamydiae. The serotype-specific antigens are protein in nature (major outer membrane protein, MOMP) and can be determined by micro immunofluorescence tests. The MOMP is encoded by *ompA* and there is considerable antigenic heterogeneity of this protein. Molecular and monoclonal antibody based techniques have identified four surface-exposed variable domains that help in serotyping. The serotype-specific antigens are important in some species like *C. trachomatis*. In *C. pneumoniae* the variable domains are not well recognized by immune system. Recently a 60-kDa cysteine-rich outer membrane protein (OmcB) is characterized from *Chlamydia* which can act as genus as well as species specific antigen. Most of the *Chlamydia* infected patients are positive for antibodies against OmcB.

There are three biovars of *C. trachomatis* - TRIC (trachoma and inclusion conjunctivitis), LGV (lymphogranuloma venereum) and MoPn (mouse pneumonia). *C. trachomatis* biovar TRIC and biovar LGV has 15 and 3 (L1, L2 and L3) serotypes, respectively. *C. psittaci* has eight serotypes - A (psittacine birds and human patients), B (cattle, pigeon, turkey), C (birds and human), D (turkeys, parakeets and human), E (human), F (parakeets), G (hares and muskrats) and H (cattle).

Toxins and virulence factors

Chlamydiae can secreate haemagglutinin and endotoxin like other Gram-negative bacteria. The haemagglutinin can facilitate attachment of the bacteria to the host cells. The endotoxin is responsible for inflammatory tissue damage during infection. However, different pro-inflammatory cytokines released during chlamydial infection may also be responsible for such tissue damage.

Chlamydia also contains several putative adhesion factors responsible for intimate attachment of the bacteria to the host cells like major outer membrane protein (MOMP), a heat labile cytadhesin, OmcB and heat shock protein (HSP).

Pathogenesis

Transmission

The respiratory, intestinal and genital tracts constitute the major reservoir of the bacteria. Infection is transmitted by direct contact and inhalation of the contaminated dust particles or droplets. In some chlamydial infections (enzootic abortion of ewes or enteritis) the transmission may occur by ingestion. Vertical transmission through the egg is possible in birds. The evidences are there that the chlamydiae may be transmitted by arthropods also.

Life cycle

The life cycle of chlamydiae is unique and it consists of biphasic developmental stages. The infectious form i.e. elementary body (EB) is extremely small (250-350 nm in diameter), pear to spherical shaped particle with electron dense irregular nucleoid. It has rigid cell wall with disulphide cross linkage among the cysteine rich amino acids of MOMP proteins. This form can survive for a long period in the environment. The infection starts with the attachment of elementary bodies to the host cell membrane. The site of predilection varies depending upon the chlamydial species and serovar. In general chlamydiae have an affinity to the mucous membrane. The attachment is mediated by specific adhesin of the pathogens and receptors on the host cells. It is assumed that the variable domains of MOMP acts as adhesin and heparan sulphate glycosaminoglycans act as specific receptors. Following attachment, the EB enters into the host cells via endocytosis. In the vesicle, the EB loses its electron dense DNA core and the cell wall loses rigidity due to breaking up of disulphide bridges. Finally, it is converted into reticulate bodies (RB). The reticulate bodies are non-infectious form, larger and metabolically active. The RBs multiply by binary fission and start genus specific protein synthesis after 18 hours of infection. The structural reorientation started and RBs are transformed into EBs after 24 hours of infection. The EB is developed within the vesicle. Thus chlamydial micro colony with 100-500 EBs within the vesicle is called 'inclusion body'. Later, by 40-70 hours the infected cells rupture and the EBs are released to attack new cells and the cycle is repeated.

Therapeutic intervention or host cell immunity is not effective enough to eliminate the infection. During the process, chlamydial organisms utilize host cell iron and tryptophan. Moreover, they also modulate respiratory burst and release of nitric oxide and superoxide radicals to prevent the cellular killing process. Thus prolonged persistence leads to chronic inflammatory reactions in the non-immune host cells and tissue damage.

Disease produced

Bacteria	Hosts	Diseases
Chlamydia trachomatis	Humans	Trachoma, sexually transmitted diseases, arthritis, conjunctivitis, pneumonia, Reiter's syndrome, lymphogranuloma venereum (LGV)
C. suis	Pigs	Conjunctivitis, rhinitis, enteritis, pericarditis, polyarthritis, pneumonia
C. muridarum	Mice, hamsters	Pneumonitis, respiratory diseases
C. abortus	Ruminants, pigs	Abortions, stillbirths
C. caviae	Guinea pig	Conjunctivitis
C. felis	Cats	Conjunctivitis, pneumonitis, rhinitis, upper respiratory tract disorders
C. pecorum	Ruminants, pigs, koala	Conjunctivitis, encephalitis, abortion, fertility, arthritis, pneumonia, encephalitis, enteritis
C. psittaci	Birds, human	**Ornithosis** and **Psittacosis**: It is characterized by inflamed eyes, conjunctivitis, airsacculitis, pneumonia, difficulty in breathing, watery droppings and green urates enteritis, myocarditis, encephalitis in human
C. pneumoniae	Human, horses, koala bears	Conjunctivitis, cystitis, Alzheimer's disease (associated cause) atherosclerosis, respiratory diseases
Parachlamydia acanthamoebae	Small ruminants	Abortion

Diagnosis

Clinical specimens: Faecal sample, conjunctival swab, nasal swab can be collected from suspected birds. Placenta, vaginal swabs, uterine cotyledons, foetal lung and liver are taken from abortion cases. Synovial fluid is the clinical specimen from arthritis patients.

Chlamydiae are relatively labile organisms and special precautions are required to avoid the chance of misdiagnosis and misinterpretation. Samples should be maintained in cold chamber and processed immediately after collection. If the samples cannot be processed within 24 hours, it should be kept at -70^{0}C. For successful isolation and culture, the clinical samples should be sent to the laboratory in special *Chlamydia* transport medium such as 2SP (0.2 M sucrose phosphate medium containing 10 µg /ml of gentamicin, 25 U of nystatin and 25 µg/ml of vancomycin) and SPG (75 g of sucrose, 0.52 g of KH_2PO_4, 1.22 g of Na_2HPO_4, 0.72 g of glutamic acid and water in 1litre, pH 7.4-7.6) supplemented with bovine serum albumin, streptomycin, vancomycin and nystatin. Broad spectrum chemotherapeutic agents like tetracycline, chloramphenicol, macrolides, sulphonamides, penicillin should not be added in the transport medium as they have anti-chlamydial effect.

Laboratory examination

Direct examination: The inclusion bodies may be demonstrated using appropriate stains. *C. trachomatis* infection can be detected by observing typical reinform inclusion bodies surrounding the nucleus following Giemsa, Castaneda or Macchiavello staining. Transmission electron microscopy (TEM) may be used for visualization of *C. psittaci* inclusion bodies containing reticulate bodies, condensing form and elementary bodies.

Staining of the sample smear can also be performed with FITC labeled antibodies against species or genus specific antigen (Figure 1). Immunofluorescence based detection has higher sensitivity as well as specificity and can be done rapidly.

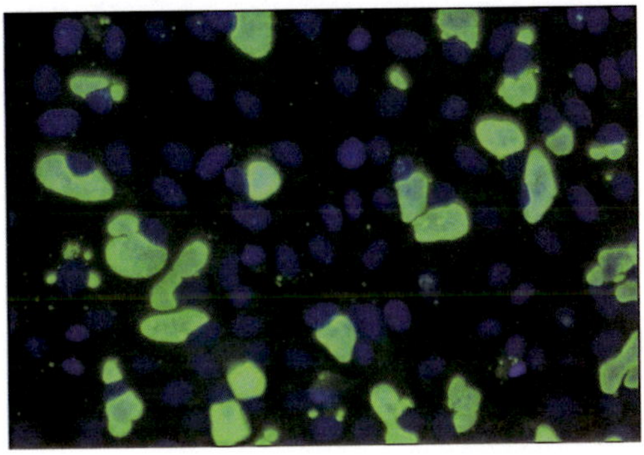

Fig. 1: FAT image of *Chlamydia abortus* (grown in HeLa cell line). The inclusions with elementary bodies produce green fluorescence (FITC) and the cellular nuclei are stained blue (DAPI, 40X) (Courtesy: Prof. Rajesh Chahota and Prof. Mandeep Sharma, Department of Veterinary Microbiology, College of Veterinary and Animal Sciences, CSK HP Agricultural University, Palampur, H.P., India)

Isolation of bacteria from clinical samples: The conditions are described earlier.

Immunological / serological tests: Enzyme linked immunossorbant assay (ELISA) has been developed to detect chlamydial antigen in vaginal discharge or to detect chlamydia specific antibodies in serum. ELISA has a comparable sensitivity and specificity with IF test. Complement fixation test (CFT) is also used to detect the rise of antibody titer against chlamydial antigen.

Frei's test: A skin test is also available using the cell mediated immune response to detect lymphogranuloma venereum (LGV) caused by *C. trachomatis*. In this test 0.1 ml of heat-inactivated LGV grown in yolk sac of embryonated egg is injected intradermally on the forearm of suspected human patients. Positive reaction is indicated by development of inflammatory nodule. The test becomes positive only 2-4 weeks of infection and remains positive for a long period. The test has lower sensitivity.

Molecular biology: In Chemiluminescence assay acridium-ester-labeled single stranded DNA probe complementary to *C. trachomatis* RNA is used to detect the labeled DNA-RNA hybrid in a luminometer to measure the light emitted by acridium ester label. Polymerase chain reaction (PCR) is used to detect the *omp1* gene encoding MOMP and 16s rRNA.

[The original chapter for the first edition of the book was contributed by Samiran Bandyopadhyay, ICAR- Indian Veterinary Research Institute, Eastern Regional Station, Kolkata, India]

Index

C

D

E

F

G

L

M

Q

R

S

T

U

V

W

X

Y

Z